ADVANCES IN BRAIN IMAGING

Edited by **Vikas Chaudhary**

Advances in Brain Imaging
Edited by Vikas Chaudhary

Published by InTech
Janeza Trdine 9, 51000 Rijeka, Croatia

Publishing Process Manager Romana Vukelic

Technical Editor Teodora Smiljanic

Cover Designer InTech Design Team

Additional hard copies can be obtained from orders@intechopen.com

Advances in Brain Imaging, Edited by Vikas Chaudhary
p. cm.
978-953-307-955-4

For EU product safety concerns:
IN TECH d.o.o., Prolaz Marije Krucifikse Kozulić 3, 51000 Rijeka, Croatia,
info@intechopen.com or visit our website at intechopen.com.

Meet the editor

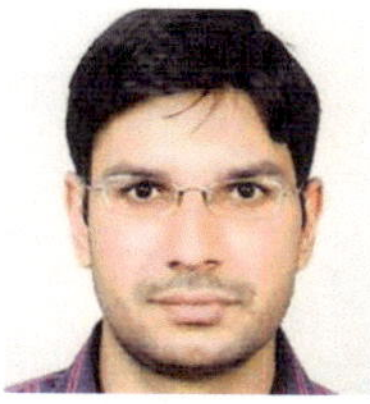

Dr Vikas Chaudhary is an Indian Radiologist who has published in many national and international publications. His other achievements include authoring chapters in other books, and reviewing articles for reputed national and international indexed journals. He was awarded Shri. M.L. Garg Memorial Medal for Best Senior Resident in Radiology at Lady Hardinge Medical College, New Delhi in 2009-2010, and was also awarded second prize for best review article with his contribution "Imaging of the Pancreas: Recent advances", during the Indian Journal of Endocrinology & Metabolism Annual Awards 2011, organised by the Endocrine Society of India at Pune, India. He has been nominated as a specialist member (subject expert) in the recruitment board for appointment of specialists, senior residents and radiographers in various ESIC Model Hospitals, and as an inspecting officer for various radiological equipments. He has received his MBBS and MD (Radiodiagnosis) from reputed Government Medical Colleges of India. During his undergraduation (MBBS), he received a Certificate of Merit in Microbiology.

Contents

Preface

Remarkable advances in medical diagnostic imaging have been made during the past few decades. The development of new imaging techniques and continuous improvements in the display of digital images have opened new horizons in the study of brain anatomy and pathology. The field of brain imaging has now become a fast-moving, demanding, and exciting multidisciplinary activity. I hope that this textbook will be useful to students and clinicians in the field of neuroscience, in understanding the fundamentals of advances in brain imaging.

We couldn't have produced the book in less than a year without the excellent team of authors. I am deeply indebted to all the authors. Their contribution and sacrifice made this a worthwhile and proud endeavour.

Special thanks to Ms. Romana Vukelic, publishing process manager for this project, for her tireless and unwavering support of the project.

We are greatly indebted to the production staff of InTech for their patience, valuable guidance and extreme professionalism.

I would also like to thank my family, friends and colleagues for their understanding and encouragement throughout the project.

Dr. Vikas Chaudhary
Department of Radiodiagnosis,
Employees' State Insurance Corporation (ESIC) Model Hospital,
India

1

Automatic Vector Seeded Region Growing for Parenchyma Classification in Brain MRI

Chuin-Mu Wang and Ruey-Maw Chen
National Chin-Yi University of Technology,
Taiwan, R.O.C.

1. Introduction

Nuclear magnetic resonance (NMR) can be used to measure the nuclear spin density, the interactions of the nuclei with their surrounding molecular environment and those between close nuclei, respectively. It produces a sequence of multiple spectral images of tissues with a variety of contrasts using several magnetic resonance parameters. When tissues are classified by means of MRI, the images are multi-spectral. Therefore, if only a single image with a certain spectrum is processed, the goal of tissue classification will not be achieved because the single image can't provide adequate information. Consequently, it is necessary to integrate the information of all the spectral images to classify tissues. Multi-spectral image processing techniques [1-3] are hence employed to collect spectral information for classification and of clinically critical values. In this paper, a new classification approach was proposed, it is called unsupervised Vector Seeded Region Growing (UVSRG). The UVSRG mainly select seed pixel vectors by means of standard deviation and relative Euclidean distance. Through the UVSRG processing, the data dimensionality of MRI can be decreased and the desired target of interest can be classified which the brain tissue and brain tumor segmentation. A series of experiments are conducted and compared to the commonly used c-means method for performance evaluation. The results show that the proposed approach is a promising and effective technique for MR image classification.

Nuclear magnetic resonance (NMR) has recently developed as a versatile technique in many fields such as chemistry, physics, engineering because its signals provide rich information about material structures that involve the nature of a population of atoms, the structure of their environment, and the way in which the atoms interact with environment1. When NMR is applied to human anatomy, NMR signals can be used to measure the nuclear spin density, the interactions of the nuclei with their surrounding molecular environment and those between close nuclei, respectively. It produces a sequence of multiple spectral images of tissues with a variety of contrasts using three magnetic resonance parameters, spin-lattice (T1), spin-spin (T2) and dual echo-echo proton density (PD). By appropriately choosing pulse sequence parameters, echo time (TE) and repetition time (TR) a sequence of images of specific anatomic area can be generated by pixel intensities that represent characteristics of different types of tissues throughout the sequence. As a result, magnetic resonance imaging (MRI) becomes a more useful image modality than X-ray computerized tomography (X-CT) when it comes to analysis of soft tissues and organs since the information about T1 and T2 offers a more precise picture of tissue functionality than that produced by X-CT2.

MRI shares many image structures and characteristics with remotely sensed imagery. They are acquired as image sequences by spectral channels at different specific wavelengths remotely. Most importantly, they produce a sequence of images which explore the spectral properties and correlation within the sequence so as to improve image analysis. One unique feature for which both multispectral MR images and remote sensing images are in common is spectral properties contained in an image pixel that are generally not explored in classical image processing. Since various material substances can be uncovered by different wavelengths, an MR or remote sensing image pixel is actually a pixel vector, of which each component represents an image pixel acquired by a specific spectral band. There are mainly four types of segmentation techniques, namely global thresholding, boundary-based segmentation, region-based segmentation, and mixed segmentation. Seeded Region Growing is an integrated method brought up by Adams and Bischof [4-13], in which few initial seeds are generated, and more similar neighboring regions are then combined to achieve region growing [14-21]. In addition, the method of unsupervised vector seeded region growing suitable for medical multi-spectral images was established. Vector seed selection mainly selects seed pixel vectors by means of standard deviation and relative Euclidean distance. Seeds emerge from even and smooth regions, so the smaller the standard deviation is, the more concentrated the data distribution is. In terms of image, it indicates that the difference between a pixel vector and the eight neighbors is smaller, and the pixel vector is suitable for the seed pixel vector. Furthermore, relative Euclidean distance is employed to more carefully select the seed pixel vector to accomplish unsupervised classification.

2. Vector seeded region growing

First of all, the multi-spectral images of a brain section were obtained. There wee five images belonging to the same section but different spectrums, respectively Band1, Band2, and Band3. When tissue classification is conducted, the characteristic information of a single image is too insufficient to achieve effects upon tissue classification if only a single image of a particular spectrum is processed. Thus, the images from Band1 to Band3 in order were combined into 3D eigenspace to acquire the 3D eigenvector of every pixel.

Vector seed selection was applied to the aforementioned eigenspace images, or multi-spectral images, to obtain initial seeds. The algorithm of seeded region growing was further adopted to divide the multi-spectral images into many small regions. The algorithm of region merging was employed to merge similar regions as well as to combine smaller regions with the nearest neighboring regions. Finally, all the regions eventually segmented by means of region growing were classified, and the algorithm of K-means clustering was used, in which it was assumed that K=3, to divide the regions into three categories. After the classification was accomplished, the regions in the same category were namely the same type of brain tissues. Figure 1 indicates the algorithmic procedures.

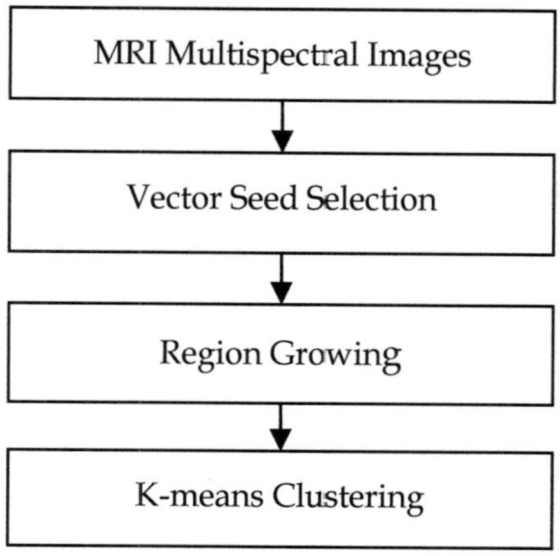

Fig. 1. Algorithmic procedures

2.1 Vector seed selection

Seeded region growing starts from seeds, and each time, it expands around at the speed of one pixel. Hence, a seed point has to be selected in the beginning. In vector seed selection, the pixel vectors which can become seeds have to possess the following characteristics:

a. There should be high similarity between a seed pixel and the neighbors.
b. There should be at least one seed in the expected region.
c. A seed should be unconnected to different regions.

The seed points can be either a single pixel vector or a group of connected pixel vectors, which will be regarded as the same region in region growing. According to the aforesaid characteristics, there are two conditions for each pixel vector in the multi-spectral images to be selected to be a seed point. One is that the similarity between one pixel vector and the eight neighbors should be higher than one threshold. The other one is that the maximum relative Euclidean distance between a seed pixel vector and its eight neighbors should be smaller than a threshold. When the above two conditions are satisfied, a pixel vector becomes a seed point.

Similarity *H*, the first condition mentioned above, calculated the similarity between each pixel vector, composed of B1~B3, and its eight neighboring points. The standard deviation of pixel vector was calculated by the following equation:

$$\begin{cases} \sigma_{B1} = \sqrt{\dfrac{1}{9}\sum_{i=1}^{9}(B1_i - \overline{B1})^2} \\ \sigma_{B2} = \sqrt{\dfrac{1}{9}\sum_{i=1}^{9}(B2_i - \overline{B2})^2} \\ \sigma_{B3} = \sqrt{\dfrac{1}{9}\sum_{i=1}^{9}(B3_i - \overline{B3})^2} \end{cases} \tag{1}$$

In the equation, $\overline{B1}$, $\overline{B2}$ and $\overline{B3}$ indicates the mean of the selected 3×3 range, calculated as follows:

$$\begin{cases} \overline{B1} = \frac{1}{9}\sum_{i=1}^{9} B1_i \\ \overline{B2} = \frac{1}{9}\sum_{i=1}^{9} B2_i \\ \overline{B3} = \frac{1}{9}\sum_{i=1}^{9} B3_i \end{cases} \tag{2}$$

The overall standard deviation is calculated as follows:

$$\sigma = \sigma_{B1} + \sigma_{B2} + \sigma_{B3} \tag{3}$$

The standard deviation was further normalized by [0, 1] as follows:

$$\sigma_N = \sigma / \sigma_{\max} \tag{4}$$

$\sigma_{\max}$ indicated the maximum standard deviation in the image. The similarity between a pixel vector and its eight neighbors was calculated as follows:

$$H = 1 - \sigma_N \tag{5}$$

Furthermore, according to the second condition, the relative Euclidean distance between each pixel vector and its eight neighboring points was calculated as follows:

$$d_i = \frac{\sqrt{(B1 - B1_i)^2 + (B2 - B2_i)^2 + (B3 - B3_i)^2}}{\sqrt{B1^2 + B2^2 + B3^2}} \quad i = 1,2,\ldots,8 \tag{6}$$

According to the experiment by Shih & Cheng [11], the efficacy of employing relative Euclidean distance is better than that of using normal Euclidean distance. Therefore, the maximum distance between each pixel and its eight neighboring points was calculated by the following equation:

$$d_{\max} = \max_{i=1}^{8}(d_i) \tag{7}$$

The two aforementioned conditions have to be satisfied in order for a pixel vector to be selected as a seed point. The first condition aims at examining whether or not there is considerably high similarity between a seed pixel vector and its neighbors whereas the second condition focuses on ensuring that a seed pixel vector is not in the boundary between two regions.

2.2 Region growing

The traditional method of region growing can not successfully classify brain tissues. Consequently, this paper modified the principle of region growing and recorded all the pixel vectors connecting with but uncovered by regions. Because the pixel vectors connecting with each other are the priority, these uncovered pixel vectors usually have the judgment upon the distance difference with the connected regions conducted to carry out region growing. It is the major reason why CSF is covered by GM and eroded. Therefore, it is necessary to modify the pixel vector, simultaneously calculate the distance difference with all the regions, and grow it into one of the regions with the minimum difference. The minimum distances were found out from the distances between the pixel vectors and all the regions, each corresponding region with the minimum distance was recorded, and the minimum distances were arranged in the order from small to large in Table T. Due to the order from small to large, the first point 'p' in Table T possessed the minimum difference and the highest similarity with the regions it connected among the pixel vectors in the rims of all the regions. Hence, p is more qualified than all the other uncovered pixel vectors to become a region.

2.3 Applying K-means to region classification

The algorithm of K-means clustering was employed to mainly classify the results of region segmentation in the previous stage. The brain MR images were classified into three categories, respectively GM, WM, and CSF. Because there were many fragmentary regions, it was necessary to classify all the regions, in which all the regions were divided into three categories, it was assumed that K=3, and the region was regarded as a unit to conduct the algorithm of K-means clustering. After the algorithm was accomplished, the regions in the same category belonged to namely the same sort of brain tissue.

3. Experimental results

The real MR images were used for performance evaluation. They were acquired from ten patients with normal physiology. One example is shown in Fig. 2(a)-(e) with the same parameter values in Table 1. Band 1 is the PD-weighted spectral image acquired by the pulse sequence TR/TE = 2500ms/25ms. Bands 2, 3 and 4 are T2-weighted spectral images were acquired by the pulse sequences TR/TE = 2500ms/50ms, TR/TE = 2500ms/75ms and TR/TE =2500ms/100ms respectively. Band 5 is the T1-weighted spectral image acquired by the pulse sequence TR/TE = 500ms/11.9ms. The tissues surrounding the brain such as bone, fat and skin, were semiautomatically extracted using interactive thresholding and masking. The slice thickness of all the MR images are 6mm and axial section were taken from GE MR 1.5T Scanner.

In this experiment, there was one type of real brain MR images. In order to evaluate the performance of the UVSRG, the widely used c-means method (also known as k-means) is used for comparative analysis. The reason to select the c-means method is because it is a spatial-based pattern classification technique. In order to make a fair comparison, the implemented c-means method always designates the desired target signature d as one of its class means with d fixed during iterations.

In order to enhance classification of these MR images, the interfering effects resulting from tissue variability and characterization must be eliminated. However, to identify the sources that cause such interference is nearly impossible unless prior information is provided. On the other hand, in many MRI applications, the three cerebral tissues, GM, WM and CSF are of major interest where their knowledge can be generally obtained directly from the images. A zero-mean Gaussian noise was added to the phantom images so as to achieve various signal-to-noise ratios (SNR) ranging from 5db to 20db. Table 1 tabulates the values of the parameters used by the MRI pulse sequence and the gray level values of the tissues of each band used as phantom in the experiments and Tables 2-5 tabulate the results for SNR = 20db, 15db, 10 and 5db respectively. In our experiments, the spectral signatures of GM, WM and CSF used for the UVSRG were extracted directly from the MR images. Fig. 3(a)-(c) show the classification results of the UVSRG using five images in Fig. 1(a)-(e). For comparison, we also applied the c-means method to Fig. 2(a)-(e) to produce Fig. 4(a)-(c) where the classification maps of GM, WM and CSF are labeled by (a), (b) and (c) respectively. Compared to Fig. 3(a)-(c), the UVSRG performed significantly better than did the c-means method. All the experimental results presented here were verified by experienced radiologists.

Band #	MRI Parameter	BKG	GM	WM	CSF
Band 1	TR/TE=2500ms/25ms	3	207	188	182
Band 2	TR/TE=2500ms/50ms	3	219	180	253
Band 3	TR/TE=2500ms/75ms	3	150	124	232
Band 4	TR/TE=2500ms/100ms	3	105	94	220
Band 5	TR/TE=500ms/11.9ms	3	95	103	42

Table 1. Gray level values used for the five bands of the test phantom

	N	$N_D(d)$	$N_F(d)$	$R_D(d)$	$R_F(d)$	R_D	R_F
GM	9040	9040	0	1	0		
WM	8745	8745	0	1	0	1	0
CSF	3282	3282	0	1	0		

Table 2. Detection results with SNR = 20 db

	N	$N_D(d)$	$N_F(d)$	$R_D(d)$	$R_F(d)$	R_D	R_F
GM	9040	9040	0	1	0		
WM	8745	8745	0	1	0	1	0
CSF	3282	3282	0	1	0		

Table 3. Detection results with SNR = 15 db

	N	$N_D(d)$	$N_F(d)$	$R_D(d)$	$R_F(d)$	R_D	R_F
GM	9040	9036	8	0.9995	0.0006		
WM	8745	8737	4	0.9990	0.0003	0.9994	0.0004
CSF	3282	3282	0	1	0		

Table 4. Detection results with SNR =10 db

	N	$N_D(d)$	$N_F(d)$	$R_D(d)$	$R_F(d)$	R_D	R_F
GM	9040	8688	455	0.9610	0.0378		
WM	8745	8290	352	0.9479	0.0285	0.9616	0.0280
CSF	3282	3282	0	1	0		

Table 5. Detection results with SNR = 5 db

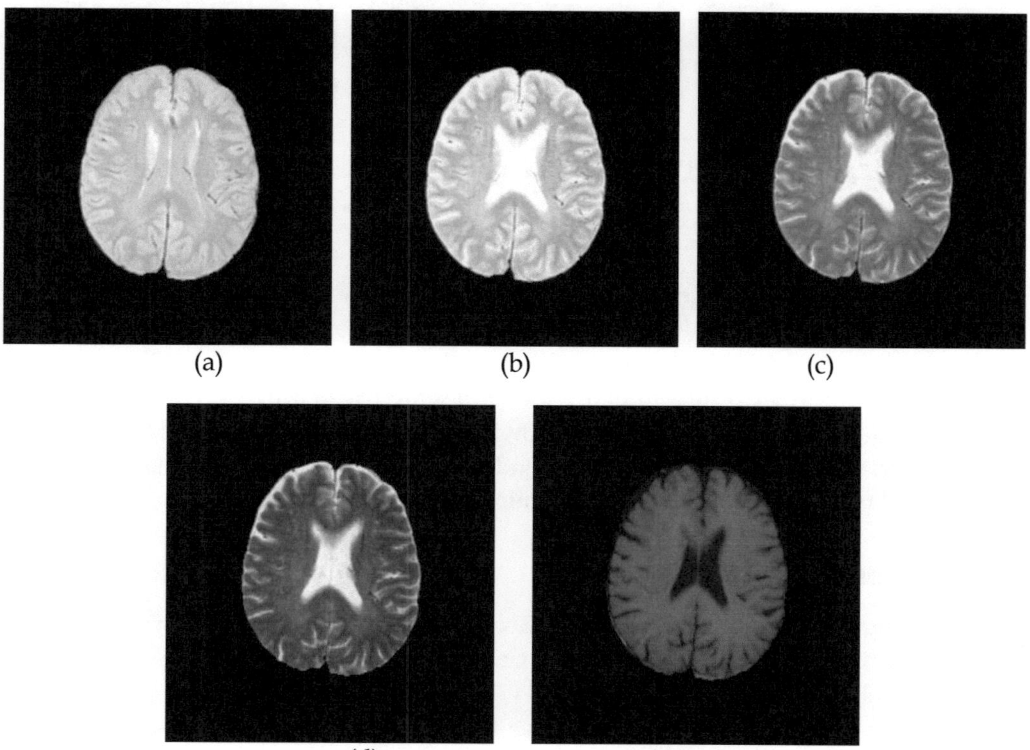

(a) (b) (c) (d) (e)

Fig. 2. Real brain MR images. (a) TR1/TE1=2500ms/25ms (b) TR2/TE2=2500ms/50ms (c) TR3/TE3=2500ms/75ms (d) TR4/TE4=2500ms/100ms (e) TR5/TE5=500ms/11.9ms

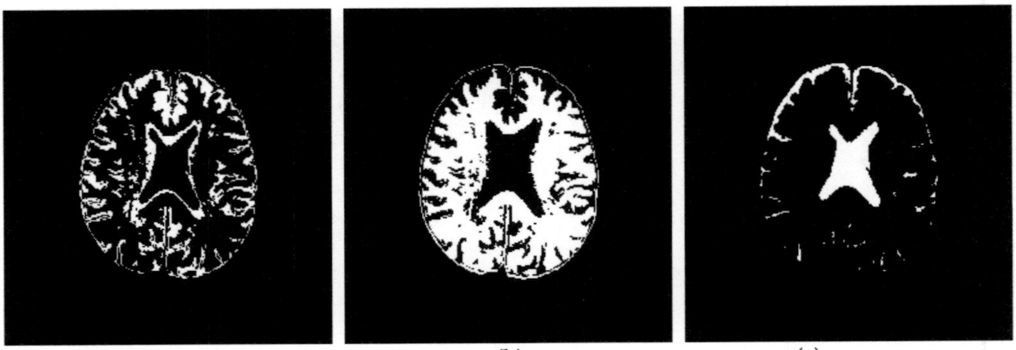

(a) (b) (c)

Fig. 3. Real Classification result of brain MR images by UVSRG. (a)GM (b)WM (c)CSF

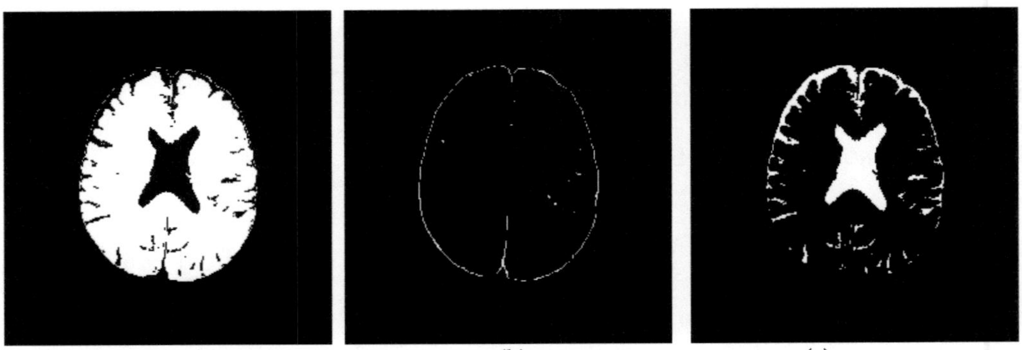

(a) (b) (c)

Fig. 4. Real Classification result of brain MR images by C-means. (a)GM (b)WM (c)CSF

4. Conclusion

Generally, real brain MR images result from the CSF near the skull, which tends to be close to the boundary in the image. In vector seed selection, seeds tend to appear in more smooth regions. Hence, seeds will not be generated from the pixel vectors in the CSF close to the boundary, which further results in that these tissues are covered by the neighboring gray-scaled tissues in the stage of region growing, and the classification is thus failed. Consequently, this paper improved the method of region growing and successfully applied vector seeded region growing to the classification of brain MR images.

5. References

[1] Di Jia, Fangfang Han, Jinzhu Yang, Yifei Zhang, Dazhe Zhao, Ge Yu, "A Synchronization Algorithm of MRI Denoising and Contrast Enhancement Based on PM-CLAHE Model", JDCTA, Vol. 4, No. 6, pp. 144 ~ 149, 2010

[2] Satish Chandra , Rajesh Bhat , Harinder Singh , D.S.Chauhan , "Detection of Brain Tumors from MRI using Gaussian RBF kernel based Support Vector Machine ", IJACT, Vol. 1, No. 1, pp. 46 ~ 51, 2009

[3] Saif D. Salman & Ahmed A. Bahrani, "Segmentation of tumor tissue in gray medical images using watershed transformation method", IJACT, Vol. 2, No. 4, pp. 123 ~ 127, 2010

[4] J. R. Jimenez-Alaniz, V. Medina-Banuelos, O. Yanez-Suarez, "Data-driven brain MRI segmentation supported on edge confidence and a priori tissue information", IEEE Transactions on Medical Imaging 25 (1) (2006) 74–83.

[5] T. Song, M. M. Jamshidi, R. R. Lee, M. Huang, "A Modified Probabilistic Neural Network for Partial Volume Segmentation in Brain MR Image", IEEE Transactions on Neural Networks 18 (5) (2007) 1424-1432.

[6] J. Tohka, E. Krestyannikov, I. D. Dinov, A. M. Graham, D. W. Shattuck, U. Ruotsalainen, A. W. Toga, "Genetic Algorithms for Finite Mixture Model Based Voxel Classification in Neuroimaging", IEEE Transactions on Medical Imaging 26 (5) (2007) 696-711.

[7] S. Duchesne, A. Caroli, C. Geroldi, C. Barillot, G. B. Frisoni, D. L. Collins, "MRI-Based Automated Computer Classification of Probable AD Versus Normal Controls", IEEE Transactions on Medical Imaging 27 (4) (2008) 509-520.

[8] J. J. Corso, E. Sharon, S. Dube, S. El-Saden, U. Sinha, A. Yuille, "Efficient Multilevel Brain Tumor Segmentation With Integrated Bayesian Model Classification", IEEE Transactions on Medical Imaging 27 (5) (2008) 629-640.

[9] A. Mayer, H. Greenspan, "An Adaptive Mean-Shift Framework for MRI Brain Segmentation", IEEE Transactions on Medical Imaging 28 (8) (2009) 1238-1250.

[10] H. Gudbjartsson, S. Patz, "The Rician distribution of noisy MRI data," Magn. Reson. Med. vol.34, no.6, pp.910–914, 1995.

[11] C. M. Wang, C. C. C. Chen, Y. N. Chung, S. C. Yang, P. C. Chung, C. W. Yang, C. I. Chang, "Detection of Spectral Signatures in Multispectral MR Images for Classification," IEEE Trans. on Medical Imaging, vol.22, no.1, pp.50-61, 2003.

[12] J. R. Jimenez-Alaniz, V. Medina-Banuelos, O. Yanez-Suarez, "Data-driven brain MRI segmentation supported on edge confidence and a priori tissue information," IEEE Trans. on Medical Imaging, vol.25, no.1, pp.74–83, 2006.

[13] R. Adams, L. Bischof, "Seeded region growing," IEEE Trans. on Pattern Analysis and Machine Intelligence, vol.16, no.6, pp.641–647, 1994.

[14] T. Pavlidis, Y.T. Liow, "Integrating region growing and edge detection," IEEE Trans. on Pattern Analysis and Machine Intelligence, vol.12, no.3, pp. 225–233, 1990.

[15] N.R. Pal, S.K. Pal, "A review on image segmentation techniques," Pattern Recognition, vol.26, no.9, pp.1277–1294, 1993.

[16] C. Chu, J.K. Aggarwal, "The integration of image segmentation maps using region and edge information," IEEE Transactions on Pattern Analysis and Machine Intelligence, vol.15, no.2, pp.1241–1252, 1993.

[17] A. Tremeau, N. Bolel, "A region growing and merging algorithm to color segmentation," Pattern Recognition, vol.30, no.7, pp.1191–1203, 1997.

[18] S.A. Hojjatoleslami, J. Kittler, "Region growing: a new approach," IEEE Trans. on Image Processing, vol.7, no.7, pp.1079–1084, 1998.

[19] J. Fan, D.K.Y. Yau, A.K. Elmagarmid, W.G. Aref, "Automatic image segmentation by integrating color-edge extraction and seeded region growing," IEEE Transactions on Image Processing, vol.10, no.10, pp.1454–1466, 2001.
[20] F. Y. Shih, S. Cheng, "Automatic seeded region growing for color image segmentation," Image and Vision Computing, vol.23, no.10, pp.877–886, 2005.
[21] R.O. Duda and P.E. Hart, "Pattern Classification and Scene Analysis," John Wiley and Sons, NY, 1973.

2

Neuroimaging and Dissociative Disorders

Angelica Staniloiu[1,2,3], Irina Vitcu[3] and Hans J. Markowitsch[1]
[1]*University of Bielefeld, Bielefeld,*
[2]*University of Toronto, Toronto,*
[3]*Centre for Addiction and Mental Health, Toronto,*
[1]*Germany*
[2,3]*Canada*

1. Introduction

Although they were for a while "dissociated" (Spiegel, 2006) from the clinical and scientific arena, dissociative disorders have in the last several years received a renewed interest among several groups of researchers, who embarked on the work of identifying and describing their underlying neural correlates. Dissociative disorders are characterized by transient or chronic failures or disruptions of integration of otherwise integrated functions of consciousness, memory, perception, identity or emotion. The DSM-IV-TR (2000) includes nowadays under the heading of dissociative disorders several diagnostic entities, such as dissociative amnesia and fugue, depersonalization disorder, dissociative identity disorder and dissociative disorder not otherwise specified (such as Ganser syndrome). In contrast to DSM-IV-TR, ICD-10 (1992) also comprises under the category of dissociative (conversion) disorder the entity of conversion disorder (with its various forms), which is in DSM-IV-TR (2000) captured under the heading of somatoform disorders (and probably will remain under the same heading in the upcoming DSM-V).

Dissociative disorders had been previously subsumed under the diagnostic construct of hysteria, which had described the occurrence of various constellations of unexplained medical symptoms, without evidence of tissue pathology that can adequately or solely account for the symptom(s). Although not the first one who used the term dissociation or who suggested a connection between (early) traumatic experiences and psychiatric symptomatology (van der Kolk & van der Hart, 1989; Breuer & Freud, 1895), it is Janet (1898, 1907) who claimed dissociation as a mechanism related to traumatic experiences that accounted for the various manifestations of hysteria.

By definition, dissociative disorders are viewed in international nosological classifications as underlain by the mechanism of dissociation; there is still debate if the mechanism of dissociation that is involved in dissociative disorders is distinct from the so-called non-pathological or normative dissociation (that includes absorption or reverie) or a continuum exists between the two (Seligman & Kirmayer, 2008). Janet had reportedly viewed on one hand, dissociation as being intrinsically pathological and causally bound to unresolved traumatic memories (Bell, Oakley, Halligan, & Deeley, 2011). On the other hand, Janet had suggested that the impact of trauma on a particular individual may depend on a variety of factors (such as the person's characteristics, prior experiences and the severity, duration and recurrence of the trauma) and might not become evident immediately, but after a certain latency period (van der Kolk & van der Hart, 1989). Janet is credited by several authors (Maldonado & Spiegel, 2008) with a superior view of dissociation that anticipated contemporaneous theories. Freud, a pupil of Charcot, proposed in collaboration with Breuer (Breuer & Freud, 1895) that the dissociative process was the result of the repression of traumatic material into unconscious (Bell et al., 2011). This process of repression was intimately connected to the one of conversion, during which the affective discomfort accompanying the repressed memories of trauma led to a conversion of the psychological emotional distress into physical symptoms (conversion hysteria). Repression, conversion and dissociation occurred without awareness or intentionality (Markowitsch, 2002), which distinguishes them from memory suppression or motivated forgetting (Anderson & Green, 2001). Later elaborations on the mechanisms of repression versus dissociation posited that they corresponded to various views of the self-one that is vertically organized (such as in the case of repression) versus one that is horizontally aligned, with areas of incompatibility separated by dissociation (Mitchell & Black, 1995). Many of Janet's ideas presented above received corroboration later from both clinical observations and neurobiological investigations and have subsequently been incorporated in contemporaneous pathogenetic models of dissociative disorders. Though some authors still dispute their legitimacy (Pope, Poliakof, Parker, Boynes, & Hudson, 2007), dissociative disorders have indeed been linked to psychological trauma or stress in a variety of cultures (Maldonado & Spiegel, 2008).

In the present chapter, after a brief description of the dissociative (conversion) disorders, we review neuroimaging data pertaining to dissociative (conversion) disorders, which were obtained with functional imaging methods performed during rest or various tasks, such as single-photon emission computed tomography (SPECT), positron emission tomography (PET), functional magnetic resonance imaging (fMRI), as well as structural imaging techniques, including newer structural imaging methods such as diffusion tensor imaging (DTI) or magnetization transfer ratio measurements. In particular, we focus on reviewing neuroimaging data from studies of patients with dissociative amnesia and fugue, dissociative identity disorder (multiple personality disorder) and Ganser syndrome (Dissociative Disorders Not Otherwise Specified [NOS]). We also review functional brain imaging studies of patients with various forms of conversion disorder (e.g. psychogenic motor or sensory changes, psychogenic blindness, pseudoseizures) as well as depersonalization disorder. As hypnotizability traits have been postulated to be associated with a higher tendency for developing dissociative symptoms, we briefly refer to functional imaging studies of hypnosis. In addition we make reference to neuroimaging investigations pertaining to dissociative symptoms of psychiatric conditions that are not categorized under the heading of dissociative (conversion) disorders, but may have dissociative symptoms as part of their clinical presentations (such as post-traumatic stress disorder or borderline personality disorder). Given that the concept of mindfulness is often viewed as being situated at the opposite pole of that of dissociation, we discuss the neuro-imaging findings of the so-called dispositional mindfulness as well as of the mindfulness-based cognitive therapy in patients with conditions that may be associated with dissociative symptoms (such as borderline personality disorder).

2. Dissociative amnesic disorders

Several dissociative disorders have as hallmark amnesia for autobiographical events. Among them, the most frequently mentioned are dissociative amnesia and its variant dissociative fugue. The inability to recall personal events is however also a common occurrence in other dissociative disorders, such as dissociative identity disorder or multiple personality disorder, a characteristic that is going to be underlined in the upcoming edition of the DSM–V. Also Ganser syndrome (see below) was initially described to feature amnesia as part of its constellation of symptoms. Dissociative amnesia has as its central symptom the inability to recall important personal information, usually from an epoch encompassing events of stressful or traumatic nature. The symptoms are not better explained by normative forgetfulness or other psychiatric or medical conditions (such as traumatic brain injury). Deliberate feigning that is consciously motivated by external incentives (such as malingering) or is prompted by psychological motivations in the absence of identifiable potential external gains (such as in Factitious Disorder) has to be ruled out. This is not always an easy task. Especially the psychologically motivated exacerbation of symptoms has been found to accompany a variety of disorders, including dissociative disorders, major depressive disorder, traumatic brain injury. The symptoms of dissociative amnesia are assumed to cause significant impairment of functioning or distress. The degree of experienced distress may, however, depend on many variables, including the cultural views of dissociative experiences, selfhood and past (Seligman & Kirmayer, 2008). While in DSM-IV-TR the preponderant contribution of psychological mechanisms to the emergence of dissociative amnesia is conveyed in a more implicit way, the ICD-10 explicitly spells out as a criterion for the diagnosis of dissociative amnesia (as well as for the other dissociative disorders) the existence of "convincing associations in time between the symptoms of the disorder and stressful events, problems or needs". The presence of amnesia (which in psychoanalytic theories is posited to have the role of covering the unfortunate past) might, however, pose a significant challenge to clinicians trying to identify the precipitating stressful events. Furthermore some cases of dissociative (psychogenic) amnesia did not occur as a result of an objective major psychological stressor, but were recorded after a seemingly objective minor stress (Staniloiu et al., 2009). In most of the latter cases, a careful history taking and collateral information gathering provided evidence for a series of stressful events often occurring since childhood or early adulthood. These observations are consistent with pathogenetic models of kindling sensitization (Post, Weiss, Smith, Rosen, & Frye, 1995), or protracted effects of early life stressful events, due to an incubation phenomenon (Lupien, McEwen, Gunnar, & Heim, 2009). Another factor that may prevent the identification of convincing associations between stressful events and onset of dissociative amnesia is the presence in some patients with dissociative amnesia of an impaired capacity for emotional processing in the face of ongoing stress (Staniloiu et al., 2009).

According to most studies dissociative amnesia affects both genders roughly equally. Dissociative amnesia is most frequently diagnosed in the third and fourth decade of life. Dissociative amnesia typically occurs as a single episode, not uncommonly after a mild traumatic brain injury, although – similarly to dissociative fugue – recurrent episodes have been reported (Coons & Milstein, 1992). Some cases of dissociative amnesia follow a chronic course, despite treatment. Comorbidities of dissociative amnesia with major depressive disorder, personality disorders, bulimia nervosa, conversion disorder and somatisation disorder have been reported (Maldonado & Spiegel, 2008). Changes in personality after the onset of dissociative amnesia in the form of changes in eating preferences, smoking or drinking habits or other engagement in various activities have also been reported (Fujiwara et al., 2008; Tramoni et al., 2009; Thomas Antérion, Mazzola, Foyatier-Michel, & Laurent, 2008).

Dissociative amnesia could be differentiated according to the degree and timeframe of impairment (global versus selective, anterograde versus retrograde) of autobiographical-episodic memory and the co-existence of deficits in autobiographical-semantic memory and general semantic knowledge. The most frequent types of dissociative amnesias are retrograde, a fact that is in fact captured by the diagnostic criteria of DSM-IV-TR (2000). The latter distinguishes between localized amnesia, selective amnesia, generalized amnesia, continuous amnesia and systematized amnesia.

Retrograde dissociative amnesia may sometimes present as an episodic-autobiographical block, which may encompass the whole past life. Affected patients otherwise have largely preserved semantic memories; they can read, write, calculate and know how to behave in social situations. Additionally, they can encode new autobiographic-episodic memories long term, though the acquisition of these new events may be less emotionally-tagged in comparison to normal probands, often lacking that feeling of warmth and first person autonoetic connection (Reinhold & Markowitsch, 2009 ; Levine, Svoboda, Turner, Mandic, & Mackey, 2009). Although anterograde memory deficits could occasionally accompany retrograde dissociative (psychogenic) amnesia, cases of dissociative (psychogenic) anterograde amnesia with preserved retrograde memory are a much rarer occurrence (for a review see Staniloiu & Markowitsch, 2010).

When retrograde dissociative amnesia is accompanied by suddenly leaving the customary environment and compromised knowledge about personal identity – the condition is named dissociative fugue. Fugues have been reported for over a century, though they were frequently erroneously associated with epilepsy (e.g., Burgl, 1900; Donath, 1899). A century ago, these conditions were named *Wanderlust* in Germany (cf e.g. Burgl, 1900). Fugue states were described to be preponderant in children and young adults (Dana, 1894; Donath, 1908). Identified precipitants included sexual assault, combat, marital and financial problems. Presentations similar to fugues have also been described in certain cultures, where they might represent idioms of distress (Maldonado & Spiegel, 2008). Most fugues were usually reported to be brief, but some prolonged courses were also described (Hennig-Fast et al., 2008). Associations between fugues and Ganser syndrome (see below) were also found.

Dissociative Identity Disorder (DID) or multiple personality disorder is assumed to have its onset in childhood, but it is usually diagnosed in the fourth decade. It affects preponderantly women and typically runs a chronic, waxing and waning course. Comorbidities with other conditions (such as mood disorders and substance abuse) and its plethora of clinical manifestations may hinder timely diagnosing. Apart from marked impairments in the sense of identity and self (in the form of the existence of two or more distinct identities or personality states), inability to recall personal information (amnesia) is a common occurrence in DID. Currently included under the separate entity of dissociative trance disorder, possession trance seems to be an equivalent of dissociative identity disorder. It involves episodes of consciousness alteration and perceived replacement of the usual identity by a new identity, which is attributed to the influence of a supernatural entity (deity, spirit, power) (DSM –IV-TR, 2000).

3. The "dissociation"of memory systems

In order to better understand the clinical manifestations and neuroimaging data of those dissociative disorders, which have as hallmark inability to recall personal past events, we will briefly review the current classifications of the long-term memory systems. Two overlapping classifications currently dominate the memory research literature – the one that was initiated by Larry Squire and the one that was advanced by Endel Tulving. In Squire's classification, a main distinction is made between declarative and non-declarative memory. Under declarative memory, episodic and semantic memories – that is (biographical) events and general facts – are listed. Non-declarative memory contains several other forms of memory, which are considered to be automatically processed.

Tulving's classification is depicted in Figure 1 and, in our opinion, offers clinicians the best framework for describing the pattern of memory impairment in amnesic conditions. Aside from short-term memory (not illustrated in Fig. 1), it contains five long-term memory systems. These memory systems are considered to build up on each other phylo- and ontogenetically. Procedural memory and priming constitute the first developing memory systems, being still devoid of the need for conscious reflection upon the environment ("anoetic"). Procedural memory is largely motor-based, but includes also sensory and cognitive skills ("routines"). Examples are biking, skiing, playing piano, or reading words presented in a mirror-image. Priming refers to a higher likelihood of re-identifying previously perceived stimuli, either identical or similar ones. An example is the repetition of an advertisement which initially may not be in the focus of attention, but may leave a prime in the brain so that its repetition will make it likely to become effective. Perceptual memory enables distinguishing an object or person on the basis of distinct features; it works on a pre-semantic, but conscious ("noetic") level. It is effective for identifying, for example, an apple as an apple, no matter what color it is or if it is half eaten or intact. It also allows distinguishing an apple from a pear or peach. Semantic memory that was also termed 'knowledge system' is context-free and refers to general facts. It is considered to be noetic as well. The episodic-autobiographical memory system is context-specific with respect to time and place. It allows subjective mental time travel and re-experiencing of the event by attaching an emotional flavor to it. Examples are events such as the last vacation or the dinner of the previous night. Tulving (2005) defined episodic –autobiographical memory as being the conjunction of autonoetic consciousness, subjective time, and the experiencing self where autonoetic consciousness represents the capacity "that allows adult humans to mentally represent and to become aware of their protracted existence across subjective time" (Wheeler, Stuss, & Tulving, 1997, p.335).

Each memory system is embedded in specific brain networks. In a simplified way, there are primarily subcortical and cortical motor-related structures for the procedural memory system, neocortical, modality-specific regions for the priming system, the neocortical association cortex for perceptual memory, and cortical and limbic regions for semantic memory. In the case of episodic-autobiographical memory system, several widespread limbic and cortical (including prefrontal) regions are of importance, rendering this memory system more susceptible to environmental insults in comparison to the other systems.

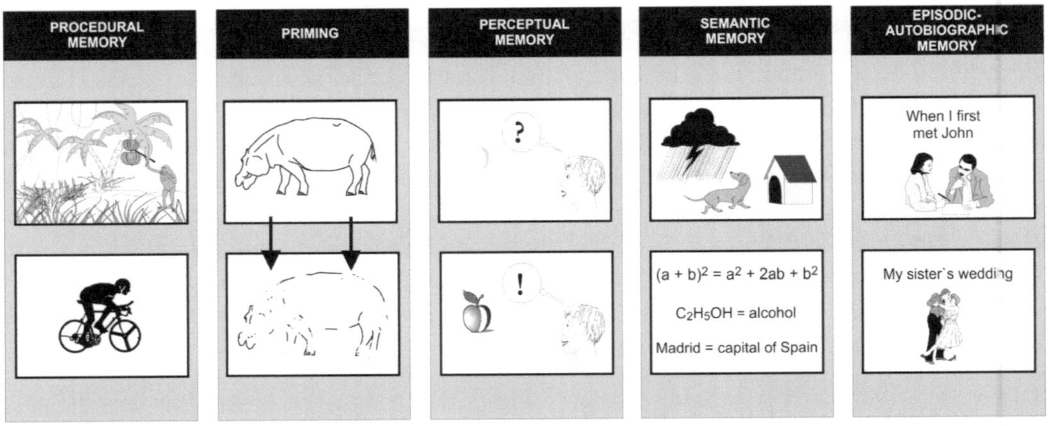

Fig. 1. The five long-term memory systems. Procedural memory is largely motor-based, but includes also sensory and cognitive skills ("routines"). Priming refers to a higher likeliness of re-identifying previously perceived stimuli. Perceptual memory allows distinguishing an object, item, or person on the basis of distinct features. Semantic memory is context-free and refers to general facts. It is termed the knowledge systems as well. The episodic-autobiographical memory system is context-specific with respect to time and place. It allows mental time travel. Examples are events such as the last vacation or the dinner of the previous night. Tulving (2005) defined it as the conjunction of autonoetic consciousness, subjective time, and the experiencing self.

A main feature of episodic-autobiographical memory is its state-dependency. This implies that episodic-autobiographical memories are best retrieved when the conditions during encoding (mood and environment) match those during retrieval. A mismatch between encoding and retrieval conditions may result in a gamut of memory retrieval disturbances, ranging from the tip-of-the-tongue phenomena to complete blockades, such as in dissociative amnesic disorders. The blockade in dissociative amnesia is posited to preponderantly reflect a desynchronization during retrieval between emotional and fact-based information processing (Markowitsch, 2002). This blockade is opined to be caused by adverse life conditions in the form of massive acute stress or chronic stress, which elicits the release of several stress hormones (O`Brien, 1997; Joels & Baram, 2009), which then bind to the amygdala and the hippocampus - areas with a high density of glucocorticod receptors (Rodriguez, LeDoux, et al., 2009). This process then may initiate changes of the morphology or functional connectivity of the above mentioned structures, which in turn may lead to severe and persisting impairments of recollecting the episodic-autobiographical material.

4. The neuroimaging of dissociative amnesia and fugue

Dissociative amnesia and fugue conditions typically occur in the absence of significant brain damage as detected by conventional structural brain imaging techniques. When some brain damage exists, the extent of amnesia cannot be accounted for by the locus and degree of brain damage and amnesia is often labeled as "disproportionate amnesia" (Piolino et al., 2005). In the last years, functional brain imaging was used with increasing frequency in patients with various forms of dissociative amnesic disorders (Figure 2). Most frequently, and particularly in the first publications, positron-emission-tomography (PET) was applied (Markowitsch, 1999; Markowitsch, Calabrese et al., 1997a; Markowitsch, Fink, Thöne, Kessler, & Heiss, 1997b; Markowitsch, Thiel, Kessler, von Stockhausen, & Heiss, 1997c; Markowitsch, Kessler, Van der Ven, Weber-Luxenburger, & Heiss, 1998; Markowitsch, Kessler et al., 2000). The studies using glucose PET attempted to find changes in cerebral metabolism associated with dissociative memory impairments, in particular persistent retrograde dissociative amnesia affecting episodic-autobiographical domain in single cases with dissociative amnesia. Markowitsch, Kessler et al. (1998, 2000), for example, found significant reductions in glucose metabolism in the brain of a patient (case A.M.N.) with dissociative (psychogenic) amnesia; these reductions were observed all over the cerebrum, but in particular in memory-processing regions of the medial temporal lobe and the diencephalon. In these regions the reductions amounted to 2/3 of the normal level in both hemispheres. A.M.N. was a 23 year- old employee of an insurance company with 11 years of education. After discovering one evening the outbreak of a fire in the cellar of his house, he immediately left the house shouting "Fire, fire" while his friend – who was in the house at the time as well – called the fire workers who immediately extinguished the fire. In the night of the event A.M.N. and his friend retired to bed as usually, but the next morning, upon waking up, A.M.N. thought that he was 17 years old only, did not remember any personal events beyond this age and also became unable to acquire new events long-term. Three weeks later he was admitted to an university clinic, where he underwent medical and laboratory work up (that included structural brain MRI, EEG, carotid arteries ultrasound, chest X-ray and ECG), which was unremarkable. After three weeks of psychotherapeutic interventions in the hospital the patient recollected one of his childhood memories. He remembered that at age 4 years he saw a car crash with another car in flames. He was then witness to the driver's death in flames. This memory was confirmed by the patient's mother, who witnessed that event as well. Since then the open fire was reportedly perceived as life threatening by him. The authors hypothesized that the witnessing of the traumatic incident at age 4 already initiated subtle biological changes and that the latter witnessing of the fire outbreak in the house triggered a magnified biological response in the form of a neurotoxic cascade-like release of stress hormones, such as glucocorticoids (O'Brien, 1997), which led to the mnestic blockade that covered his last 6 years of life. The fact that the blockade of his conscious memories for personal events spanned the last 6 years of his life may have been accounted for by several experiences he had during that time, which had an intense and negative emotional connotation: he disclosed to his parents and his entourage his sexual preferences, he experienced conflicts with parents and ended up leaving both school and his parents' house. In a subsequent paper from 2000 the authors could demonstrate that, after combined psycho-pharmaceutical (antidepressant medication treatment) and psychotherapeutic interventions, memory recovered and the brain's glucose level returned to normal values in all areas. Probably this was the first paper that provided objective evidence via brain imaging for functional brain changes paralleling successful combined psychiatric treatment.

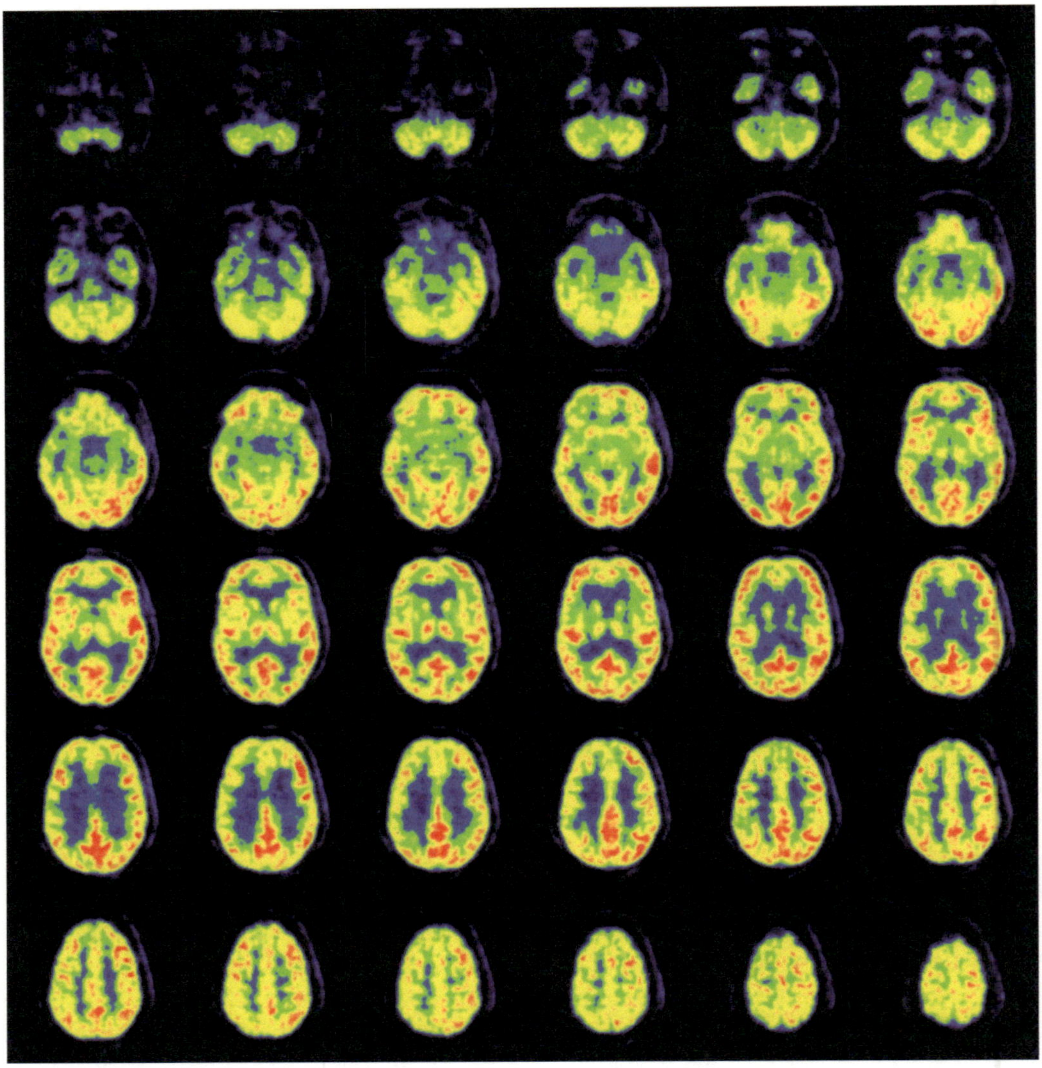

Fig. 2. Example of reduced regional cerebral glucose metabolism in the anterior temporo-frontal cortices in a patient with dissociative amnesia.

In likely the first paper on functional brain imaging in a variant of dissociative amnesia (dissociative fugue condition), Markowitsch, Fink et al. (1997b) used water-PET in order to find out whether the retrogradely amnesic patient showed any differences in functional activations in comparison to controls (Fink et al., 1996) when confronted with episodes from his personal past. Indeed, the patient's brain showed markedly different activations in comparison to that of the normals: While the normal probands had predominantly right temporo-frontal activation (Fink et al., 1996), the patient had a left-hemispheric activation of these regions. In light of other data on brain activations during memory retrieval (e.g., Reinhold, Kühnel, Brand, & Markowitsch, 2006; LaBar & Cabeza, 2006), this finding was interpreted as suggesting that the patient perceived his own episodic-autobiographical episodes as if they were belonging to a third, neutral person.

In a paper in which glucose-PET data from 14 patients with dissociative amnesia and severe episodic-autobiographical memory deficits were analyzed in combination, it was found that again the right temporo-frontal region was hypometabolic in a significant number of patients, with a significant reduction in the right inferolateral prefrontal cortex (Brand et al., 2009). This finding has possible therapeutic implications. It suggests that if the brain regions of the right temporofrontal cortex, which are interconnected by the uncinate fascicle, were brought to normal metabolic activity via environmental manipulations, the patients' ability to recollect personal events from the past might be reinstated. A kind of confirmation and extension of these results came in same year from the work of Tramoni et al. (2009), who in a patient with dissociative ("functional") amnesia performed magnetization transfer ratio measurement and MR spectroscopic imaging - methods sensitive to microstructural and metabolic brain changes. They found evidence of significant metabolic changes and subtle structural alterations of the white matter in the right prefrontal region.

In other reports on patients with dissociative amnesia glucose-PET, single photon emission computed tomography (SPECT) or fMRI, or combinations of several of these methods were used (Sellal, Manning, Seegmuller, Scheiber, & Schoenfelder, 2002, Glisky et al., 2004; Botzung, Denkova, & Manning, 2007; Hennig-Fast et al., 2008; Serra, Fadda, Buccione, Caltagirone, & Carlesimo, 2007; Stracciari, Fonti, & Guarino, 2008; Yang et al., 2005; Piolino et al., 2005; Yasuno et al., 2000; Thomas- Antérion, Guedj, Decousous, & Laurent, 2010 ; Arzy, Collette, Wissmeyer, Lazeyras, Kaplan, & Blanke, in press; Kikuchi et al., 2010). In most cases brain metabolic and functional changes were found, which involved areas that are agreed upon to play crucial roles in mnemonic processing. The differences in the localization and nature of the changes, which were at times reported, might be accounted for by several factors, such as the individual characteristics of the patients, the lack of control for variables, such as sex, differences in methodology (types of imaging methods used, the performance of functional imaging during rest versus administration of various tasks, differences in the task paradigms employed etc). In the case report of Thomas- Antérion , Guedj, Decousous and Laurent (2010), FDG-PET in resting state was performed in a right handed 30-40 year old male of probably Chinese origin who spoke French and had retrograde dissociative amnesia with personal identity loss approximately 15 months after he had been found in a French city. The PET scan demonstrated major hypometabolism, especially in left medial temporal lobe and insular/opercular area. The hypometabolism affected areas in termporal polar cortex, the amygdala, the hippocampus, the parahippocampus and the fusiform gyrus. The structural MRI was found to be within normal limits. Three years later, the patient still showed retrograde amnesia and loss of personal identity. In the paper of Glisky, Ryan, Reminger, Hardt, Hayes, and Hupbach (2004) a patient with a psychogenic fugue condition is presented, who lost conscious access to his autobiography together with native German language, while his implicit memory and knowledge of German grammar structure remained intact. Neuroimaging data revealed a reduced prefrontal metabolism, which was in conformity with his poor performance on tests of executive functions.

5. The neuroimaging of dissociative identity disorder

Research on structural brain changes in patients with dissociative identity disorder produced non-uniform results. One study reported volumetric decreases in amygdala and hippocampus in patients with dissociative identity disorder (Vermetten et al., 2006), while another yielded negative results (Weniger, Lange, Sachsse, & Irle, 2008). The non-homogeneity of these results may partly be understood in the light of new research data, which suggest that the impact of stress on structures involved in mnemonic processing (such as hippocampus and amygdala) has a differentiated response, which is modulated by the existence of certain developmental windows of vulnerability (Lupien et al., 2009). Several researchers investigated patients with dissociative identity disorder via functional imaging. Saxe, Vasile, Hill, Bloomingdale and van der Kolk (1992) found in a study using single emission computerized tomography (SPECT) that changes in personality state in a patient with DID were associated with significant fluctuations in the right temporal lobe blood flow. Sar, Unal, Kiziltan, Kundakci, and Ozturk (2001) and Sar, Unal, and Ozturk (2007) studied brain perfusion in a considerable number of patients (15 in one study, 21 in the other) with DID. Regional cerebral blood flow was found to be decreased in the left and right orbitofrontal cortex of the DID patients and increased in their left (dominant) lateral temporal (Sar et al., 2001) or bilaterally in the occipital cortex (Sar et al., 2007).

Two interesting studies were performed by Simone Reinders from the Netherlands (Reinders et al., 2003, 2006). Together with her colleagues she studied patients with DID. Using fMRI she found different brain activations when the patients where in distinct mental states of self-awareness, each with its own access to autobiographical trauma-related memory. As in many other studies, the medial prefrontal cortex was related to these self-states and the ability of conscious reflection. Verbal working memory was investigated in 16 patients with the diagnoses DID or Dissociative Disorder - not otherwise specified (DD-NOS) (Elzinga et al., 2007). They found that the patients and 16 matched normal subjects activated similar brain regions , which are typically involved in working memory (especially dorsolateral prefrontal and parietal cortex); however, the patients showed a higher activation in these areas and made fewer errors with increasing task load compared to the healthy individuals (though they felt more anxious and less able to concentrate).

6. Ganser syndrome and neuroimaging

A particular form of dissociative disorder is the Ganser syndrome. The syndrome has been submitted to several diagnostic revisions and debates over the years (Cocores, Santa, & Patel, 1984). In comparison to previous DSM editions, where Ganser syndrome was presented as a Factitious Disorder, Ganser syndrome is currently included under the category of Dissociative Disorders NOS (Not Otherwise Specified) in DSM-IV-TR (2000) and it is simply defined by giving approximate answers to questions (*vorbeireden*). Ganser's (1898, 1904) original description of the syndrome was, however, much broader than the current DSM-IV-TR one. It featured a hysterical semitrance characterized by a tendency to give approximate answers, amnesia and hallucinations. Though initially linked to forensic background, Ganser syndrome was also reported in non-forensic contexts. The syndrome was found to affect preponderantly young men with a mean age of 35 years, although there were case-reports in women and children as well (Nardi & Di Scipio, 1977). The onset of Ganser syndrome is usually acute in nature, often with a picture suggestive of a hysterical pseudo-dementia. Its course can be transient or chronic. A higher incidence of Ganser syndrome in patients with immigrant background or ethnic minorities has also been suggested (Staniloiu et al., 2009).

Comorbidity with other psychiatric (such as major depressive disorder, conversion disorder) or neurological conditions (e.g. mild traumatic brain injury) are very common, which may make imaging data more difficult to interpret. Functional imaging data in patients with Ganser syndrome is however very scant. So far, we have been aware of only two studies: one performed by Markowitsch and co-workers (described in Staniloiu & Markowitsch, 2010) and an older report by Snyder and co-workers (1998). Snyder, Monte, Buchsbaum and Krishnab (1998) described the case of a 32 year old man of Spanish origin who since age 9 had been raised bilingually in both Spanish and English and while recovering from an asthma attack presented with conversion symptoms (psychogenic blindness), Ganser-like presentation (approximate answers), memory difficulties, naming and calculation difficulties and a lack of concern about his symptoms - "la belle indifference" (Janet, 1907). Head CT scan without contrast was within normal limits. MRI without contrast revealed a signal abnormality in the right parietal cortex. Cerebral angiogram was within normal limits. Glucose PET revealed severe bilateral hypometabolic regions in the posterior cortex. His visual symptoms disappeared 37 days after the asthma attack, but 83 days after the attack he continued to have naming difficulties.

Markowitsch and co-workers described two male patients in their 30's with this syndrome, one with a clear forensic background (Staniloiu and Markowitsch, 2010) and one without (Staniloiu et al., 2009). In the patient without forensic background, the condition emerged after a mild traumatic brain injury and was accompanied by symptoms of major depressive disorder. Both patients showed in addition to symptoms of *vorbeireden* (giving approximate answers) a global deterioration of their intellectual capacities suggestive of a pseudo-dementic picture as well as conversion symptoms. One for example exhibited psychogenic urinary retention. Their clinical presentation followed a chronic course that extended beyond two years, despite treatment.

Although in both cases of Ganser syndrome the structural brain imaging investigations were not indicative of organic impairment, in the patient where additional functional imaging (glucose PET) was performed, a global significant reduction in the brain metabolism was visualized. The mentioned functional imaging result and the chronic course of the above mentioned two patients are relevant, in the light of findings from previous studies. Some of those studies pointed to a possible organic basis to the psychiatric presentation of the Ganser syndrome that can especially become apparent over time. For example, Ladowsky-Brooks and Fischer (2003) described a patient, who presented with features of Ganser syndrome and severe cognitive deficits in other domains. However, the individual's cognitive decline over a period of a year, in combination with findings from functional imaging, led to a diagnosis of fronto-temporal dementia.

7. Depersonalization disorder and neuroimaging

The manifestations and courses of dissociative disorders vary widely (Priebe & Schmahl, 2009). Depersonalization disorder involves a dissociation of perceptions (e.g. feeling detached from own body or mental activity, like in a dreaming state or like an outsider observer), in the absence of significant impairment of reality testing. It is characterized by an alteration of the subjective experience of self. Its onset dates back to adolescence or adult life. Comorbidity with other mood or anxiety disorders is common and may hinder its timely diagnosis, promoting therefore a chronic course of the illness. While several imaging studies of depersonalization focused on targeting the neural correlates of depersonalization as a symptom of other disorder (Lanius et al., 2005) or a symptom that was induced via various environmental manipulations (Blanke & Metzinger, 2009; Mathew et al., 1999) only a few studies looked at the neural correlates of depersonalization disorders. Simeon et al. (2000) investigated 8 subjects with depersonalization disorder and 24 healthy matched-controls with both structural (MRI) and functional imaging (FDG-PET). During the PET scanning the subjects were given a variant of California Verbal Learning Test modified for use in imaging study. The depersonalization disorder group showed significantly lower metabolic rates in areas belonging to the right superior temporal gyrus and middle temporal gyrus. In addition, they showed higher metabolic rates in parietal lobe in comparison to normal probands. In occipital lobes, left Brodmann area 19 was significantly more active in the depersonalization group. The authors concluded that depersonalization disorder is associated with functional abnormalities in sensory cortex (visual, auditory and somatosensory) as well as areas that are important for body schema (such as parietal cortex).

8. Conversion disorder and neuroimaging

Other dissociative disorders are those which present with impairments of perceptual or motor functions that cannot be explained by medical or neurological conditions (Stone, Vuilleumier, & Friedman, 2010).They are subsumed under dissociative (conversion) disorders in ICD-10, but belong to the category of somatoform disorders in DSM-IV-TR. Although Sigmund Freud described "Die psychogene Sehstörung in psychoanalytischer Auffassung" [Psychogenic visual disturbance in psychoanalytic view] already in 1910, data on functional imaging in this condition is scant. Apart from the glucose PET study of the Ganser-like presentation with accompanying psychogenic blindness presented above (Snyder et al., 1998) we found one functional magnetic resonance imaging study on visual symptomatologies in dissociative patients. Werring, Weston, Bullmore, Plant, and Ron (2004) observed reduced activation in visual cortical areas during flicker-light stimulation and decreased anterior cingulate activation. The posterior cingulate cortex on the other hand showed increased activity, as did the insula, the temporopolar areas, striatum, and thalamus. The data were interpreted as demonstrating visual blocking via limbic activation.

For somatosensory and motor disturbances, on the other hand, first studies using SPECT started in 1995 in a patient with hemisensory disturbances and revealed some qualitative changes in fronto-parietal regions (Tiihonen, Kuikka, Viinamäki, Lehtonen, & Partanen, 1995). Three years later, another study (Yazici & Kostakoglu, 1998) investigated five patients with more heterogeneous symptomatologies and more heterogeneous reductions in brain perfusion, in particular in left temporo-parietal regions. In 2006, Ghaffar and his co-workers (Ghaffar, Staines, & Feinstein, 2006) assessed three individuals with unexplained sensory loss using fMRI during unilateral and bilateral vibrotactile stimulation. They found that stimulation of the affected limb did not produce activation of the contralateral primary sensory cortex, while this was elicited with bilateral stimulation. The authors emphasized the role of attention mechanisms in the conversion disorder (Bell et al., 2011).

Movement-related conversion disorders (unilateral limb weaknesses) were studied with functional brain imaging in more detail (Cojan, Waber, Carruzzo, & Vuilleumier, 2009; Stone et al., 2007; Vuilleumier et al., 2001; Spence, Crimlisk, Cope, Ron, & Grasby, 2000) . In the SPECT study published in 2001 by Vuilleumier and co-workers (Vuilleumier et al., 2001), the authors used three different conditions: a baseline resting condition, a passive activation condition, and vibrotactile stimulation of the affected and unaffected limbs (for some patients after the motor symptoms had recovered). Vibrotactile compared to baseline condition activated frontal and parietal regions related to somatosensory and motor functions. A further comparison in the recovered patients revealed in the hemisphere contralateral to the motor deficits basal ganglia and thalamus decreases when the deficit was present.

Burgmer et al. published in 2006 a report on patients who due to psychic changes were unable to lift their hands. The authors used fMRI to study their brain activations, when the patients either tried to lift their hands or observed other persons lifting their hands. Main results were that when normal subjects lifted hands or observed others lifting theirs, the hand region of their motor cortex was activated; in the case of the patients this activation failed to occur. The authors interpreted their findings as suggesting that in normal individuals mirror neurons (or the so-called mirror system) "mimic" the action of the other, while in the brains of patients with movement-related dissociative disorders, no such activity occurs.

An unusual case of conversion disorder is that of a woman with spatial neglect due to conversion disorder (Saj et al., 2009), who presented with left spatial neglect as assessed by line- bisection and bell-cancellation tests. Findings from fMRI pointed to selective activation of the posterior or parietal cortex, primarily in the right side when comparing lines with deviated bisection relative to centered bisection (which was similar to those from normal probands performing comparable tests), together with increased activity in the anterior cingulate cortex. The results were interpreted as supporting the impaired access to conscious control in patients with conversion disorder and extending the findings about the role of anterior cingulate cortex in conversion disorder, which may relate to the anterior cingulate's functions in attention and inhibitory processes.

Psychogenic non-epileptic seizures are also possible manifestations of conversion disorder. The differential diagnosis of these conditions might pose a variety of challenges , given that psychogenic non-epileptic seizures might at times occur after traumatic brain injury, neurosurgery or in patients with an already diagnosed epileptic condition. Several methods have been used to distinguish psychogenic non-epileptic seizures from true epileptic seizures. Among them, the performance of interictal SPECT might be a useful tool (Scevola et al., 2009).

9. Imaging the symptom of dissociation

Various dissociative symptoms can accompany a number of psychiatric diagnostic entities (other than dissociative or conversion disorders) and have been targeted by several functional imaging studies (Kraus et al., 2009; Ludaescher et al., 2010). For example dissociative amnesia can occur as a symptom in certain anxiety disorders, such as acute stress disorder and post-traumatic stress disorder (PTSD) or in the DSM-IV-TR described somatization disorder or in borderline personality disorder (Zanarini, Frankenburg, Jager-Hyman, Reich, & Fitzmaurice, 2008).

PTSD conditions which are accompanied by "positive" dissociative symptoms such as flashbacks and intrusions seem to engage different neural networks than PTSD conditions that are accompanied by "negative" dissociative symptoms such as amnesia (Oakley, 1999). Lanius, Williamson et al. (2005) found that in general a network of prefronto-temporo-parietal areas was engaged in all patients, but that the group with "positive" symptoms had - compared to normal subjects - in addition a greater covariation with the right insula and right visual association cortex (compared to the reference in the left ventrolateral thalamus). Between the two groups, that with "negative" symptoms of dissociation showed - compared to the "positive" (flashbacks) group - a more significant covariation in the left inferior frontal gyrus, while vice versa the "positive" symptoms group had more significant covariations with posterior cingulate/precuneus regions, the right middle temporal and the left inferior frontal gyri. In a recent review arguments were made for a mechanism of undermodulation of emotion via failure of prefrontal inhibition of limbic regions (such as amygdala) underlying the re-experiencing/hyperarousal PTSD subtype and one of overmodulation of the emotional limbic reactions in the ("negative") dissociative PTSD subtype (Lanius et al., 2010).

10. Imaging and hypnosis

Hypnotizability traits have been postulated to be associated with a higher tendency for developing dissociative symptoms (Maldonado & Spiegel, 2008). Recently, we have witnessed an increase in studies investigating the relationship between trait hypnotizability and risk for developing various dissociative (conversion) disorders. As Bell et al. (2011) pointed to in a recent comprehensive review article, the results are mixed. Despite this, several studies tried to model various dissociative (conversion) symptoms via hypnotic suggestions. One functional MRI study employed hypnosis to affect memories for scenes of a movie when a posthypnotic cue was given (Mendelsohn, Chalamish, Solomonovich, & Dudai, 2008). The study compared three groups: one group that scored high on hypnotizability, another group that was characterized by low hypnotizability traits and a group that was asked to simulate high hypnotizability. According to the findings of the study, only the group with high hypnotizability traits manifested impaired recall. The latter was associated with diminished functional brain activity particularly in the left extrastriate occipital lobe and left temporal pole and heightened activity in the left rostro-lateral prefrontal cortex. Following the reversal of 'forget' suggestion and normalization of memory performance, an increase in brain activity was observed in several regions, including areas in the occipital, parietal and dorso-lateral frontal regions. This result was interpreted (Bell et al., 2011) as being in the line with the advanced model of exaggerated inhibition in psychogenic (dissociative) amnesia (Kopelman, 2000; Anderson & Green, 2001). This model proposes that the inability to retrieve personal events in psychogenic (dissociative) amnesia reflects an increase in the activity of inhibitory regions of the prefrontal cortex coupled with a subsequent decrease in the activity of hippocampus, similar to the one that occurs in suppression or motivated forgetting. The other main model of dissociative amnesia (which we already described above) posits that the recollection deficit in dissociative amnesia reflects a stress hormone-triggered and -mediated memory blockade, underpinned by a desynchronization during retrieval between a frontal lobe system, important for autonoetic consciousness, and a temporo-amygdalar system, important for emotional processing and colorization (Markowitsch, 2002).

11. Mindfulness versus dissociation

The concept of mindfulness is often viewed as being situated at the opposite pole of that of dissociation. In a simplified way, Kabat-Zinn refers to mindfulness as moment-to-moment awareness (Kabat-Zinn, 2005). This awareness arises through intentionally attending to one's moment to moment experience in a non-judgmental and accepting way (Shapiro, Oman, Thoresen, Plante, & Flinders, 2008). Mindfulness is considered an inherent human capacity that can however be enhanced through training and practice through meditation techniques. In the recent past, there has been an increased interest in integrating the ancient Buddhist practice of mindfulness meditation (MM) with current psychological and medical practice as means to treat a variety of psychological and physical disorders (Baer, 2003; Grossman et al., 2004), to reduce stress in healthy individuals and to enhance the well being and overall health. Mindfulness based interventions (MBI), which include, but are not limited to mindfulness-based stress reduction (MBSR) and mindfulness-based cognitive therapy (MBCT) have flourished from the fertile ground of mindfulness meditation (Grossman, Niemann, Schmidt, & Walach, 2004). Both MM and MBIs aim to reduce the onset and maintenance of negative emotions such as anger while enhancing happiness and compassion (Chiesa & Malinowski, 2011; Sharot, Riccardi, Raio, & Phelps, 2007).

Numerous studies evaluated mindfulness' effects on well-being. Imaging techniques were employed to unveil the neuronal circuitry underlying the neurobiological mechanism, as well as the structural changes occurring in the brain during mindfulness meditation or any derivates of this technique, however, their review is beyond our scope. We will instead focus on available evidence from neuroimaging on identifying the neural correlates of dispositional mindfulness and the clinical application of MBCT to conditions that might be accompanied by dissociative symptoms such as BPD (borderline personality disorder) and PTSD (post traumatic stress disorder).

MBCT is a 8-week training program rooting from MM and CBT with direct application as additive therapy to prevent relapses in major depression, anxiety disorders and bipolar disorder. Attempts have been made to use this technique in BPD (Sachse, Keville, & Feigenbaum, in press) with the conclusion that further exploring may be worthwhile due to the observed effects of MBCT on mindfulness, experiential avoidance, state anxiety, and somatoform dissociation. However, to our knowledge there are no functional imaging data available to further support these findings.

With respect to the potential impact of MBCT on mechanisms that might perpetuate/exacerbate recollection impairment in dissociative amnesia, such as cognitive avoidance (Fujiwara et al., 2008), one study is worthwhile to be mentioned (Williams, Teasdale, Segal, & Soulsby, 2000). The authors of this study used MBCT in patients who recovered from major depressive disorder - a condition characterized by episodic-autobiographical memory impairments in the form of overgeneralized memory that may persist beyond the recovery of classical depressive symptoms (Williams & Scott, 1988). They showed that in comparison to controls (recovered depressed patients who received no MBCT), patients with recovered major depression who received MBCT experienced a reduction in their overgeneralized autobiographical memories. (People are considered to have overgeneralized autobiographical memories when in response to a verbal cue they retrieve generic summaries of their personal past rather than specific events.) Again no functional imaging paradigm was employed in this study.

Five main meditation practices are identified (Ospina et al., 2007).

- Mantra meditation (Transcendental meditation, relaxation response, clinically standardized meditation);
- Mindfulness meditation (Vipassana, Zen, MBSR);
- Yoga;
- Tai-chi and
- Qi Gong.

In order to attain the "meditative" state two main approaches are employed: focused attention FA (direct and sustained attention on a selected object, detecting distractions and disengagement of attention from distractions with cognitive reappraisal of the distracter) and objective monitoring OM (non reactive cognitive monitoring and awareness of sensory, perceptual and endogenous (Lutz, Slagter, Dunne, & Davidson, 2008).

Evidence on the EEG profile supports differences in the frequency bands between the two approaches as follows: FA is associated with beta 1 and gamma frequency bands while OM (Vipassana, Zen), with theta frequency bands. There is also evidence for a third type of frequency band, alpha1, associated with an automatic self-transcending encountered during Transcendental Meditation (Travis & Shear, 2010).

An fMRI study contrasted FA and OM meditation forms in expert meditators versus novices (Manna et al., 2010) and concluded that experienced meditators control cognitive engagement in conscious processing of sensory-related, thought and emotion contents by massive self regulation in fronto-parietal and insular areas in the left hemisphere in a meditative state when compared with rest. They also concluded based on their findings that the anterior cingulate and dorso-lateral prefrontal cortex seem to play antagonist roles in the executive control of the attention setting during meditation task. This in their opinion reconciled findings of transient hypofrontality in meditation with evidence of activation of executive brain areas during meditation. They proposed that the practice of mediation leads to a functional reorganization of activity of prefrontal cortex and insula. Insula is a structure that has been hypothesized to sustain the so-called "sentient" (feeling) self (Craig, 2009). It has recently received an increased interest in stress related disturbances of self and consciousness (Lanius et al., 2005, 2010), including the ones accompanying the dissociative memory "loss" (Thomas-Anterion et al., 2010; Brand et al., 2009). Hidden in the Sylvian sulcus in the triangle of frontal, parietal, and temporal cortex, the insula is connected to numerous brain regions, including inferior frontal gyrus, septum and amygdala (Markowitsch, Emmans, Irle, Streicher, & Preilowski, 1985, Augustine. 1996). It sends projections to hippocampus and receives efferents from the entorhinal cortex. The most anterior and ventral portion of the insula that is close to the frontal operculum contains the so-called Von Economo neurons (VEN) (Allman, Watson, Tetreault, & Hakeem, 2005). The VEN neurons, which are also present in the anterior cingular cortex (ACC), might play functions in consciousness and emotional awareness (Allman et al., 2005). Insula has also been assigned functions in verbal memory tasks, inner speech, time perception , self projection (Arzy et al., 2009) , drug smoking cravings , eating regulation, taste, pain and temperature perception. In normal subjects increased activations of the insula have been evidenced in tasks involving self versus other conditions (Schilbach et al., 2006) and the right insula was found to be activated during self face recognition (Devue et al., 2007).

As mentioned above the insula has bilateral connections with the amygdala. The amygdala is a structure involved in integrating emotions with cognition and is connected with the prefrontal cortex via uncinate fascicle and other fiber bundles. Interestingly, the uncinate fascicle has a temporal, frontal and insular part and was ascribed functions in memory and emotional processing (Markowitsch, 1995). The ventromedial portion of uncinate fascicle primarily connects the amygdala and uncus with the gyrus rectus and the subcallosal area (Ebeling & von Cramon, 1992). Associating events mindfully to oneself appears to be one of the major functions of amygdaloid neurons in the human brain (Stein, Ives-Deliperi, & Thomas, 2008). Furthermore, traits like the optimism bias were suggested to be underpinned by the strength of the connectivity between the rostral anterior cingulate cortex and amygdala (Sharot, Riccardi, Raio & Phelps, 2007). An fMRI study that investigated the neural correlates of dispositional mindfulness during affect labelling found strong negative associations between areas of prefrontal cortex and right amygdala in subjects with high mindfulness, but not in participants low in mindfulness (Creswell, Way, Eisenberger & Lieberman, 2007).

The pathophysiological changes associated with different mindfulness-based practices and various meditation practices and the biological mechanisms through which mindfulness - based practices may prevent, alleviate or undo various dissociative symptoms remain a topic for future research. There is however preliminary evidence from various sources that these mechanisms might involve biological changes related to modulation of hormonal stresses responses such via alterations of the function of hypothalamic-pituitary-adrenal (HPA) axis (Vera et al., 2009; Infante et al., 1998).

12. Conclusions

Dissociative disorders have been linked to psychological trauma and stress in a variety of cultures. The advent of functional brain imaging techniques and newer sophisticated structural brain imaging methods has considerably improved and will continue to further our understanding of the neurobiological underpinnings of these conditions. The use of these techniques has shown that environmentally-driven alterations of cognition, perception, behavior and self-related processing are accompanied by metabolic and probably even structural brain changes. These findings have called into questioning the strict traditional dichotomy between neurological-organic and psychiatric-mind based illnesses and prompted several researchers and clinicians from both psychiatry and neurology fields to advocate for moving beyond this dichotomy, by abandoning the organic-functional distinction from formal classification systems or everyday medical jargon. As Pietro Pietrini stated in 2003 in the *American Journal of Psychiatry* (p. 1908): "It was not long ago that psychiatric disorders were grossly classified as 'organic' and 'functional' according to whether there was a known brain structural alteration (e.g., dementia) or not (e.g., depression or schizophrenia). This merely reflected our inability to go beyond what could be visible to the naked eye in the brain. Functional brain studies ... have given us a powerful microscope to dissect the intimate molecular aspects of brain function."

13. References

Allman, J. M., Watson, K. K., Tetreault, N. A., & Hakeem, A. Y. (2005). Intuition and autism: a possible role for Von Economo neurons. *Trends in Cognitive Sciences, 9*, 367-373.

Arzy, S., Collette, S., Wissmeyer, M., Lazeyras, F., Kaplan, P. W., & Blanke, O. (2011) Psychogenic amnesia and self-identity: a multimodal functional investigation. *European Journal of Neurology, 18*, 1422-1425..

Arzy, S., Collette, S., Ionta, S., Fornari, E., & Blanke, O. (2009). Subjective mental time: the functional architecture of projecting the self to past and future. *European Journal of Neuroscience, 30*, 2009-2017.

Anderson, M. C., & Green, C. (2001). Suppressing unwanted memories. *Nature*, 410, 366-369.

Augustine, J. R. (1996). Circuitry and functional aspects of the insular lobe in primates including humans. *Brain Research Reviews, 22*, 229-244.

Bell, V., Oakley, D. A., Halligan, P. W., & Deeley, Q. (2011). Dissociation in hysteria and hypnosis: evidence from cognitive neuroscience. *Journal of Neurology, Neurosurgery, and Psychiatry, 82*, 332-339.

Blanke, O., & Metzinger, T. (2009). Full-body illusions and minimal phenomenal selfhood. *Trends in Cognitive Sciences, 13*, 7-13.

Bluhm, R. L., Wiliamson, P. C., Osuch, E. A., Frewen, P. A., Stevens, T. K., Boksman, K., et al. (2009). Alterations in default network connectivity in posttraumatic stress disorder related to early-life trauma. *Journal of Psychiatry and Neuroscience, 34*, 187-194.

Botzung, A., Denkova, E., & Manning, L. (2007). Psychogenic memory deficits associated with functional cerebral changes: An fMRI study. *Neurocase, 13*, 378-384.

Brand, M., Eggers, C., Reinhold, N., Fujiwara, E., Kessler, J., Heiss, W.-D., & Markowitsch, H. J. (2009). Functional brain imaging in fourteen patients with dissociative amnesia reveals right inferolateral prefrontal hypometabolism. *Psychiatry Research: Neuroimaging Section, 174*, 32-39.

Breuer, J., & Freud, S. (1895). *Studien über Hysterie [Studies on hysteria]*. Wien: Deuticke.

Burgl, G. (1900). Eine Reise in die Schweiz im epileptischen Dämmerzustande und die transitorischen Bewusstseinsstörungen der Epileptiker vor dem Strafrichter [A journey to Switzerland done in epileptic somnolence and the transitory disturbances of consciousness before the criminal judge]. *Münchener medizinische Wochenschrift, 37*, 1270-1273.

Burgmer, M., Konrad, C., Jansen, A., Kugel, H., Sommer, J., Heindel, W., et al. (2006). Abnormal brain activation during movement observation in patients with conversion paralysis. *Neuroimage, 29*(4), 1336-1343.

Chiesa, A., & Malinowski, P. (2011). Mindfulness-based approaches: are they all the same? *Journal of Clinical Psychology, 67*, 404-424.

Cocores, J. A., Santa, W. G., & Patel, M. D. (1984). The Ganser syndrome: Evidence suggesting its classification as a dissociative disorder. *International Journal of Psychiatry in Medicine, 14*, 47-56.

Cojan, Y., Waber, L., Carruzzo, A., & Vuilleumier, P. (2009). Motor inhibition in hysterical conversion paralysis. *Neuroimage, 47*, 1026-1037.

Coons, P. M., & Milstein, V. (1992). Psychogenic amnesia: A clinical investigation of 25 cases. *Dissociation, 5*, 73-79.

Craig, A. D. (2009). How do you feel - now? The anterior insula and human awareness. *Nature Reviews Neuroscience, 10*, 59-70.

Creswell, J. D., Way, B. M., Eisenberger, N. I., & Lieberman, M. D. (2007). Neural correlates of dispositional mindfulness during affect labeling. *Psychosomatic Medicine, 69*, 560-565.

Dana, C. L. (1894). The study of a case of amnesia or 'double consciousness'. *Psychological Review, 1,* 570-580.

Devue, C., Collette, F., Balteau, E., Degueldre, C., Luxen, A., Maquet, P., et al. (2007). Here I am: the cortical correlates of visual self-recognition. *Brain Research, 1143,* 169-182.

Donath, J. (1899). Der epileptische Wandertrieb (Poriomanie) [The epileptic drive to wander (poriomania)]. *Archiv für Psychiatrie und Nervenkrankheiten, 32,* 335-355.

Donath, J. (1908). Ueber hysterische Amnesie [On hysterical amnesia]. *Archiv für Psychiatrie und Nervenkrankheiten, 44,* 559-575.

DSM-IV-TR. (2000). *Diagnostic and statistical manual of mental disorders* (4th ed.). Washington, DC: American Psychiatric Association.

Ebeling, U., & von Cramon, D. (1992). Topography of the uncinate fascicle and adjacent temporal fiber tracts. *Acta Neurochirurgica (Wien), 115,* 143-148.

Elzinga, B. M., Ardon, A. M., Heijnis, M. K., de Ruiter, M. B., van Dyck, R., & Veltman, D. J. (2007). Neural correlates of enhanced working-memory performance in dissociative disorder: a functional MRI study. *Psychological Medicine, 37,* 235-245.

Fink, G. R., Markowitsch, H. J., Reinkemeier, M., Bruckbauer, T., Kessler, J., & Heiss, W.-D. (1996). Cerebral representation of one's own past: neural networks involved in autobiographical memory. *Journal of Neuroscience, 16,* 4275-4282.

Freud, S. (1910). Die psychogene Sehstöung in psychoanalytischer Auffassung [Psychogenic visual disturbance in psychoanalytic view]. *Ärztliche Fortbildung (Beiheft zu Ärztliche Standesbildung), 9,* 42-44.

Fujiwara, E., Brand, M., Kracht, L., Kessler, J., Diebel, A., Netz, J., Markowitsch, H. J., (2008). Functional retrograde amnesia: a multiple case study. *Cortex. 44,* 29-45.

Ganser, S. J. (1898). Ueber einen eigenartigen hysterischen Dämmerzustand [On a peculiar hysterical state of somnolence]. *Archiv für Psychiatrie und Nervenkrankheiten, 30,* 633-640.

Ganser, S. J. (1904). Zur Lehre vom hysterischen Dämmerzustande [On the theory of the hysterical state of somnolence]. *Archiv für Psychiatrie und Nervenkrankheiten, 38,* 34-46.

Ghaffar, O., Staines, W. R., & Feinstein, A. (2006). Unexplained neurologic symptoms: an fMRI study of sensory conversion disorder. *Neurology, 67,* 2036-2038.

Hennig-Fast, K., Meister, F., Frödl, T., Beraldi, A., Padberg, F., Engel, R. R., Reiser, M., Möller, H.-J., & Meindl, T. (2008). A case of persistent retrograde amnesia following a dissociative fugue: Neuropsychological and neurofunctional underpinnings of loss of autobiographical memory and self-awareness. *Neuropsychologia, 46,* 2993-3005.

ICD-10. (1992). *Classification of mental and behavioral disorders: Clinical descriptions and diagnostic guidelines.* Geneva: World Health Organization.

Infante, J. R., Peran, F., Martinez, M., Roldan, A., Poyatos, R., Ruiz, C., et al. (1998). ACTH and beta-endorphin in transcendental meditation. *Physiology and Behavior, 64,* 311-315.

Janet, P. (1898). *Nevroses et idees fixes* (Vols. 1, 2). Paris, Felix Alcan. [cited after van der Kolk & van der Hart, 1989].

Janet, P. (1907). *The major symptoms of hysteria: fifteen lectures given in the Medical School of Harvard University.* New York: Macmillan.

Joels, M., & Baram, T. Z. (2009). The neuro-symphony of stress. *Nature Reviews Neuroscience, 10*, 459-466.

Kabat-Zinn, J. (2005). Full catastrophe living: using the wisdom of your body and mind to face stress, pain, and illness. New York: Bantam Dell, a division of Random House Inc.

Kikuchi, H., Fujii, T., Abe, N., Suzuki, M., Takagi, M., Mugikura, S., Takahashi, S., & Mori, E. (2010). Memory repression: brain mechanisms underlying dissociative amnesia. *Journal of Cognitive Neuroscience, 22*, 602-613.

Kopelman, M. D. (2000). Focal retrograde amnesia and the attribution of causality: An exceptionally critical review. *Cognitive Neuropsychology*, 17, 585–621, 2000.

Kraus, A., Esposito, F., Seifritz, E., Di Salle, F., Ruf, M., Valerius, G., Ludaescher, P., Bohus, M, & Schmahl, C., (2009). Amygdala deactivation as a neural correlate of pain processing in patients with borderline personality disorder and co-occurrent posttraumatic stress disorder. *Biological Psychiatry, 65*, 819-822.

LaBar, K. S., & Cabeza, R. (2006). Cognitive neuroscience of emotional memory. *Nature Reviews Neuroscience, 7*, 54-64.

Ladowsky-Brooks, R. L., & Fischer, C. E. (2003). Ganser symptoms in a case of frontal-temporal lobe dementia: Is there a common neural substrate? *Journal of Clinical and Experimental Neuropsychology, 25*, 761–768.

Lanius, R. A., Hopper, J. W., & Menon, R. S. (2003). Individual differences in a husband and wife who developed PTSD after a motor vehicle accident: A functional MRI case study. *American Journal of Psychiatry, 160*, 667-669.

Lanius, R. A., Vermetten, E., Loewenstein, R. J., Brand, B., Schmahl, C., Bremner, J. D., & Spiegel, D. (2010). Emotion modulation in PTSD: Clinical and neurobiological evidence for a dissociative subtype. *American Journal of Psychiatry, 167*, 640-647.

Lanius, R. A., Williamson, P. C., Bluhm, R. L., Densmore, M., Boksman, K., Neufeld, R. W., Gati, J. S., & Menon, R. S. (2005). Functional connectivity of dissociative responses in posttraumatic stress disorder: a functional magnetic resonance imaging investigation. *Biological Psychiatry, 57*, 873-884.

Levine, B., Svoboda, E., Turner, G. R., Mandic, M., & Mackey, A. (2009). Behavioral and functional neuroanatomical correlates of anterograde autobiographical memory in isolated retrograde amnesic patient M.L. *Neuropsychologia, 47*, 2188-2196.

Ludascher, P., Valerius, G., Stiglmayr, C., Mauchnik, J., Lanius, R. A., Bohus, M., & Schmahl, C. (2010). Pain sensitivity and neural processing during dissociative states in patients with borderline personality disorder with and without comorbid posttraumatic stress disorder: a pilot study. *Journal of Psychiatry and Neuroscience, 35*, 177-184.

Lupien, S. J., McEwen, B. S., Gunnar, M. R., & Heim, C. (2009). Effects of stress throughout the lifespan on the brain, behaviour and cognition. *Nature Reviews Neuroscience, 10*, 434-445.

Lutz, A., Slagter, H. A., Dunne, J. D., & Davidson, R. J. (2008). Attention regulation and monitoring in meditation. *Trends in Cognitive Sciences, 12*, 163-169.

Maldonado, J. R., & Spiegel, D. (2008). Dissociative disorders. In R. E. Hales, S. C. Yudofsky, & G. O. Gabbard (Eds.), *The American psychiatric publishing textbook of psychiatry* (5th ed.) (pp. 665-710). Arlington, VA: American Psychiatric Publ.

Manna, A., Raffone, A., Perrucci, M. G., Nardo, D., Ferretti, A., Tartaro, A., et al. (2010). Neural correlates of focused attention and cognitive monitoring in meditation. *Brain Research Bulletin, 82*(1-2), 46-56.

Markowitsch, H. J. (1995). Which brain regions are critically involved in the retrieval of old autobiographic memory? *Brain Research Reviews, 21*, 117-127.

Markowitsch, H. J. (1999). Neuroimaging and mechanisms of brain function in psychiatric disorders. *Current Opinion in Psychiatry, 12*, 331-337.

Markowitsch, H. J., Calabrese, P., Fink, G. R., Durwen, H. F., Kessler, J., Härting, C., König, M., Mirzaian, E. B., Heiss, W.-D., Heuser, L., & Gehlen, W. (1997a). Impaired episodic memory retrieval in a case of probable psychogenic amnesia. *Psychiatry Research: Neuroimaging Section, 74*, 119-126.

Markowitsch, H. J., Fink, G. R., Thöne, A. I. M., Kessler, J., & Heiss, W.-D. (1997b). Persistent psychogenic amnesia with a PET-proven organic basis. *Cognitive Neuropsychiatry, 2*, 135-158.

Markowitsch,H. J., Kessler, J., Van der Ven, C., Weber-Luxenburger, G., & Heiss, W.-D. (1998). Psychic trauma causing grossly reduced brain metabolism and cognitive deterioration. *Neuropsychologia, 36*, 77-82.

Markowitsch, H. J., Kessler, J., Weber-Luxenburger, G., Van der Ven, C., Albers, M., & Heiss, W. D. (2000). Neuroimaging and behavioral correlates of recovery from mnestic block syndrome and other cognitive deteriorations. *Neuropsychiatry Neuropsychology and Behavioral Neurology, 13*, 60-66.

Markowitsch, H. J., Thiel, A., Kessler, J., von Stockhausen, H.-M., & Heiss, W.-D. (1997c). Ecphorizing semi-conscious episodic information via the right temporopolar cortex - a PET study. *Neurocase, 3*, 445-449.

Markowitsch, H. J. (2002). Functional retrograde amnesia - mnestic block syndrome. *Cortex, 38*, 651-654.

Markowitsch, H. J., Emmans, D., Irle, E., Streicher, M., & Preilowski, B. (1985). Cortical and subcortical afferent connections of the primate's temporal pole: A study of rhesus monkeys, squirrel monkeys, and marmosets. *Journal of Comparative Neurology, 242*, 425-458.

Mathew, R. J., Wilson, W. H., Chiu, N. Y., Turkington, T. G., Degrado, T. R., & Coleman, R. E. (1999). Regional cerebral blood flow and depersonalization after tetrahydrocannabinol administration. *Acta Psychiatrica Scandinavica, 100*, 67-75.

Mendelsohn, A., Chalamish, Y., Solomonovich, A., & Dudai, Y. (2008). Mesmerizing memories: brain substrates of episodic memory suppression in posthypnotic amnesia. *Neuron, 57*(1), 159-170.

Nardi, T. J., & Di Scipio, W. J. (1977). The Ganser syndrome in an adolescent Hispanic-black female. *American Journal of Psychiatry, 134*, 453-454.

Oakley, D. A. (1999). Hypnosis and conversion hysteria: a unifying model. *Cognitive Neuropsychiatry, 4*, 243-265.

O'Brien, J. T. (1997). The 'glucocorticoid cascade' hypothesis in man. *British Journal of Psychiatry, 170*, 199-201.

Ospina, M. B., Bond, K., Karkhaneh, M., Tjosvold, L., Vandermeer, B., Liang, Y., et al. (2007). Meditation practices for health: state of the research. *Evidence Report /Technology Assessment (Full Rep)*(155), 1-263.

Pietrini, P. (2003). Toward a biochemistry of mind? *American Journal of Psychiatry, 160,* 1907-1908.

Piolino, P., Hannequin, D., Desgranges, B., Girard, C., Beaunieux, H., Gittard, B., et al. (2005). Right ventral frontal hypomeabolism and abnormal sense of self in a case of disproportionate retrograde amnesia. *Cognitive Neuropsychology, 22,* 1005-1034.

Pope, H. G., Jr., Poliakoff, M. B., Parker, M. P., Boynes, M., & Hudson, J. I. (2007). Is dissociative amnesia a culture-bound syndrome? Findings from a survey of historical literature. *Psychological Medicine, 37,* 225-233.

Post, R. M., Weiss, S. R., Smith, M., Rosen, J., & Frye, M. (1995). Stress, conditioning, and the temporal aspects of affective disorders. *Annals of the New York Academy of Sciences, 771,* 677-696.

Priebe, K., & Schmahl, C. (2009). Dissoziative Störungen [Dissociative disorders]. *Fortschritte der Neurologie- Psychiatrie, 77,* 595-603; quiz 604.

Reinders, A. A. T. S., Nijenhuis, E. R. S., Paans, A. M. J., Korf, J., Willemsen, A. T. M., & den Boer, J. A. (2003). One brain, two selves. *NeuroImage, 20,* 2119-2125.

Reinders, A. A., Nijenhuis, E. R., Quak, J., Korf, J., Haaksma, J.,Paans, A. M.,Willemsen, A. T., & den Boer, J. A. (2006). Psychobiological characteristics of dissociative identity disorder: a symptom provocation study. *Biological Psychiatry, 60,* 730-740.

Reinhold, N., Kühnel, S., Brand, M., & Markowitsch, H. J. (2006). Functional neuroimaging in memory and memory disturbances. *Current Medical Imaging Reviews, 2,* 35-57.

Reinhold, N., & Markowitsch, H. J. (2009). Retrograde episodic memory and emotion: a perspective from patients with dissociative amnesia. *Neuropsychologia, 47,* 2197-2206.

Rodriguez, S. M., LeDoux, J. E., & Sapolsky, R. M. (2009). The influence of stress hormones on fear circuitry. *Annual Reviews of Neuroscience, 32,* 289-313.

Sachse, S., Keville, S., & Feigenbaum, J. A feasibility study of mindfulness-based cognitive therapy for individuals with borderline personality disorder. *Psychology and Psychotherapy, in press.*

Saj, A., Arzy, S., & Vuilleumier, P. (2009). Functional brain imaging in a woman with spatial neglect due to conversion disorder. *Journal of the American Medical Association, 302,* 2552-2554.

Sar, V., Unal, S. N., Kiziltan, E., Kundakci, T., & Ozturk, E. (2001). HMPAO SPECT study of regional cerebral blood flow in dissociative identity disorder. *Journal of Trauma & Dissociation, 2,* 5-25.

Sar, V., Unal, S. N., & Ozturk, E. (2007). Frontal and occipital perfusion changes in dissociative identity disorder. *Psychiatry Research: Neuroimaging, 156,* 217-223.

Saxe, G. N., Vasile, R. G., Hill, T. C., Bloomingdale, K., & Van Der Kolk, B. A. (1992). SPECT imaging and multiple personality disorder. *Journal of Nervous and Mental Diseases, 180,* 662-663.

Scevola, L., D'Alessio, L., Saferstein, D., Centurion, E., Consalvo, D., & Kochen, S. Article ID 712813. Psychogenic nonepileptic seizures after head injury: a case report. *Case Reports in Medicine, 2009.*

Schilbach, L., Wohlschlaeger, A. M., Kraemer, N. C., Newen, A., Shah, N. J., Fink, G. R., & Vogeley, K. (2006). Being with virtual others: Neural correlates of social interaction. *Neuropsychologia, 44,* 718-730.

Sellal, F., Manning, L., Seegmuller, C., Scheiber, C., & Schoenfelder, F. (2002). Pure retrograde amnesia following a mild head trauma: a neuropsychological and metabolic study. *Cortex, 38*, 499-509.

Seligman, R., & Kirmayer, L. J. (2008). Dissociative experience and cultural neuroscience: narrative, metaphor and mechanism. *Culture, Medicine and Psychiatry, 32*, 31-64.

Serra, L., Fadda, L., Buccione, I., Caltagirone, C., & Carlesimo, G. A. (2007). Psychogenic and organic amnesia: a multidimensional assessment of clinical, neuroradiological, neuropsychological and psychopathological features. *Behavioural Neurology, 18*, 53-64.

Shapiro, S. L., Oman, D., Thoresen, C. E., Plante, T. G., & Flinders, T. (2008). Cultivating mindfulness: effects on well-being. *Journal of Clinical Psychology, 6*, 840-862.

Sharot, T., Riccardi, A. M., Raio, C. M., & Phelps, E. A. (2007). Neural mechanisms mediating optimism bias. *Nature, 450*, 102-105.

Simeon, D., Guralnik, O., Hazlett, E. A., Spiegel-Cohen, J., Hollander, E., & Buchsbaum, M. S. (2000). Feeling unreal: a PET study of depersonalization disorder. *American Journal of Psychiatry, 157*, 1782-1788.

Snyder, S. L., Buchsbaum, M. S., & Krishna, R. C. (1998). Unusual visual symptoms and Ganser-like state due to cerebral injury: a case study using (18)F-deoxyglucose positron emission tomography. *Behavioural Neurology, 11*, 51-54.

Spence, S. A., Crimlisk, H. L., Cope, H., Ron, M. A., & Grasby, P. M. (2000). Discrete neurophysiological correlates in prefrontal cortex during hysterical and feigned disorder of movement. *Lancet, 355*, 1243-1244.

Spiegel, D. (2006). Recognizing traumatic dissociation. *American Journal of Psychiatry, 163*, 4.

Staniloiu, A., Bender, A., Smolewska, K., Ellis, J., Abramowitz, C., & Markowitsch, H. J. (2009). Ganser syndrome with work–related onset in a patient with a background of immigration. *Cognitive Neuropsychiatry, 14*, 180–198.

Staniloiu, A., & Markowitsch, H. J. (2010). Searching for the anatomy of dissociative amnesia. *Journal of Psychology, 218*, 96-108.

Stein, D. J., Ives-Deliperi, V., & Thomas, K. G. (2008). Psychobiology of mindfulness. *CNS Spectrums, 13*, 752-756.

Stone, J., Vuilleumier, P., & Friedman, J. H. (2010). Conversion disorder: separating "how" from "why". *Neurology, 74*, 190-191.

Stone, J., Zeman, A., Simonotto, E., Meyer, M., Azuma, R., Flett, S., et al. (2007). FMRI in patients with motor conversion symptoms and controls with simulated weakness. *Psychosomatic Medicine, 69*, 961-969.

Thomas-Antérion, C., Guedj, E., Decousus, M., & Laurent, B. (2010) Can we see personal identity loss? A functional imaging study of typical 'hysterical amnesia'. *Journal of Neurology, Neurosurgery , and Psychiatry, 81*, 468-469.

Thomas-Antérion, C., Mazzola, L., Foyatier-Michel, N., & Laurent, B. (2008). À la recherche de la mémoire perdue: nature des troubles et mode de récupération d'un cas d'amnésie rétrograde pure. *Revue Neurologique, 164*, 271-277.

Tiihonen, J., Kuikka, J., Viinamäki, H., Lehtonen, J., & Partanen, J. (1995). Altered cerebral blood flow during hysterical paresthesia. *Biological Psychiatry, 37*, 134-135.

Tramoni, E., Aubert-Khalfa, S., Guye, M., Ranjeva, J. P., Felician, O., & Ceccaldi, M. (2009). Hypo-retrieval and hyper-suppression mechanisms in functional amnesia. *Neuropsychologia, 47*, 611-624.

Travis, F., & Shear, J. (2010). Focused attention, open monitoring and automatic self-transcending: Categories to organize meditations from Vedic, Buddhist and Chinese traditions. *Consciousness and Cognition, 19,* 1110-1118.

Tulving, E., & Markowitsch, H. J. (1998). Episodic and declarative memory: Role of the hippocampus. *Hippocampus, 8,* 198-204.

Tulving, E. (2005). Episodic memory and autonoesis: Uniquely human? In H. S. Terrace & J. Metcalfe (Eds.), *The missing link in cognition: Self-knowing consciousness in man and animals* (pp. 3-56). NewYork: Oxford University Press.

Yang, J. C., Jeong, G. W., Lee, M. S., Kang, H. K., Eun, S. J., Kim, Y. K., & Lee, Y. H.(2005). Functional MR imaging of psychogenic amnesia: a case report. *Korean Journal of Radiology, 6*(3), 196-199.

Yasuno, F., Nishikawa, T., Nakagawa, Y., Ikejiri, Y., Tokunaga, H., Mizuta, I., Shinozaki, K., Hashikawa, K., Sugita, L., Nishimura, T., & Takeda, M. (2000). Functional anatomical study of psychogenic amnesia. *Psychiatry Research, 99*(1), 43-57.

Yazici, K. M., & Kostakoglu, L. (1998). Cerebral blood flow changes in patients with conversion disorder. *Psychiatry Research: Neuroimaging Section, 83,* 163-168.

van der Kolk, B. A., & van der Hart, O. (1989). Pierre Janet and the breakdown of adaptation in psychological trauma. *American Journal of Psychiatry, 146,* 1530-1540.

Vera, F. M., Manzaneque, J. M., Maldonado, E. F., Carranque, G. A., Rodriguez, F. M., Blanca, M. J., et al. (2009). Subjective sleep quality and hormonal modulation in long-term yoga practitioners. *Biological Psychology, 81,* 164-168.

Vermetten, E., Schmahl, C., Lindner, S., Loewenstein, R. J., & Bremner, J. D. (2006). Hippocampal and amygdalar volumes in dissociative identity disorder. *American Journal of Psychiatry, 163,* 630-636.

Vuilleumier, P., Chichério, C., Assal, F., Schwartz, S., Slosman, D., & Landis, T. (2001). Functional neuroanatomical correlates of hysterical sensorimotor loss. *Brain, 124,* 1077-1090.

Weniger, G., Lange, C., Sachsse, U., & Irle, E. (2008). Amygdala and hippocampal volumes and cognition in adult survivors of childhood abuse with dissociative disorders. *Acta Psychiatrica Scandinavica, 118*(4), 281-290.

Werring, D. J., Weston, L., Bullmore, E. T., Plant, G. T., & Ron, M. A. (2004). Functional magnetic resonance imaging of the cerebral response to visual stimulation in medically unexplained visual loss. *Psychological Medicine, 34,* 583-589.

Wheeler, M. A., Stuss, D. T., & Tulving, E. (1997). Towards a theory of episodic memory. The frontal lobes and autonoetic consciousness. *Psychological Bulletin, 121,* 331-354.

Williams, J. M., Teasdale, J. D., Segal, Z. V., & Soulsby, J. (2000). Mindfulness-based cognitive therapy reduces overgeneral autobiographical memory in formerly depressed patients. *Journal of Abnormal Psychology, 109,* 150-155.

Williams, J. M., & Scott, J. (1988). Autobiographical memory in depression. *Psychological Medicine, 18,* 689-695.

Zanarini, M. C., Frankenburg, F. R., Jager-Hyman, S., Reich, D. B., & Fitzmaurice, G. (2008). The course of dissociation for patients with borderline personality disorder and axis II comparison subjects: a 10-year follow-up study. *Acta Psychiatrica Scandinavica, 118,* 291-296.

3

Neural Mechanisms for Dual-Process Reasoning: Evidence from the Belief-Bias Effect

Takeo Tsujii and Kaoru Sakatani
Nihon University School of Medicine,
Japan

1. Introduction

Recent neuroimaging studies have increasingly focused on the neural mechanisms of human deductive reasoning (see Goel, 2006 for recent review). Deductive reasoning is the cognitive process of drawing valid conclusions from a given set of premises. Although it should be performed independently of prior knowledge and intuitive beliefs, actual human reasoning often relies on them. Sometimes such beliefs provide valid solutions to problems, though they can also bias our judgment. This tendency toward bias in human reasoning has been experimentally studied through the demonstration of belief-bias effect in syllogistic reasoning (De Neys, 2006a, 2006b; Tsujii et al., 2006).

Belief-bias effect refers to the tendency of subjects to be more likely to accept the conclusion to a syllogism if they find it believable than if they disbelieve it, irrespective of its actual logical validity (De Neys, 2006a, 2006b; Tsujii et al., 2006). The experiment of belief-bias effect includes two types of syllogisms: one in congruent trials, in which the logical conclusion is consistent with beliefs about the world (valid-believable and invalid-unbelievable), the other in incongruent trials, in which the logical conclusion is inconsistent with beliefs (valid-unbelievable and invalid-believable). A typical material design was presented in Fig.1. Belief-bias thus facilitates logical responses in congruent trials, while it opposes logically correct responses in incongruent trials (De Neys et al., 2008; De Neys & van Gelder, 2009b; Goel & Dolan, 2003; Tsujii & Watanabe, 2009, 2010; Tsujii et al., 2010a, 2010b, 2011).

One explanation for the belief-bias effect is offered by the dual-process theory of reasoning, which proposes the existence of two different human reasoning systems (Evans, 2003, 2008; De Neys, 2006a, 2006b). The first system, often called the heuristic system, tends to solve problems by relying on prior knowledge and belief. The second system, often called the analytic system, engages in reasoning according to logical standards. The schematic representation of the dual-process theory was presented in Fig. 2. The heuristic default system is assumed to operate rapidly and automatically, whereas operations of the analytic system are believed to be slow and heavily demanding of computational resources (De Neys, 2006a, 2006b; Tsujii & Watanabe, 2009, 2010). The aim of this chapter was to summarize the recent neuroimaging findings which supported the dual-process account of deductive reasoning, focusing on studies of the belief-bias effect.

Reasoning:

Belief:	Valid	Invalid
Believable	No mammals are birds. All dogs are mammals. ------------------------------ No dogs are birds.	No pigeons are mammals. All pigeons are birds. ------------------------------ No birds are mammals.
Unbelievable	No mammals are birds. All pigeons are mammals. ------------------------------ No pigeons are birds.	No birds are dogs. All birds are mammals. ------------------------------ No mammals are dogs.

☐ **CON** (congruent) ☐ **INC** (incongruent)

Fig. 1. Material design of the belief-bias effect

Several neuroimaging studies using functional magnetic resonance imaging (fMRI) have examined the neural mechanisms of belief-bias reasoning (Goel, 2007). These studies reported that the belief-bias effect was associated with right inferior frontal cortex (IFC) activity (De Neys et al., 2008; Goel & Dolan, 2003). Right IFC activity was enhanced when subjects could respond correctly to incongruent reasoning trials. The authors of these studies claimed that the right IFC plays a role in inhibiting the default heuristic system for successful logical reasoning (De Neys et al., 2008; Goel & Dolan, 2003).

In general, the right IFC activity is known to play a central role in inhibitory function (Aron et al., 2004, 2007). For example, response inhibition has been found to be associated with the right IFC activity in several tasks, including the go/no-go task (Chikazoe et al., 2007, 2009; Chiu et al., 2008; Rubia et al., 2001; Tsujii et al., 2011b) and the stop-signal task (Aron and Poldrack, 2006; Hampshire et al., 2010; Rubia et al., 2001, 2003). Furthermore, when subjects changed from one task to another (task-set switching), the right IFC activity was also enhanced (Cools et al., 2002; Smith et al., 2004, 2006; Xue et al., 2008). In addition, other studies have suggested that the right IFC deficit may underlie the impaired response inhibition in patients with attention-deficit hyperactivity disorder (Durston et al., 2006, 2011; Rubia et al., 2005, 2010). These observations are consistent with the claims of dual-process theory that the right IFC plays a functional role in inhibiting the default heuristic system to enable analytic logical reasoning system activity (De Neys et al., 2008; Goel, 2007; Goel & Dolan, 2003). In the present paper, we further presented recent studies in our laboratory which examined the attention-demanding and time-consuming properties of the right IFC activity in belief-bias reasoning (Tsujii & Watanabe, 2009, 2010).

While most of the neuroimaging studies of deductive reasoning have used fMRI (Goel et al., 2000; Goel and Dolan, 2001, 2003; Knauff et al., 2002, 2003; Monti et al., 2007, 2009; Reverbeli et al., 2007, 2009, 2010), our laboratory utilized two relatively new imaging technique: one is functional near-infrared spectroscopy (fNIRS) and the other is repetitive transcranial magnetic stimulation (rTMS). fNIRS is the imaging technique for investigating cortical hemodynamic responses by measuring changes in the attenuation of near-infrared light passing through tissue. Since oxygenated hemoglobin (oxy-Hb) and deoxygenated hemoglobin (deoxy-Hb) have different absorption spectra in the infrared range, changes in concentrations of oxy- and deoxy-Hb can be calculated by detecting infrared light at two different wavelengths on the skull (approximately 787 and 827 nm). In general, enhanced oxy-Hb and reduced deoxy-Hb are associated with regional cortical activation. NIRS is non-invasive, robust against body movement and has been validated as a suitable technique for investigating neural mechanisms in psychological experiments (Tsujii et al., 2007, 2009a, 2009b, 2010b, 2010c, 2011b).

Although fMRI and fNIRS studies have provided interesting findings of the neural mechanisms of deductive reasoning, they can only examine correlations between cortical areas and a type of behaviour. The second aim of the present study was to demonstrate recent findings of rTMS studies in our laboratory which elucidated the roles of the inferior frontal cortex (IFC) and the superior parietal lobule (SPL) in human deductive reasoning (Tsujii et al., 2010a, 2011a). Especially, we adopted an off-line rTMS method in which low-frequency rTMS is delivered to a specific brain area over several minutes to disrupt normal functioning of this area transiently after stimulation (Devlin et al., 2003; Hamidi et al., 2008, 2009; Hilgetag et al., 2001; Miller et al., 2008; Robertson et al., 2003). We investigated the effect of off-line rTMS of IFC and SPL on subsequent reasoning performance of congruent and incongruent trials. The rTMS approach can establish the causal relationships between brain and behaviour more directly compared with fMRI and fNIRS.

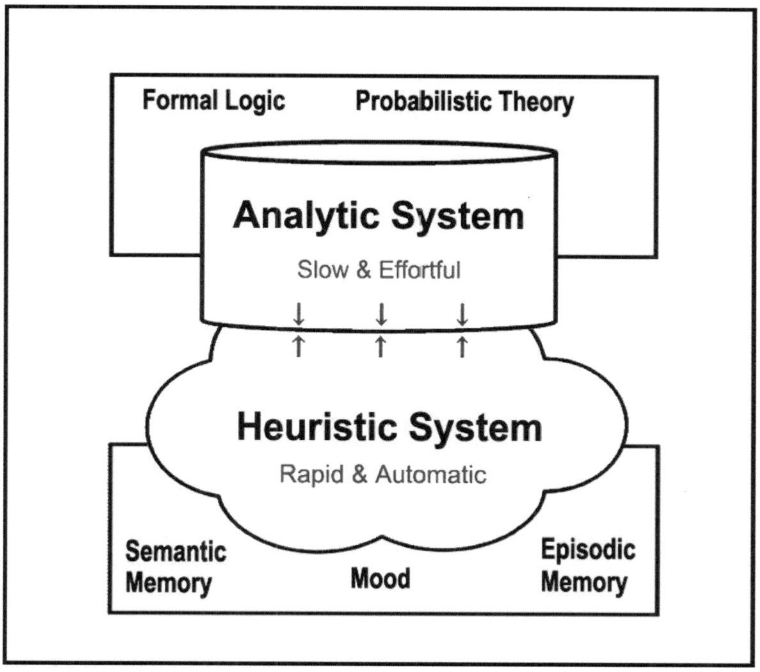

Fig. 2. Schematic illustration of the dual-process theory

2. fNIRS studies: Dual-task and time-pressure effects on reasoning

The dual-process theory claimed that the heuristic default system is assumed to operate rapidly and automatically, whereas operations of the analytic system are believed to be slow and heavily demanding of computational resources. Although these claims were supported by behavioural findings (De Neys, 2006a, 2006b), the neural correlates of dual-task and time-pressure effect on belief-bias reasoning was unknown. Thus, a series of fNIRS studies in our laboratory examined the attention-demanding and time-consuming properties of the analytic reasoning system and IFC activity using fNIRS (Tsujii & Watanabe, 2009, 2010). In addition, we examined the aging effect on hemispheric asymmetry in IFC activity using fNIRS (Tsujii et al., 2010b).

2.1 Dual-task effect on belief-bias reasoning

Tsujii & Watanabe (2009) examined the relationship between dual-task effect and IFC activity during belief-bias reasoning by fNIRS. Previous behavioural studies demonstrated that subjects with poor working memory capacity exhibited larger belief-bias effect than those with rich working memory capacity (De Neys, 2006a, 2006b; Stanovich & West, 2000). More directly, De Neys (2006a) found that attention-demanding concurrent tasks impaired incongruent but not congruent reasoning trials. These findings suggest that the analytic system is attention-demanding, and that when attention is divided by a concurrent task, individuals tend to rely on the automatic heuristic system, resulting in belief-bias responses. Although these behavioural findings are important, the neural correlates of dual-task reasoning are still unclear.

Tsujii & Watanabe (2009) therefore examined the neural correlates of the dual-task effect on IFC activity in belief-bias reasoning using fNIRS approach. Subjects were asked to perform a syllogistic reasoning task, involving congruent and incongruent trials, while responding to attention-demanding secondary tasks, in which a white square stimulus appeared at one of the four corners of a black screen throughout the experiment (Fig. 3). In the low-load condition, subjects were required to respond whenever the stimulus was in a predetermined location (e.g. upper-left position). In the high-load condition, subjects were asked to respond when the current stimulus was in the same location as the stimulus two trials previously (2-back).

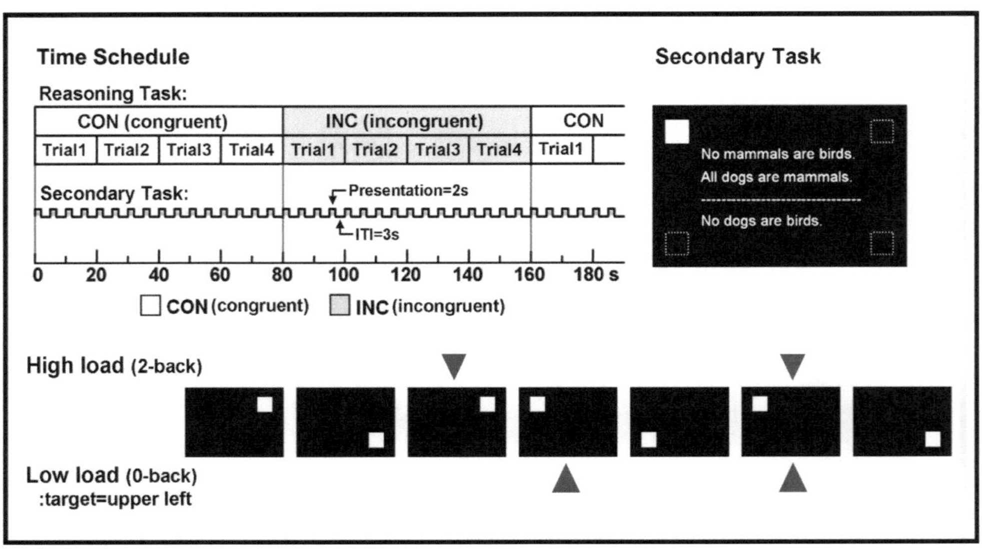

Fig. 3. Time schedule and schematic drawings of the secondary task.

Behavioural analysis showed that the high-load secondary task impaired only incongruent reasoning performance. NIRS analysis found that the high-load secondary task decreased right IFC activity during incongruent trials. Correlation analysis showed that subjects with enhanced right IFC activity could perform better in the incongruent reasoning trials, though subjects for whom right IFC activity was impaired by the secondary task could not maintain better reasoning performance. These findings suggest that the right IFC may be responsible for the dual-task effect in conflicting reasoning processes. When secondary tasks impair right IFC activity, subjects may rely on the automatic heuristic system, which results in belief-bias responses. Tsujii & Watanabe (2009) therefore offer the first demonstration of neural correlates of dual-task effect on IFC activity in belief-bias reasoning.

2.2 Belief-bias reasoning under time-pressure

Tsujii & Watanabe (2010) addressed the difference in speed between the heuristic and analytic reasoning systems. The dual-process theory of reasoning explained the belief-bias effect by proposing a belief-based fast heuristic system and a logic-based slow analytic system. Although the claims were supported by behavioural findings that the belief-bias effect was enhanced when subjects were not given sufficient time for reasoning (De Neys, 2006b; Evans & Curtis-Holmes, 2005), the neural correlates were still unknown. Tsujii & Watanabe (2010), thus, examined the neural correlates of the time-pressure effect on the IFC activity in belief-bias reasoning using fNIRS. Subjects were asked to perform a syllogistic reasoning task, involving congruent and incongruent trials, both in long-span (20 s) and short-span conditions (10 s).

Behavioural analysis found that only incongruent reasoning performance was impaired by the time-pressure of short-span trials. NIRS analysis found that the time-pressure decreased right IFC activity during incongruent trials. Correlation analysis showed that subjects with enhanced right IFC activity could perform better in incongruent trials, while subjects for whom the right IFC activity was impaired by the time-pressure could not maintain better reasoning performance. These findings suggest that the right IFC may be responsible for the time-pressure effect in conflicting reasoning processes. When the right IFC activity was impaired in the short-span trials in which subjects were not given sufficient time for reasoning, the subjects may rely on the fast heuristic system, which result in belief-bias responses. Tsujii & Watanabe (2010) therefore offer the first demonstration of neural correlates of time-pressure effect on the IFC activity in belief-bias reasoning.

2.3 Aging and belief-bias reasoning

Behavioural Tsujii et al. (2010b) examined the difference in neural activity associated with deductive reasoning processes between young and older adults. Some behavioural studies reported that older adults exhibited a larger belief-bias effect than young adults (De Neys & Van Gelder, 2009), though the neural correlates of the aging effect on belief-bias reasoning remained unknown. Therefore, Tsujii et al. (2010b) examined IFC activity differences in belief-bias reasoning between young (mean age, 21.50 years) and older subjects (mean age, 68.53 years) using fNIRS.

Behavioural analysis found that older adults exhibited a larger belief-bias than young adults. Although the belief-bias effect was significant in both age groups, the size of the effect was significantly larger for older than young adults. In the belief-bias reasoning paradigm, automatic semantic processing interferes with reasoning performance in incongruent trials. Subjects were thus required to inhibit irrelevant semantic processing to resolve the conflicting reasoning. However, it is generally known that older adults are less able to inhibit task-irrelevant information processing than young adults. This may be one of the reasons that older adults exhibited a larger belief-bias effect in deductive reasoning.

NIRS analysis showed that the right IFC was more activated than the left IFC in young adults, while there was no significant difference between the right and left IFCs in older adults. That is, hemispheric asymmetry of IFC activation (right-lateralization) was only observed in young subjects. In addition, the reduced lateralization of older adults was not due to reduction of right IFC activity, but due to enhancement of left IFC activity. These results are in line with numerous fMRI findings that showed age-related reduction of hemispheric asymmetry and over-recruitment in prefrontal activity in several tasks (Cabeza et al., 1997, 2002, 2004; Langenecker et al., 2004, 2007; Nielson et al., 2002, 2004; Rajah & McIntosh, 2008; Rympa & D'Esposito, 2000). For example, older adults often show bilateral activation in tasks associated with left-lateralized activity in young adults, such as verbal working memory and semantic processing tasks (Bergerbest et al., 2009; Rajah & McIntosh, 2008; Rympa & D'Esposito, 2000). Likewise, older adults often show bilateral activation in tasks associated with right-lateralized activity in young adults such as episodic retrieval and response inhibition tasks (Langenecker & Nielson, 2003; Nielson et al., 2002, 2004).

With regard to the function of age-related lateralization reduction, two main interpretations have been proposed: the compensatory and dedifferentiation hypotheses. The compensation hypothesis considers that older adults recruit more areas of the contralateral hemisphere than younger adults in order to achieve or attempt to achieve the same levels of performance (Reuter-Lorenz et al., 2000). In contrast, the dedifferentiation hypothesis considers that the additional recruitment reflects a generalized spreading of activity due to reduced specialization of function, regardless of whether it has a compensatory effect (Logan et al., 2002). Tsujii et al. (2010b) conducted the correlation analysis which revealed that the positive correlation between reasoning accuracy and IFC activation was significant in both hemispheres for older subjects, while a significant correlation was only found in the right hemisphere for young subjects. These findings are consistent with the compensatory hypothesis that older adults may recruit the left IFC to compensate for the age-related decline of inhibitory control functions.

2.4 Utility of fNIRS in reasoning studies

In the present chapter, we introduced fNIRS approach to elucidate the neural mechanisms of deductive reasoning processes, although most of the previous studies used fMRI technique (Goel et al., 2000; Goel and Dolan, 2001, 2003; Knauff et al., 2002, 2003; Monti et al., 2007, 2009; Stavy et al., 2006). Certain shortcomings of the NIRS technique thus need to be mentioned. First, NIRS can detect hemodynamic changes only at the surface of the brain (about 2 cm beneath the skull). Subcortical responses thus cannot be examined using NIRS. In particular, activity in the anterior cingulate cortex, which is known to be associated with conflict detection and is probably an important neural locus of belief-bias reasoning (Goel, 2007; De Neys et al., 2008), cannot be examined by NIRS. Second, NIRS features relatively low spatial resolution compared with fMRI, making precise analysis with it difficult.

Despite these shortcomings, use of NIRS is becoming increasingly common in recent neuroimaging studies, because of its advantages, such as exceptional safety, low cost and robustness against body movement. Indeed, recent NIRS studies have established the utility of NIRS in various cognitive tasks involving working memory (Ehlis et al., 2008; Tsujii et al. 2007, 2009b, 2010c), response inhibition (Boecker et al., 2007; Tsujii et al., 2011b), and semantic memory retrieval (Herrmann et al., 2003, 2004; Tsujii et al., 2009a). We believe that NIRS will improve understanding of the neural substrates of reasoning processes.

fNIRS is also expected to facilitate the investigation of wide subject populations, including young children (Minagawa-Kawai et al., 2008; Tsujii et al., 2009b) and the elderly (Herrmann et al., 2006; Kameyama et al., 2004). Children and elderly subjects have been found to exhibit a larger belief-bias effect than young adults (De Neys and Van Gelder, 2009). It is thus important to examine the neural mechanisms in these subject populations in reasoning research. In deed, we successfully demonstrated the hemispheric difference of IFC activity between young and older adults in the belief-bias reasoning task (Tsujii et al. 2010b). We believe that fNIRS will improve understanding of the neural substrates of reasoning processes.

3. TMS study in deductive reasoning

Although neuroimaging studies, such as fMRI and fNIRS, have provided useful insights of the neural mechanisms of deductive reasoning, they can only examine correlations between cortical areas and a type of behaviour. In contrast, the rTMS approach can establish the causal relationships between brain and behaviour more directly compared with fMRI and fNIRS. In our laboratory, an off-line method of rTMS was adopted to examine the neural correlates of deductive reasoning. In the off-line method, low-frequency rTMS is delivered to a specific brain area over several minutes to disrupt normal functioning of this area transiently after stimulation (see Robertson et al., 2003 for detailed review). For example, Devlin et al. (2003) delivered low-frequency (1Hz) magnetic stimulation at IFC region for 10 min and found that the semantic processing was disrupted in a semantic decision task. In the first experiment, we examine the effect of low-frequency magnetic stimulation at IFC region on performance of congruent and incongruent reasoning performance (Tsujii et al., 2010a). In the second experiment (Tsujii et al., 2011a), we investigated the effect of rTMS at SPL (superior parietal lobule) on the performance of abstract reasoning in which semantic content was lacking (e.g., "All P is B"). The stimulation sites of IFC and SPL were presented in Fig. 4.

3.1 The role of IFC in belief-bias reasoning

Tsujii et al. (2010a) examined the role of IFC in belief-bias reasoning using rTMS approach. Subjects participated in a belief-bias reasoning task for 10 min (pre-test), then received low-frequency (1 Hz) rTMS in the left or right IFC for 10 min, and finally performed a reasoning task again for 10 min (post-test). The reasoning task included congruent and incongruent trials. For control conditions, we used a specially designed sham coil with the same visual appearance and same audible clicking sound as the TMS coil but without production of any magnetic field. There was no significant difference between TMS and sham condition in the pre-test. Our interest was the TMS effect on performance of congruent and incongruent reasoning trials in the post-test.

We found that right IFC stimulation significantly impaired reasoning performance in incongruent but not congruent trials, enhancing the belief-bias effect. This is consistent with the findings of previous neuroimaging studies using fMRI and fNIRS. In the belief-bias reasoning paradigm, semantic information processing should interfere with reasoning performance in incongruent trial, while facilitating it in congruent trials. Subjects were therefore required to inhibit semantic processing to resolve the conflicts in reasoning. When rTMS inhibited the inhibitory function of the right IFC, subjects could not respond correctly in incongruent trials, enhancing belief-bias responses.

De Neys & Franssens (2009) recently investigated the detailed nature of the inhibition process in belief-bias reasoning. In their experiments, subjects performed a lexical decision task after solving the deductive reasoning task which involved congruent and incongruent trials. They found that incongruent reasoning delayed lexical decisions regarding the target word that were relevant to the cued heuristic beliefs. Interestingly, no significant difference was apparent between congruent and incongruent reasoning trials for unrelated words. That is, the accessibility of unrelated words was unaffected. This suggests that the inhibition process is focused in nature and is specifically targeted at cued beliefs, not at semantic processing in general.

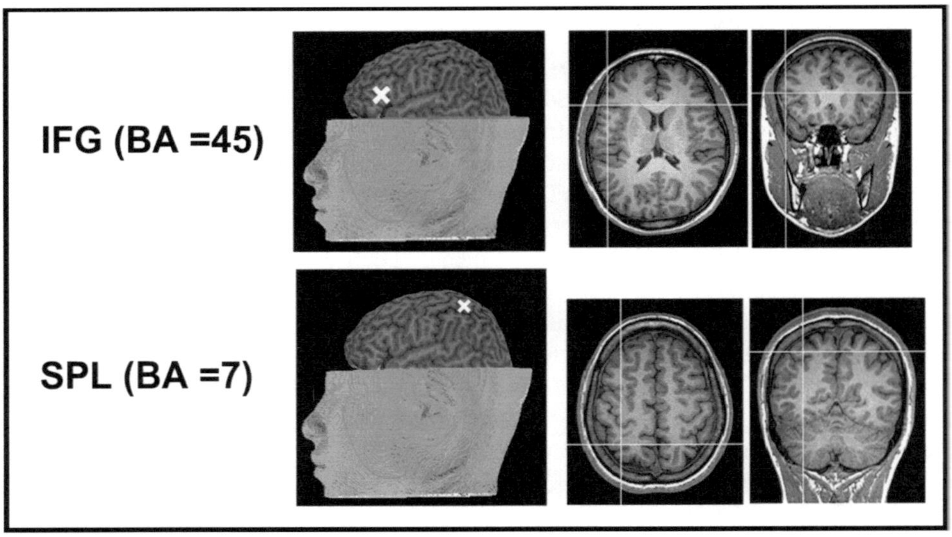

Fig. 4. Stimulation sites in rTMS experiments (IFG: inferior frontal gyrus, SPL: superior parietal lobule, BA: Broadman area).

In contrast, left IFC stimulation impaired congruent reasoning performance, while paradoxically facilitating incongruent reasoning performance. As a result, the belief-bias effect was eliminated. The left IFC is generally known to be associated with verbal or semantic processing in a wide variety of tasks, including the semantic decision task (Devlin et al., 2003), verbal fluency task (Costafreda et al., 2006), and sentence comprehension task (Zhu et al., 2009). Subjects whose left IFC was impaired by rTMS did not suffer from interference by irrelevant semantic processing, resulting in elimination of belief-bias effect. This study thus demonstrated for the first time the roles of the left and right IFC in belief-bias reasoning using an rTMS approach.

3.2 The role of SPL in abstract reasoning

Tsujii et al. (2011a) examined the effect of IFC stimulation on abstract reasoning trials in which semantic content was lacking (e.g. "All P are B"), as well as content reasoning trials which involved the congruent and incongruent trials. In contrast of the incongruent reasoning performance, we did not find the significant IFC stimulation effect on abstract reasoning performance. Right IFC stimulation impaired only incongruent trials. These findings suggest that the right IFC may not the neural locus of the analytic reasoning system. Rather, the right IFC may play a role in blocking the belief-based heuristic system (left IFC) in solving incongruent reasoning trials. On the other hand, individuals need not actively inhibit the heuristic processing on abstract trials, so right IFC stimulation did not significantly affect abstract reasoning trials.

So, where is the neural locus responsible for abstract reasoning performance? Tsujii et al (2011a) magnetically stimulated SPL (superior parietal lobule: BA = 7). In contrast to the IFC stimulation, bilateral SPL stimulation significantly impaired abstract reasoning performance. This is consistent with previous fMRI studies which showed that the abstract reasoning performance significantly activated the SPL region (Goel et al., 2000; Goel & Dolan, 2001; Knauff et al., 2002, 2003). In general, SPL is associated with spatial processing based on evidence from fMRI (Takahama et al., 2010; Thakral & Slotnick, 2009), neurological patients (Ferber & Danckert, 2006; Shinoura et al., 2009) and TMS studies (Hamidi et al., 2008, 2009). Some authors have claimed that cognitive processes of constructing and manipulating spatially organized mental models are essential for deductive reasoning (Johnson-Laird, 1999, 2001). The mental models are a form of representation that can be spatial but more abstract. Phenomenological reports in the reasoning literature often have suggested that subjects may solve abstract syllogisms through the use of mental images of Venn diagrams and Euler circles (Goel et al., 2000; Goel & Dolan). Stimulation of SPL may thus have impaired abstract and incongruent reasoning by disrupting spatial processing. In contrast, congruent reasoning performance where semantic-based heuristics are sufficient to solve the problem was unimpaired.

The findings are largely consistent with the dual-process theory of reasoning, which proposes the existence of two different reasoning systems in humans: a belief-based heuristic system; and a logic-based analytic system. In our study, the left IFG appears to correspond to the heuristic system, while bilateral SPLs are part of the analytic system. The right IFG may play a role in blocking the belief-based heuristic system (left IFG) in solving incongruent reasoning trials. So, our rTMS study could offer an insight about functional roles of distributed brain systems in human deductive reasoning by utilizing the rTMS approach.

4. Conclusion

In the present chapter, we briefly reviewed recent neuroimaging studies of human deductive reasoning, especially focusing on relatively new imaging technique: functional near-infrared spectroscopy (fNIRS) and repetitive transcranial magnetic stimulation (rTMS). A series of studies in our laboratory successfully provided evidence which is consistent with recent dual-process theory of reasoning. The dual-process theory proposed belief-based heuristic system and a logic-based analytic system. The heuristic system is assumed to operate rapidly and automatically, whereas operations of the analytic system are believed to be slow and demanding of computational resources. Our fNIRS findings could demonstrate the attention-demanding and time-consuming properties of the right IFC activities. In addition, our rTMS studies showed that the left IFG appears to correspond to the heuristic system, while bilateral SPLs are part of the analytic system. The right IFG may play a role in blocking the belief-based heuristic system (left IFG) in solving incongruent reasoning trials. Although there are several limitations of fNIRS and rTMS, we believe they are useful to examine the neural substrates of logical reasoning process.

5. Acknowledgment

Funding for this study was provided by the fund of Grant-in-Aid for Young Scientists (B) from the Ministry of Education, Culture, Sports, Science, and Technology (MEXT) of Japan, the fund of Center of Developmental Education and Research (CODER) of Japan, and the fund for Japan Science and Technology Agency (JST), under the Strategic Promotion of Innovative Research and Development Program.

6. References

Aron, A.R., Robbins, T.W. & Poldrack, R.A. (2004). Inhibition and the right inferior frontal cortex. *Trends in Cognive Sciences,* Vol.8, No.4 (April 2004), pp.170-177, ISSN: 1364-6613

Aron, A.R., & Poldrack, R.A. (2006). Cortical and subcortical contributions to Stop signal response inhibition: role of the subthalamic nucleus. *Journal of Neuroscience,* Vol.26, No.9 (March 2006), pp.2424-33, ISSN: 1364-6613

Aron, A.R., Behrens, T.E., Smith, S., Frank, M.J. & Poldrack, R.A. (2007). Triangulating a cognitive control network using diffusion-weighted magnetic resonance imaging (MRI) and functional MRI. *Journal of Neuroscience.* Vol.27, No.14 (April 2007), pp.3743-3752, ISSN: 0270-6474

Bergerbest, D., Gabrieli, J.D., Whitfield-Gabrieli, S., Kim, H., Stebbins, G.T., Bennett, D.A., Fleischman, D.A. Age-associated reduction of asymmetry in prefrontal function and preservation of conceptual repetition priming. *Neuroimage,* Vol.45, No.1 (March 2009), pp.237-246, ISSN: 1053-8119

Boecker, M., Buecheler, M.M., Schroeter, M.L. & Gauggel, S. (2007). Prefrontal brain activation during stop-signal response inhibition: an event-related functional near-infrared spectroscopy study. *Behavioural Brain Research,* Vol.176, No.2 (January 2007), pp.259-266, ISSN: 0166-4328

Cabeza, R., Grady, C.L., Nyberg, L., McIntosh, A.R., Tulving, E., Kapur, S., Jennings, J.M., Houle, S. & Craik, F.I. (1997). Age-related differences in neural activity during memory encoding and retrieval: a positron emission tomography study. *Journal of Neuroscience,* Vol.17, No.1 (January 1997), pp.391-400, ISSN: 0270-6474

Cabeza, R., Anderson, N.D., Locantore, J.K. & McIntosh, A.R. (2002). Aging gracefully: compensatory brain activity in high-performing older adults. *Neuroimage,* Vol.17, No.3 (November 2002), pp.1394-1402, ISSN: 1053-8119

Cabeza, R., Daselaar, S.M., Dolcos, F., Prince, S.E., Budde, M. & Nyberg, L. (2004). Task-independent and task-specific age effects on brain activity during working memory, visual attention and episodic retrieval. *Cerebral Cortex*, Vol.14, No.4 (April 2004), pp.364-375, ISSN: 1047-3211

Chikazoe, J., Konishi, S., Asari, T., Jimura, K. & Miyashita, Y. (2007). Activation of right inferior frontal gyrus during response inhibition across response modalities. *Journal of Cognive Neuroscience*, Vol.19, No.1, (January 2007), pp.69-80.

Chikazoe, J., Jimura, K., Asari, T., Yamashita, K., Morimoto, H., Hirose, S., Miyashita, Y. & Konishi, S. (2009). Functional dissociation in right inferior frontal cortex during performance of go/no-go task. *Cerebral Cortex*, Vol.19, No.1 (January 2009), pp.146-152.

Chiu, P.H., Holmes, A.J. & Pizzagalli D.A. (2008). Dissociable recruitment of rostral anterior cingulate and inferior frontal cortex in emotional response inhibition. *Neuroimage*, Vol.42, No.2 (August 2008), 988-997.

Cools, R., Clark, L., Owen, A.M. & Robbins, T.W. (2002). Defining the neural mechanisms of probabilistic reversal learning using event-related functional magnetic resonance imaging. *Journal of Neuroscience*, Vol.22, No.11, (June 2002), 4563-4567.

Costafreda, S.G., Fu, C.H., Lee, L., Everitt, B., Brammer, M.J. & David, A.S. (2006). A systematic review and quantitative appraisal of fMRI studies of verbal fluency: role of the left inferior frontal gyrus. *Human Brain Mapping*, Vol.27, No.10 (October 2006), pp.799-810, ISSN: 1065-9471

De Neys, W. (2006a). Dual processing in reasoning: two systems but one reasoner. *Psychological Science*, Vol.17, No.5 (May 2006), pp.428-433, ISSN: 0956-7976

De Neys, W. (2006b). Automatic-heuristic and executive-analytic processing during reasoning: Chronometric and dual-task considerations. *Quarterly Journal of Experimental Psychology*. Vol.59, No.6 (June 2006), pp.1070-1100, ISSN: 0272-4987

De Neys, W., Vartanian, O. & Goel, V. (2008). Smarter than we think: when our brains detect that we are biased. *Psychological Science*. Vol.19, No.5 (May 2008), pp.483-489, ISSN: 0956-7976

De Neys, W. & Franssens, S. (2009a). Belief inhibition during thinking: not always winning but at least taking part. *Cognition*, Vol.113, No.1 (October 2009), pp.45-61. ISSN: 0010-0277

De Neys, W. & Van Gelder, E. (2009b). Logic and belief across the lifespan: the rise and fall of belief inhibition during syllogistic reasoning. *Developmental Science*, Vol.12, No.1 (January 2009), pp.123-130, ISSN: 1363-755X

Devlin, J.T., Matthews, P.M. & Rushworth, M.F. (2003). Semantic processing in the left inferior prefrontal cortex: a combined functional magnetic resonance imaging and transcranial magnetic stimulation study. *Journal of Cognitive Neuroscience*, Vol.15, No.1, (January 2003), pp.71-84, ISSN: 0898-929X.

Durston, S., Mulder, M., Casey, B.J., Ziermans, T. & van Engeland, H. (2006). Activation in ventral prefrontal cortex is sensitive to genetic vulnerability for attention-deficit hyperactivity disorder. *Biological Psychiatry*, Vol.60, No.10 (November 2006), pp.1062-1070, ISSN: 0006-3223

Durston, S., van Belle, J. & de Zeeuw, P. (2011). Differentiating frontostriatal and fronto-cerebellar circuits in attention-deficit/hyperactivity disorder. *Biological Psychiatry*, Vol.69, No.12 (June, 2011), pp.1178-1184, ISSN: 0006-3223

Ehlis, A.C., Bahne, C.G., Jacob, C.P., Herrmann, M.J. & Fallgatter, A.J. (2008). Reduced lateral prefrontal activation in adult patients with attention-deficit/hyperactivity disorder (ADHD) during a working memory task: a functional near-infrared spectroscopy (fNIRS) study. *Journal of Psychiatry Research*, Vol.42, No.13 (October 2008), pp.1060-1067, ISSN: 0022-3956

Evans, J.S. (2003). In two minds: dual-process accounts of reasoning. *Trends in Cognitive Sciences*, Vol.7, No.10 (October 2003), pp.454-459, ISSN: 1364-6613

Evans, J.S. (2008). Dual-processing accounts of reasoning, judgment, and social cognition. *Annual Review of Psychology*, Vol.59 (2008), pp.255-278, ISSN: 0066-4308

Evans, J.S., & Cutis-Holmes, J. (2005). Rapid responding increases belief-bias: evidence for the dual process theory fo reasoning. *Thinking & Reasoning*, Vol.11, No.3 (September 2005), pp.382-389, ISSN: 1464-0708

Ferber, S. & Danckert, J. (2006). Lost in space--the fate of memory representations for non-neglected stimuli. *Neuropsychologia*, Vol.44, No.2 (June 2006), pp.320-325, ISSN: 0028-3932

Goel, V., Buchel, C., Frith, C. & Dolan, R.J. (2000). Dissociation of mechanisms underlying syllogistic reasoning. *Neuroimage*, Vol.12, No.5 (November 2000), pp.504-514, ISSN: 1053-8119

Goel, V. & Dolan, R.J. (2001). Functional neuroanatomy of three-term relational reasoning. Neuropsychologia. 2001;Vol.39, No.9 (May 2001), pp.901-909, ISSN: 0028-3932

Goel, V., & Dolan, R.J. (2003). Explaining modulation of reasoning by belief. *Cognition*, Vol.87, No.1 (February, 2003), pp.B11-22, ISSN: 0010-0277

Goel, V. (2007). Anatomy of deductive reasoning. *Trends in Cognitive Sciences*, Vol.11, No.10 (October 2007), pp.435-441, ISSN: 1364-6613

Goel, V., Stollstorff, M., Nakic, M., Knutson, K. & Grafman, J. (2009). A role for right ventrolateral prefrontal cortex in reasoning about indeterminate relations. *Neuropsychologia*, Vol.47, No.13 (November, 2009), pp.2790-2797, ISSN: 0028-3932

Hamidi, M., Tononi, G. & Postle, B.R. (2008). Evaluating frontal and parietal contributions to spatial working memory with repetitive transcranial magnetic stimulation. *Brain Research*, Vol.1230 (September 2008), pp.202-210, ISSN: 0006-8993

Hamidi, M., Tononi, G. & Postle B.R. (2009). Evaluating the role of prefrontal and parietal cortices in memory-guided response with repetitive transcranial magnetic stimulation. *Neuropsychologia*, Vol.47, No.2 (January 2009), pp.295-302, ISSN: 0028-3932

Hampshire, A., Chamberlain, S.R., Monti, M.M., Duncan, J. & Owen, A.M. (2010). The role of the right inferior frontal gyrus: inhibition and attentional control. *Neuroimage*, Vol.50, No.3 (April 2010), pp.1313-1319.

Herrmann, M.J., Walter, A., Ehlis, A.C. & Fallgatter, A.J. (2006). Cerebral oxygenation changes in the prefrontal cortex: effects of age and gender. *Neurobiology & Aging*, Vol.27, No.6, (June 2006), pp.888-94.f

Herrmann, M.J., Ehlis, A.C. & Fallgatter, A.J. (2004). Bilaterally reduced frontal activation during a verbal fluency task in depressed patients as measured by near-infrared spectroscopy. *Journal of Neuropsychiatry and Clinical Neuroscience*, Vol.16, No.2, (Spring 2004), pp.170-175.

Herrmann, M.J., Ehlis, A.C. & Fallgatter, A.J. (2003). Frontal activation during a verbal-fluency task as measured by near-infrared spectroscopy. *Brain Research Bulletin*, Vol.61, No.1 (June 2003), pp.51-56.

Hilgetag, C.C., Theoret, H. & Pascual-Leone, A. (2001). Enhanced visual spatial attention ipsilateral to rTMS-induced 'virtual lesions' of human parietal cortex. *Nature Neuroscience*, Vol.4, No.9 (September 2001), pp.953-957, ISSN: 1471-0048

Johnson-Laird, P.N. (1999). Deductive reasoning. *Annual Review of Psychology*, Vol.50 (1999), pp.109-135, ISSN: 0066-4308.

Johnson-Laird, P.N. (2001). Mental models and deduction. *Trends in Cognitive Sciences*, Vol.5, No.10 (October, 2001), pp.434-442, ISSN: 1364-6613

Kameyama, M., Fukuda, M., Uehara, T. & Mikuni, M. (2004). Sex and age dependencies of cerebral blood volume changes during cognitive activation: a multichannel near-infrared spectroscopy study. *Neuroimage*, Vol.22, No.4 (August 2004), pp.1715-1721.

Knauff, M., Mulack, T., Kassubek, J., Salih, H.R. & Greenlee, M.W. (2002). Spatial imagery in deductive reasoning: a functional MRI study. *Brain Research*, Vol.13, No.2(May 2002), pp.203-212, ISSN: 0006-8993.

Knauff, M., Fangmeier, T., Ruff, C.C., & Johnson-Laird, P.N. (2003). Reasoning, models, and images: behavioral measures and cortical activity. *Journal of Cognitive Neuroscience*, Vol.15, No.4 (May 2003), pp.559-573, ISSN: 0898-929X.

Langenecker, S.A. & Nielson, K.A. (2003). Frontal recruitment during response inhibition in older adults replicated with fMRI. *Neuroimage*, Vol.20, No.2 (October 2003), pp.1384-1392, ISSN: 1053-8119

Langenecker, S.A., & Nielson, K.A. & Rao, S.M. (2004). fMRI of healthy older adults during Stroop interference. *Neuroimage*, Vol.21, No.1 (January 2004), pp.192-200, ISSN: 1053-8119

Langenecker, S.A., Briceno, E.M., Hamid, N.M. & Nielson, K.A. (2007). An evaluation of distinct volumetric and functional MRI contributions toward understanding age and task performance: a study in the basal ganglia. *Brain Research*, Vol.1135, No.1 (March 2007), pp.58-68, ISSN: 0006-8993

Logan, J.M., Sanders, A.L., Snyder, A.Z., Morris, J.C. & Buckner, R.L. (2002). Under-recruitment and nonselective recruitment: dissociable neural mechanisms associated with aging. *Neuron*, Vol.33, No.5 (February 2002), pp.827-840, ISSN: 0896-6273

Miller, B.T., Verstynen, T., Johnson, M.K. & D'Esposito, M. (2008). Prefrontal and parietal contributions to refreshing: an rTMS study. *Neuroimage*, Vol.39, No.1 (January 2008), pp.436-440, ISSN: 1053-8119.

Minagawa-Kawai, Y., Mori, K., Hebden, J.C. & Dupoux, E. (2008). Optical imaging of infants' neurocognitive development: recent advances and perspectives. Developmental Neurobiology, Vol.68, No.6 (May 2008), pp.712-728, ISSN: 1932-8451

Monti, M.M., Osherson, D.N., Martinez, M.J., & Parsons, L.M. (2007) Functional neuroanatomy of deductive inference: a language-independent distributed network. *Neuroimage*, Vol.37, No.3 (September 2007), pp.1005-1016, ISSN: 1053-8119

Monti, M.M., Parsons, L.M. & Osherson, D.N. The boundaries of language and thought in deductive inference. *Proceedings of National Academy of Sciences USA*, Vol.106, No.30, (July 2009), pp.12554-12559, ISSN: 1091-6490

Nielson, K.A., Langenecker, S.A., Ross, T.J., Garavan, H., Rao, S.M. & Stein, E.A. (2004). Comparability of functional MRI response in young and old during inhibition. *Neuroreport*, Vol.15, No.1, (January 2004), pp.129-133, ISSN: 0959-4965

Nielson, K.A., Langenecker, S.A. & Garavan, H. (2002). Differences in the functional neuroanatomy of inhibitory control across the adult life span. *Psychology & Aging*, Vol.17, No.1 (March 2002), pp.56-71, ISSN: 0882-7974

Rajah, M.N. & McIntosh, A.R. (2008). Age-related differences in brain activity during verbal recency memory. *Brain Research*, Vol.1199, No.111-125 (March 2008), pp.111-125, ISSN: 0006-8993

Reuter-Lorenz, P.A., Jonides, J., Smith, E.E., Hartley, A., Miller, A., Marshuetz, C. & Koeppe, R.A. Age differences in the frontal lateralization of verbal and spatial working memory revealed by PET. *Journal of Cognitive Neuroscience*, Vol.12, No.1 (January 2000), pp.174-187, ISSN: 0898-929X

Reverberi, C., Cherubini, P., Rapisarda, A., Rigamonti, E., Caltagirone, C., Frackowiak, R.S, Macaluso, E. & Paulesu, E. (2007). Neural basis of generation of conclusions in elementary deduction. *Neuroimage*, Vol.38, No.4 (December 2007), pp.752-762, ISSN: 1053-8119

Reverberi, C., Shallice, T., D'Agostini, S., Skrap, M. & Bonatti, L.L. (2009). Cortical bases of elementary deductive reasoning: inference, memory, and metadeduction. *Neuropsychologia*, Vol.47, No.4 (March 2009), pp.1107-1116, ISSN: 0028-3932

Reverberi, C., Cherubini, P., Frackowiak, R.S., Caltagirone, C., Paulesu, E. & Macaluso, E. (2010). Conditional and syllogistic deductive tasks dissociate functionally during premise integration. *Human Brain Mapping*, Vol.31, No.9 (September, 2010), pp.1430-45, ISSN: 1065-9471

Robertson, E.M., Theoret, H. & Pascual-Leone, A. (2003). Studies in cognition: the problems solved and created by transcranial magnetic stimulation. *Journal of Cognitive Neuroscience*, Vol.15, No.7 (October 2003), pp.948-60, ISSN: 0898-929X.

Rubia, K., Russell, T., Overmeyer, S., Brammer, M.J., Bullmore, E.T., Sharma, T., Simmons, A., Williams, S.C., Giampietro, V., Andrew, C.M. & Taylor, E. (2001). Mapping motor inhibition: conjunctive brain activations across different versions of go/no-go and stop tasks. *Neuroimage*, Vol.13, No.2 (February, 2001), pp.250-261, ISSN: 1053-8119

Rubia, K., Smith, A.B., Brammer, M.J. & Taylor, E. (2003). Right inferior prefrontal cortex mediates response inhibition while mesial prefrontal cortex is responsible for error detection. *Neuroimage*, Vol.20, No.1 (September, 2003), pp.351-358, ISSN: 1053-8119

Rubia, K., Smith, A.B., Brammer, M.J., Toone, B. & Taylor, E. (2005). Abnormal brain activation during inhibition and error detection in medication-naive adolescents with ADHD. *American Journal of Psychiatry*, Vol.162, No.6 (June, 2005), pp.1067-1075, ISSN: 0002-953X

Rubia, K., Halari, R., Cubillo, A., Mohammad, A.M., Scott, S. & Brammer, M. (2010). Disorder-specific inferior prefrontal hypofunction in boys with pure attention-deficit/hyperactivity disorder compared to boys with pure conduct disorder during cognitive flexibility. *Human Brain Mapping*, Vol.31, No.12 (December, 2010), pp.1823-1833, ISSN: 1065-9471

Rypma, B. & D'Esposito, M. (2000). Isolating the neural mechanisms of age-related changes in human working memory. *Nature Neuroscience*, Vol.3, No.5 (May 2000), pp.509-515, ISSN: 1471-0048

Shinoura, N., Suzuki, Y., Yamada, R., Tabei, Y., Saito, K. & Yagi, K. (2009). Damage to the right superior longitudinal fasciculus in the inferior parietal lobe plays a role in spatial neglect. *Neuropsychologia*, Vol.47, No.12 (October 2009), pp.2600-2603.

Smith, A.B., Taylor, E., Brammer, M. & Rubia, K. (2004). Neural correlates of switching set as measured in fast, event-related functional magnetic resonance imaging. *Human Brain Mapping*, Vol.21, No.4 (April 2004), pp.247-256, ISSN: 1065-9471

Smith, A.B., Taylor, E., Brammer, M., Toone, B. & Rubia, K. (2006). Task-specific hypoactivation in prefrontal and temporoparietal brain regions during motor inhibition and task switching in medication-naive children and adolescents with attention deficit hyperactivity disorder. *American Journal of Psychiatry*, Vol.163, No.6 (June 2006), pp.1044-1051, ISSN: 0002-953X

Stanovich, K.E. & West, R.F. (2000). Individual differences in reasoning: implications for the rationality debate? *Behavioural Brain Science*, Vol.23, No.5 (October 2000), pp.645-665.

Stavy, R., Goel, V., Critchley, H., & Dolan, R. (2006). Intuitive interference in quantitative reasoning. *Brain Research*, Vol.1073-1074 (February 2006), pp.383-388, ISSN: 0006-8993

Takahama, S., Miyauchi, S. & Saiki, J. (2010). Neural basis for dynamic updating of object representation in visual working memory. *Neuroimage*, Vol.49, No.4 (Feburuary 2010), 3394-3f403.

Thakral, P.P. & Slotnick, S.D. (2009). The role of parietal cortex during sustained visual spatial attention. *Brain Research*, Vol.1302 (December 2009), pp.157-166.

Tsujii, T., Okada, M. & Watanabe, S. (2006). Cognitive neuroscience for deductive reasoning and inhibitory mechanism: on the belief-bias effect In: *Reasoning and Cognition, Interdisciplinary Conference Series on Reasoning Studies*, Vol.2, Adler, D., Ogawa, Y., Okada, M., & Watanabe, S. (Ed.), 53-61, Keio University Press, ISBN 978-4-7664-1332-8, Tokyo, Japan.

Tsujii, T., Yamamoto, E., Ohira, T., Saito, N. & Watanabe, S. (2007). Effects of sedative and non-sedative H1 antagonists on cognitive tasks: behavioral and near-infrared spectroscopy (NIRS) examinations. *Psychopharmacology*, Vol.194, No.1, (September 2007), pp. 83-91, ISSN: 0033-3158

Tsujii, T. & Watanabe, S. (2009). Neural correlates of dual-task effect on belief-bias syllogistic reasoning: a near-infrared spectroscopy study. *Brain Research*, Vol. 1287 , pp. 118-125, ISSN 0006-8993

Tsujii, T., Masuda, S., Yamamoto, E., Ohira, T., Akiyama, T., Takahashi, T. & Watanabe, S. (2009a). Effects of sedative and nonsedative antihistamines on prefrontal activity during verbal fluency task in young children: a near-infrared spectroscopy (NIRS) study. *Psychopharmacology*, Vol.207, No.1 (November 2009), pp. 127-132, ISSN: 0033-3158

Tsujii, T., Yamamoto, E., Masuda, S., Watanabe, S. (2009b). Longitudinal study of spatial working memory development in young children. *Neuroreport*. Vol.20, No.8 (May 2009), pp.759-763, ISSN: 0959-4965

Tsujii, T., & Watanabe, S. (2010). Neural correlates of belief-bias reasoning under time pressure: a near-infrared spectroscopy study. *Neuroimage*, Vol.50, No.3 (April 2010), pp.1320-1326, ISSN: 1053-8119.

Tsujii, T., Masuda, S., Akiyama, T. & Watanabe, S. (2010a). The role of inferior frontal cortex in belief-bias reasoning: an rTMS study. *Neuropsychologia*, Vol.48, No.7 (June 2010), pp.2005-2008, ISSN: 0028-3932

Tsujii, T., Okada, M. & Watanabe, S. (2010b). Effects of aging on hemispheric asymmetry in inferior frontal cortex activity during belief-bias syllogistic reasoning: a near-infrared spectroscopy study. *Behavioural Brain Research*, Vol.210, No.2 (July 2010), pp.178-183, ISSN: 0166-4328

Tsujii, T., Yamamoto, E., Ohira, T., Takahashi, T. & Watanabe, S. (2010d). Antihistamine effects on prefrontal cortex activity during working memory process in preschool children: a near-infrared spectroscopy (NIRS) study. *Neuroscience Research*. 2010 May; Vol.67, No.1 (May 2010), pp.80-85, ISSN: 0168-0102

Tsujii, T., Sakatani, K., Masuda, S., Akiyama, T., & Watanabe, S. (2011a). Evaluating the roles of the inferior frontal gyrus and superior parietal lobule in deductive reasoning: An rTMS study. *Neuroimage*, Vol.58, No.2 (September 2011), pp.640-646, ISSN: 1053-8119

Tsujii, T., Sakatani, K., Nakashima, E., Igarashi, T., & Katayama, Y. (2011b). Characterization of the acute effects of alcohol on asymmetry of inferior frontal cortex activity during a Go/No-Go task using functional near-infrared spectroscopy. *Psychopharmacology*, Vol.217, No.4 (October 2011), pp.595-603, ISSN: 0033-3158

Xue, G., Aron, A.R. & Poldrack, R.A. (2008). Common neural substrates for inhibition of spoken and manual responses. *Cerebral Cortex*, Vol.18, No.8 (August 2008), 1923-1932.

Zhu, Z., Zhang, J.X., Wang, S., Xiao, Z., Huang, J. & Chen, H.C. (2009). Involvement of left inferior frontal gyrus in sentence-level semantic integration. *Neuroimage*, Vol.47, No.2 (August 2009), pp.756-763.

4

Functional Near Infrared Spectroscopy and Diffuse Optical Tomography in Neuroscience

Matteo Caffini[1], Davide Contini[1], Rebecca Re[1], Lucia M. Zucchelli[1], Rinaldo Cubeddu[1], Alessandro Torricelli[1] and Lorenzo Spinelli[2]
[1]*Dipartimento di Fisica - Politecnico di Milano, Milano*
[2]*CNR - Istituto di Fotonica e Nanotecnologie, Milano*
Italy

1. Introduction

Neuroimaging is the branch of medicine whose purpose is to provide visual information about the structure and the anatomy of the brain. The main techniques in clinics are: *Computed Tomography* (CT), *Magnetic Resonance Imaging* (MRI), *Diffuse Optical Tomography* (DOT), *Positron Emission Tomography* (PET) and *Single Photon Emission Computed Tomography* (SPECT).

CT scanning uses X-rays crossing the sample to image sections of the specimen in study. Specimen can be a living being, a part of if (e.g. the abdomen, a knee, the head, ...) or whatever non-living object. X-rays travel ballistically inside most of the materials (living tissue included), so measuring absorption of X-rays we can guess the composition of the sample we are measuring. Changing the direction of injection of the X-rays and merging absorption data coming from multiple directions makes a planar reconstruction of the examined section of the sample possible. CT is invasive in the sense that irradiates the patient with ionizing radiation. A little dose is given to the patient during a single CT session, anyway. CT scanning of the head is typically used to detect skull fractures, brain injuries, aneurysms, strokes, brain tumors and arteriovenous malformations in the brain.

MRI is based on nuclear magnetic resonance principles. It uses a strong static magnetic field to align the nuclear magnetization of hydrogen atoms of water in the body and then radio frequency fields are generated to alter this magnetization alignment. Several coils mounted on the scanner are then able to detect the magnetic field produced by the altered hydrogen atom magnetization and to relate the recovery time of these short-lasting magnetic fields to the environment in which resonant hydrogen atoms lie. MRI, using non-ionizing radiation, is generally considered non-invasive for the patient and provides greater contrast between different soft tissues than CT does. Magnetic resonance images of the head are mostly used to detect brain tumors.

PET and SPECT are nuclear medicine techniques and they are used in cancer localization. A radionuclide is injected in the body via blood flow and then tracked with detectors placed around the patient.

Functional neuroimaging is a particular way to perform medical neuroimaging focused more on functionality rather than just resolve anatomical features. The goal of functional neuroimaging is to detect *spatial* and *temporal* changes of activated areas of the brain, by measuring related physiological or physical features. The most common techniques are *functional Magnetic Resonance Imaging* (fMRI), *Electroencephalography* (EEG), *Magnetoencephalography* (MEG) and, recently, *functional Near InfraRed Spectroscopy* (fNIRS) and *Diffuse Optical Tomography* (DOT). PET and SPECT can be considered functional images as they use a radionuclide concentration to distinguish between healthy tissue and tumoral tissue.

Usually functional neuroimaging techniques are divided into two main classes: those with high spatial resolution ($\sim$ 1 cm or less) and those with high time resolution ($\sim$ 1 s or less).

- High spatial resolution and poor time resolution techniques (fMRI, PET and SPECT).
- High time resolution and poor spatial resolution techniques (EEG and MEG).

Having good time resolution and sufficient spatial resolution, DOT lays between the two classes and it is often considered the optimal compromise for functional neuroimaging studies. Spatial resolution in DOT is not an intrinsic feature, being the technique diffusion-limited. Nevertheless, in brain activation studies, integrating optical data and *a priori* anatomic data from MRI scans, brings to huge enhancements in spatial localization.

2. Functional near infraRed spectroscopy (fNIRS)

The simplest way to perform tissue oximetry using harmless electromagnetic radiation is to shine the tissue by means of a continuous beam of infrared light and to collect the re-emitted or transmitted light.

Hemoglobin is the key: oxygenated and deoxygenated states have considerably different absorption spectra and it turns out that, in first approximation, oxyhemoglobin and deoxyhemoglobin also are the two main chromophores in tissues into the InfraRed window. Because the underlining hypothesis states the presence of two chromophores, we need to inject radiation at two different wavelengths, possibly chosen where the spectra have the greatest differences (see Fig. 1). This spectroscopic technique uses constant light intensity and is known in literature as *Continuous Wave Near InfraRed Spectroscopy* (CW-NIRS) The most diffused wavelengths for CW-NIRS are 690 nm and 820 nm.

2.1 Absorption spectroscopy

Spectroscopy is the study of the interaction between radiation and matter, in particular absorption spectroscopy measures the absorption of radiation, in a selected range of frequency, in radiation-matter interaction. It is largely employed in analytical chemistry to check for the presence of elements or substances, being the absorption spectrum a sort of fingerprint and so characteristic of the substances. The simplest application is the detection of the amount of the substance present.

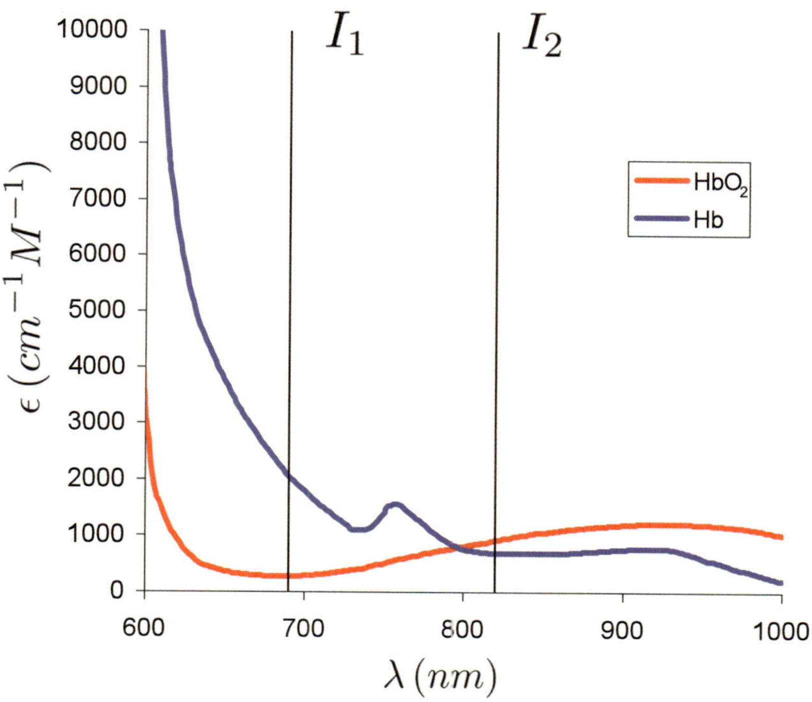

Fig. 1. The absorption spectrum, that is the molar extinction coefficient vs. the wavelength, of the oxygenated (red) and deoxygenated (blue) states of the hemoglobin. I_1 and I_2 are the chosen wavelengths for Near InfraRed Spectroscopy measurements.

When a radiation beam of known intensity I_0 crosses a layer of known width L of a certain medium (chromophore), part of the radiation is absorbed by the medium and the rest is transmitted on the other side of the layer (Fig. 2). Modeling this phenomenon supposing that each infinitesimal layer absorbs an amount of radiation $\mathrm{d}I$ and that this absorption is proportional to radiation intensity, brings to the following mathematical model. Calling μ_a the absorption coefficient and z the radiation beam direction, the radiation intensity I measured is modeled by the *Lambert-Beer law*:

$$\mathrm{d}I = -\mu_a I \mathrm{d}z \tag{1}$$

$$\int_{I_0}^{I} \frac{\mathrm{d}I}{I} = \int_0^L (-\mu_a)\,\mathrm{d}z \tag{2}$$

$$I = I_0 e^{-\mu_a L} \tag{3}$$

The absorption coefficient is measured in m^{-1} and has a straightforward interpretation: $l_a = \frac{1}{\mu_a}$ is the mean free path a photon travels prior to being absorbed. Moreover, it can be decomposed into two distinct factors: the absorbent medium concentration and its molar extinction coefficient ϵ:

$$\mu_a = [c]\,\varepsilon \tag{4}$$

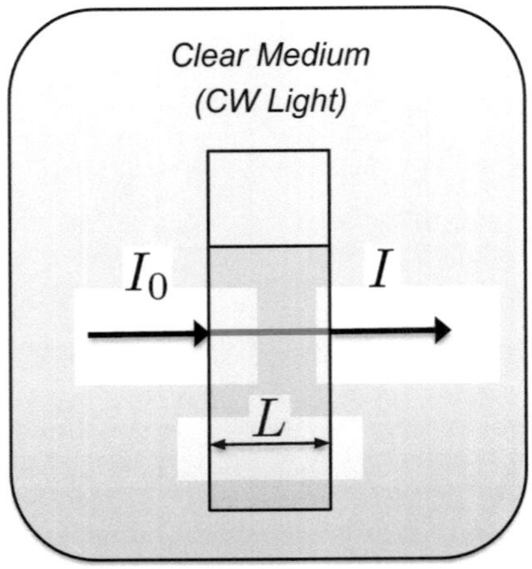

Fig. 2. Absorption Spectroscopy in the most simple geometry. Radiation is injected in the sample from one side and radiation intensity is measure on the other side. The Lambert-Beer law then allows to compute the chromophore concentration.

The extinction coefficient depends on the radiation wavelength: $\epsilon = \epsilon(\lambda)$ and so the absorption coefficient $\mu_a = \mu_a(\lambda)$. Such a functional dependence constitutes the *absorption spectrum* of the substance considered[1]. When more than a chromophore is present, each contribute is summed:

$$\mu_a = [c_1]\,\epsilon_1 + [c_2]\,\epsilon_2 + [c_3]\,\epsilon_3 + \cdots = \sum_i [c_i]\,\epsilon_i \tag{5}$$

Media for which this model holds are non-diffusing media, often called *clear media* and concentration measurements are easily conducted knowing the extinction coefficient of the chromophore and the length of the path traveled by the radiation. In the many chromophore experiment, performing multiple sessions, changing the radiation wavelength, allows to write a linear system and to obtain the unknown concentration of each chromophore.

Performing the same experiment described before using different media, it is found that for a vast class of substances this model is not accurate, as it doesn't take into account for the diffusion of radiation within the medium (Fig. 3(a)). Scattering events are due to discontinuities in dielectric properties of the medium and can be modeled as collisions between the photons of the radiation and particles in the medium. Many scattering models have been developed in physics: in classical electromagnetism by Rutherford, Thomson and Mie and in quantum physics by Compton and Raman [Feynman et al. (1964); Mie (1908); Rutherford (1911)]. A second important class of media then have to be described, media often called *turbid media*. Living tissues belong to this second class.

The Lambert-Beer model is still valid for this media, but the absorption coefficient alone is no more enough to describe the intensity drop found. A second coefficient μ_s, called *scattering*

[1] In many cases the absorption spectrum is given with respect to the frequency $\nu = \frac{c}{n\lambda}$, being c the speed of light and n the refraction index of the medium.

coefficient, is then introduced. The Lambert-Beer law it is written as follows:

$$I = I_0 e^{-(\mu_a + \mu_s)L} \tag{6}$$

The scattering coefficient here defined has a similar interpretation as the absorption coefficient: $l_s = \frac{1}{\mu_s}$ is the mean free path between two scattering events. Within this class of substances, absolute concentration measurements are possible only for thin samples (for thicker samples more complicated approaches are necessary, see section 2.3.1). Incidentally it can be noticed that this disturbing factor provides a helpful effect. Radiation scatters statistically in every direction, even backwards. It is then possible to collect radiation from the same side of the sample used for the radiation injection and to design experiments in reflectance geometry (Fig. 3(b)).

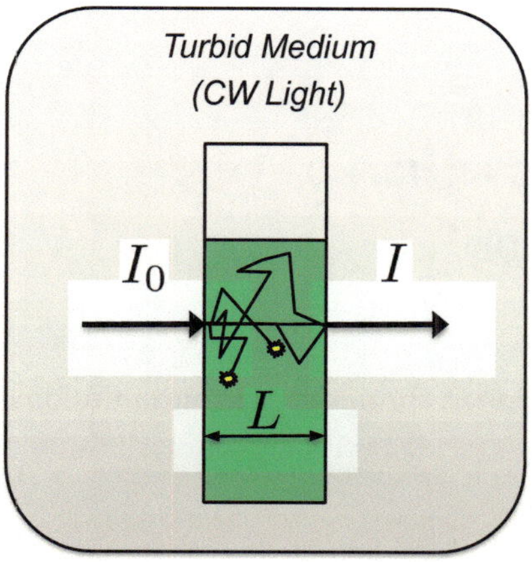

(a) Absorption Spectroscopy using a turbid medium does not allow to compute the chromophore concentration within the sample because of scattering contributes to intensity attenuation.

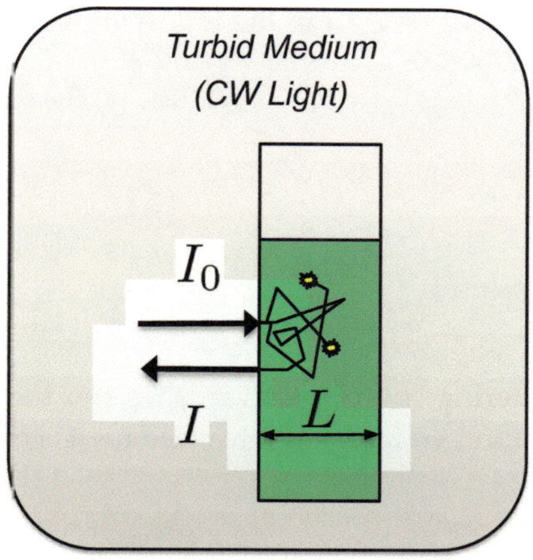

(b) When using turbid media experiments in reflection geometry are possible. Scattering provides a positive probability to have radiation traveling backwards after encountering scattering centers in the medium.

Fig. 3. Absorption spectrocopy in turbid medium in trasmission geometry (Fig. 3(a)) and reflection geometry (Fig. 3(b)).

A different approach is to irradiate the sample with a non-constant light intensity, but it becomes necessary to develop a more general model for light traveling inside turbid media. This will be done in section 2.3. First a simpler way to separate scattering contributes is explained.

In eq. 6 it has been seen that both absorption and scattering take part in the same way to radiation attenuation and that is not trivial to discriminate between the two distinct contributions. There's at least a case in which a simple way the separation is easily done. Suppose to have a medium in which the chromophore concentration $[c(t)]$ slightly varies in time and suppose to sample spectroscopic data in reflection geometry for a certain time interval. This case is not that far from reality as it may seem at first sight, for example in biological tissues chromophores concentrations change in time because of blood flow. Then for each instant t_n a Lambert-Beer equation can be written as follow:

$$I(t_n) = I_0 e^{-([c(t_n)]\epsilon DL+G)} \tag{7}$$

where scattering contribution $\mu_s L$ has been grouped into the term G and the *differential pathlength factor* D has been introduced to take into account that photon travel paths longer than the source-detector separation because they penetrate inside the medium, scatters multiple times and then a little part reaches the detector traveling backwards. The differential pathlength factor depends only on the mean refractive index of the crossed medium. Hypothesizing that G doesn't vary in time and is constant for small variations of chromophore concentrations and introducing the physical quantity *absorbance* $A = \ln \frac{I}{I_0} = -([c]\,\epsilon DL + G)$, we can compute the variation in chromophore concentration between measurement collected at time t_n and time t_m in the following way:

$$\Delta A_{mn} = A_m - A_n \tag{8}$$

$$= -c_m \epsilon DL - G + c_n \epsilon DL + G \tag{9}$$

$$= -(c_m - c_n)\epsilon DL \tag{10}$$

$$= -\Delta c_{mn} \epsilon DL \tag{11}$$

The scattering contributes vanishes and the variation in chromophore concentration depends only on the two intensity measurements collected:

$$\Delta c_{mn} = -\frac{\Delta A_{mn}}{\epsilon DL} \tag{12}$$

$$= \frac{1}{\epsilon DL}(A_n - A_m) \tag{13}$$

$$= \frac{1}{\epsilon DL}\left(\ln \frac{I_n}{I_0} - \ln \frac{I_m}{I_0}\right) \tag{14}$$

$$= \frac{1}{\epsilon DL} \ln\left(\frac{I_n}{I_m}\right) \tag{15}$$

Most of times a reference measurement is conducted and all the concentration values are then computed as variation from the reference value.

2.2 Continuous wave NIRS (CW-NIRS)

Hemodynamic activity of the brain is related through metabolic processes to the electrical activity of the neurons, then, performing hemoglobin concentration measurements on the cortical tissues, it is possible to obtain information about spatial localization and temporal behavior of neuronal activity. The spectroscopic tools described in section 2.1 provide a straightforward way to do this. It is possible to inject radiation into the tissues and collect the photons coming out, for example using a reflectance geometry. The usefulness of this technique would be to measure what happens within the blood flow, neglecting the contributes from the surrounding environment.

Collecting data at different times and then computing the absorbance variation values ΔA_{λ_1} and ΔA_{λ_2}, it is possible to write the following system of equations:

$$\begin{cases} \Delta A_{\lambda_1} = \left(\epsilon_{Hb,\lambda_1} \Delta\,[\mathrm{Hb}] + \epsilon_{\mathrm{HbO_2},\lambda_1} \Delta\,[\mathrm{HbO_2}]\right) D_{\lambda_1} L \\ \Delta A_{\lambda_2} = \left(\epsilon_{Hb,\lambda_2} \Delta\,[\mathrm{Hb}] + \epsilon_{\mathrm{HbO_2},\lambda_2} \Delta\,[\mathrm{HbO_2}]\right) D_{\lambda_2} L \end{cases} \tag{16}$$

In matrix form it becomes:

$$\begin{bmatrix} \frac{\Delta A_{\lambda_1}}{D_{\lambda_1} L} \\ \frac{\Delta A_{\lambda_2}}{D_{\lambda_2} L} \end{bmatrix} = \begin{bmatrix} \epsilon_{Hb,\lambda_1} & \epsilon_{\mathrm{HbO_2},\lambda_1} \\ \epsilon_{Hb,\lambda_2} & \epsilon_{\mathrm{HbO_2},\lambda_1} \end{bmatrix} \begin{bmatrix} \Delta\,[\mathrm{Hb}] \\ \Delta\,[\mathrm{HbO_2}] \end{bmatrix} \tag{17}$$

and finally:

$$\begin{bmatrix} \Delta\,[\mathrm{Hb}] \\ \Delta\,[\mathrm{HbO_2}] \end{bmatrix} = \begin{bmatrix} \epsilon_{Hb,\lambda_1} & \epsilon_{\mathrm{HbO_2},\lambda_1} \\ \epsilon_{Hb,\lambda_2} & \epsilon_{\mathrm{HbO_2},\lambda_1} \end{bmatrix}^{-1} \begin{bmatrix} \frac{\Delta A_{\lambda_1}}{D_{\lambda_1} L} \\ \frac{\Delta A_{\lambda_2}}{D_{\lambda_2} L} \end{bmatrix} \tag{18}$$

Being this a two equations systems with the two unknowns $\Delta\,[\mathrm{Hb}]$ and $\Delta\,[\mathrm{HbO_2}]$, a solution to the linear system is possible and the oxyhemoglobin and deoxyhemoglobin concentration variations with respect to a reference value can be computed (Eq. 18). If data are sampled for an interval of time, solving the linear system for each time sample, the time course of the concentrations is given.

Derived quantities such as total hemoglobin [tHb] are often plotted vs. time in order to improve the data visualization.

$$\Delta\,[\mathrm{tHb}] = \Delta\,[\mathrm{Hb}] + \Delta\,[\mathrm{HbO_2}] \tag{19}$$

An important limitation of CW-NIRS is the possibility to obtain just concentration variations. Having absolute concentration values, hemoglobin saturation sO_2 could be calculated:

$$\mathrm{sO_2} = \frac{[\mathrm{HbO_2}]}{[\mathrm{tHb}]} \tag{20}$$

In principle there is no depth sensitivity with a single source-detector pair in CW-NIRS. Information on the composition of the media crossed by the CW light can be measured as an average. To increase light penetration large source-detector separation have been used (4-5 cm) with the obvious consequence of increasing the sampling volume and thus worsening the spatial resolution. Increasing the complexity of the system, the use of multi-source and multi-detector tomographic or topographic arrangements could overcome this limitation and better depth sensitivity [Boas et al. (2004); Strangman et al. (2002)].

Laboratory prototypes and commercial instrumentations have been developed through the years to measure oxygenation of the muscles and of the cortical regions of the brain. A comprehensive list can be found in Wolf et al. (2007).

2.3 Photon migration approach

A different way to deal with diffusion and discriminate between scattering and absorption contributes is to use non-constant light intensities in the injected radiation. A possible way to describe the physics of the problem is to start from the electric and magnetic fields associated with the radiation and to develop a rigorous mathematical theory, taking into account scattering, diffraction and interference. This is quite complicated, especially because of multiple scattering.

A more practical physical model of photon propagation into diffuse media based on energy flow is the *Radiative Transfer Equation* (RTE). This model was first developed to describe the non-interacting neutrons diffusion in nuclear reactors [Sanchez & McCormick (1982)]. The hypothesis of non-interacting particles reasonably applies to photons in multiple elastic scattering regime. The RTE model neglects polarization effects. This is not a problem though, because even if light coherence exists, this is going to be completely lost after a few scattering events.

2.3.1 The radiative transfer equation

The average power that at position $\boldsymbol{r}$ and time t flows through the unit area oriented in the direction of the unit vector $\hat{\boldsymbol{s}}$, due to photons within a unit frequency band centered at ν, that are moving within the unit solid angle around $\hat{\boldsymbol{s}}$ is the *spectral radiance* $I_s(\boldsymbol{r},\hat{\boldsymbol{s}},t,\nu)$. Thus at time t through the unit area $\mathrm{d}\Sigma$ lying in $\boldsymbol{r}$, oriented as $\hat{\boldsymbol{s}}$, within the unit solid angle $\mathrm{d}\Omega$ and in the frequency interval $[\nu,\nu+\mathrm{d}\nu]$ flows a power $\mathrm{d}P$ given by:

$$\mathrm{d}P = I_s(\boldsymbol{r},\hat{\boldsymbol{s}},t,\nu)\,|\hat{\boldsymbol{n}}\cdot\hat{\boldsymbol{s}}|\mathrm{d}\Sigma\mathrm{d}\Omega\mathrm{d}\nu \tag{21}$$

Energy density $\frac{\mathrm{d}E}{\mathrm{d}V}$ is simply related to spectral radiance. The energy $\mathrm{d}E$ per unit frequency and per unit solid angle that crossed the area $\mathrm{d}\Sigma$ oriented as $\hat{\boldsymbol{s}}$, in the time interval $\mathrm{d}t$ is:

$$\frac{\mathrm{d}E}{\mathrm{d}V} = \frac{I_s\mathrm{d}\Sigma\mathrm{d}t}{\mathrm{d}\Sigma v\mathrm{d}t} = \frac{I_s}{v} \tag{22}$$

Where v is the speed of radiation in the medium, $v=\frac{c}{n}$. Energy density is the number of photons and so I_s is proportional to the number of photons in the unit volume, with frequency ν, that at time t are moving in the direction $\hat{\boldsymbol{s}}$. As we deal with media in which the radiation frequency doesn't change during propagation (elastic scattering), we can integrate I_s over the frequency ν and obtain the *radiance* $I(\boldsymbol{r},\hat{\boldsymbol{s}},t)$.
Integrating also over the solid angle and dividing by v gives the quantity $u(\boldsymbol{r},t) = \frac{\int_{4\pi} I(\boldsymbol{r},\hat{\boldsymbol{s}},t)\mathrm{d}\Omega}{v}$, measured in $\left[\mathrm{Jm}^{-3}\right]$, that represents the energy density at position $\boldsymbol{r}$ and time t. Finally the photon density can be obtained dividing the energy density by the energy of a single photon:

$$n(\boldsymbol{r},t) = \frac{u(\boldsymbol{r},t)}{h\nu} \tag{23}$$

The RTE is an integro-differential equation stating the balance of the incoming and outgoing radiation along the direction $\hat{\boldsymbol{s}}$, at the time t, inside the volume element $\mathrm{d}V$ at the position $\boldsymbol{r}$

[Ishimaru (1978); Martelli et al. (2010)]:

$$\frac{1}{v}\frac{\partial I}{\partial t} = -\hat{\boldsymbol{s}} \cdot \nabla I - (\mu_a + \mu_s) I + \mu_s \int_{4\pi} p\left(\hat{\boldsymbol{s}}, \hat{\boldsymbol{s}}'\right) I\left(\boldsymbol{r}, \hat{\boldsymbol{s}}', t\right) \mathrm{d}\Omega' + q \tag{24}$$

Each term appearing has a precise significance:

- $\frac{1}{v}\frac{\partial I}{\partial t} \Rightarrow$ temporal change of energy.
- $-\hat{\boldsymbol{s}} \cdot \nabla I \Rightarrow$ change due to energy flow.
- $-(\mu_a + \mu_s) I \Rightarrow$ energy drop due to absorption and scattering.
- $+\mu_s \int_{4\pi} p\left(\hat{\boldsymbol{s}}, \hat{\boldsymbol{s}}'\right) I\left(\boldsymbol{r}, \hat{\boldsymbol{s}}', t\right) \mathrm{d}\Omega' \Rightarrow$ energy gain from radiation coming from every direction, but scattered into the direction $\hat{\boldsymbol{s}}$, being $p\left(\hat{\boldsymbol{s}}, \hat{\boldsymbol{s}}'\right)$ the *phase function*, that is the probability that a photon flowing in the direction $\hat{\boldsymbol{s}}$ is scattered into the direction $\hat{\boldsymbol{s}}'$.
- $q = q\left(\boldsymbol{r}, \hat{\boldsymbol{s}}, t\right) \Rightarrow$ Radiation source inside $\mathrm{d}V \left[\mathrm{Wm}^{-3}\mathrm{sr}^{-1}\right]$.

The RTE has two immediate properties:

1. If I_0 is a solution for a non-absorbing medium with time impulsive source term $q\left(\boldsymbol{r}, \hat{\boldsymbol{s}}, t\right) = q_0\left(\boldsymbol{r}, \hat{\boldsymbol{s}}\right) \delta(t)$, then if the absorption coefficient is μ_a the solution is:

$$I = I_0 e^{-\mu_a v t} \tag{25}$$

   This property is a generalization of the Lambert-Beer law [Sassaroli & Fantini (2004); Tsuchiya (2001)].

2. If I is the Green function for a medium having extinction coefficient $\mu_t = \mu_a + \mu_s$ and albedo $a = \frac{\mu_s}{\mu_t}$, then for a medium having extinction coefficient μ_t^* and the same albedo, the solution is scaled in this way:

$$I\left(\boldsymbol{r}^*, \hat{\boldsymbol{s}}, t^*\right) = \left(\frac{\mu_t^*}{\mu_t}\right)^3 I\left(\boldsymbol{r}, \hat{\boldsymbol{s}}, t\right) \qquad \begin{cases} \mathbf{r}^* = \left(\frac{\mu_t}{\mu_t^*}\right) \mathbf{r} \\ t^* = \left(\frac{\mu_t}{\mu_t^*}\right) t \end{cases} \tag{26}$$

   This scaling property is known as the *similarity principle* [Zege et al. (1991)].

Because of the high complexity of the RTE, no analytical solutions are available and approximation methods are then applied. Numerical methods like the *Finite Difference Method* or the *Finite Elements Method* (FEM) require a large amount of computational power, but are often applied [Arridge (1995); Arridge et al. (2000); Arridge & Hebden (1997); Arridge & Schweiger (1995); Arridge et al. (1993)]. Stochastic methods like the *Monte Carlo* are widely used in many biological applications [Boas et al. (2002); Fang & Boas (2009)].

2.3.2 The P_N approximation

Many ways to simplify the RTE have been developed through the years, but most methods are based on the *P_N approximation.* Two derived quantities of interest are the *photon fluence* Φ

and the *photon flux* $\boldsymbol{J}$:

$$\Phi(\boldsymbol{r},t) = \int_{4\pi} I(\boldsymbol{r},\hat{\boldsymbol{s}},t)\,\mathrm{d}\Omega \tag{27}$$

$$\boldsymbol{J}(\boldsymbol{r},t) = \int_{4\pi} I(\boldsymbol{r},\hat{\boldsymbol{s}},t)\,\hat{\boldsymbol{s}}\mathrm{d}\Omega \tag{28}$$

Radiance and source term are expanded in spherical harmonics [Boas (1996); Jackson (1999)]:

$$I(\boldsymbol{r},\hat{\boldsymbol{s}},t) = \sum_{l=0}^{+\infty}\sum_{m=-l}^{l}\sqrt{\frac{2l+1}{4\pi}}\phi_{l,m}(\boldsymbol{r},t)\,Y_{l,m}(\hat{\boldsymbol{s}}) \tag{29}$$

$$q(\boldsymbol{r},\hat{\boldsymbol{s}},t) = \sum_{l=0}^{+\infty}\sum_{m=-l}^{l}\sqrt{\frac{2l+1}{4\pi}}q_{l,m}(\boldsymbol{r},t)\,Y_{l,m}(\hat{\boldsymbol{s}}) \tag{30}$$

Phase function is expanded in spherical harmonics too, but first the reasonable hypothesis that the scattering amplitude is only dependent on the change in direction of the photon is made. With this assumption the probability of scattering from a direction $\hat{\boldsymbol{s}}$ into a direction $\hat{\boldsymbol{s}}'$ depends only on the angle between $\hat{\boldsymbol{s}}$ and $\hat{\boldsymbol{s}}'$:

$$p(\hat{\boldsymbol{s}}\cdot\hat{\boldsymbol{s}}') = \sum_{l=0}^{+\infty}\frac{2l+1}{4\pi}g_l P_l(\hat{\boldsymbol{s}}\cdot\hat{\boldsymbol{s}}') \tag{31}$$

$$= \sum_{l=0}^{+\infty}\sum_{m=-l}^{l} g_l Y^*_{l,m}(\hat{\boldsymbol{s}}')\,Y_{l,m}(\hat{\boldsymbol{s}}) \tag{32}$$

Where P_l is the Legendre polynomial of order l and the angular addition rule has been used [Jackson (1999)]. The normalization factors $\sqrt{\frac{2l+1}{4\pi}}$ and $\frac{2l+1}{4\pi}$ are introduced for convenience.

Truncating the series at the $l = N$ term brings to the P_N approximation of the RTE [Arridge (1999)]. In the P_1 approximation the radiance[2], source and phase function reduce to:

$$I(\boldsymbol{r},\hat{\boldsymbol{s}},t) = \frac{1}{4\pi}\Phi(\boldsymbol{r},t) + \frac{3}{4\pi}\boldsymbol{J}(\boldsymbol{r},t)\cdot\hat{\boldsymbol{s}} \tag{33}$$

$$q(\boldsymbol{r},\hat{\boldsymbol{s}},t) = \frac{1}{4\pi}q_0(\boldsymbol{r},t) + \frac{3}{4\pi}\boldsymbol{q_1}(\boldsymbol{r},t)\cdot\hat{\boldsymbol{s}} \tag{34}$$

$$p(\hat{\boldsymbol{s}}\cdot\hat{\boldsymbol{s}}') = \frac{1}{4\pi}g_0 + \frac{3}{4\pi}g_1\hat{\boldsymbol{s}}\cdot\hat{\boldsymbol{s}}' \tag{35}$$

Where we used the definition of fluence 27 and flux 28, obtaining:

$$\Phi(\boldsymbol{r},t) = \phi_{0,0}(\boldsymbol{r},t) \tag{36}$$

$$\boldsymbol{J}(\boldsymbol{r},t) = \begin{pmatrix} \frac{1}{\sqrt{2}}\left(\phi_{1,-1}(\boldsymbol{r},t) - \phi_{1,1}(\boldsymbol{r},t)\right) \\ \frac{1}{i\sqrt{2}}\left(\phi_{1,-1}(\boldsymbol{r},t) + \phi_{1,1}(\boldsymbol{r},t)\right) \\ \phi_{1,0}(\boldsymbol{r},t) \end{pmatrix} \tag{37}$$

[2] As will be realized soon, this brings to assume the radiance to be nearly isotropic. This is a good approximation for biological tissues and in general for high-albedo media, because of the few absorption events relative to the scattering events.

For the source term approximation the quantities monopole moment q_0 and dipole moment $\boldsymbol{q_1}$ have been introduced:

$$q_0(\boldsymbol{r},t) = q_{0,0}(\boldsymbol{r},t) \tag{38}$$

$$\boldsymbol{q_1}(\boldsymbol{r},t) = \begin{pmatrix} \frac{1}{\sqrt{2}}\left(q_{1,-1}(\boldsymbol{r},t) - q_{1,1}(\boldsymbol{r},t)\right) \\ \frac{1}{i\sqrt{2}}\left(q_{1,-1}(\boldsymbol{r},t) + q_{1,1}(\boldsymbol{r},t)\right) \\ q_{1,0}(\boldsymbol{r},t) \end{pmatrix} \tag{39}$$

Normalizing g_0 to unity, g_1 is the average cosine of the scattering angle:

$$g_0 = 1 \tag{40}$$

$$g_1 = <\hat{\boldsymbol{s}} \cdot \hat{\boldsymbol{s}'}> \tag{41}$$

Finally, substituting these approximated expressions into 24, we obtain:

$$\frac{1}{v}\frac{\partial \Phi(\boldsymbol{r},t)}{\partial t} = -\mu_a \Phi(\boldsymbol{r},t) - \nabla \cdot \boldsymbol{J}(\boldsymbol{r},t) + q_0(\boldsymbol{r},t) \tag{42}$$

$$\frac{1}{v}\frac{\partial \boldsymbol{J}(\boldsymbol{r},t)}{\partial t} = -\left(\mu_a + \mu_s'\right)\boldsymbol{J}(\boldsymbol{r},t) - \frac{1}{3}\nabla\Phi(\boldsymbol{r},t) + \boldsymbol{q_1}(\boldsymbol{r},t) \tag{43}$$

Where we made use of the definition of reduced scattering coefficient μ_s':

$$\mu_s' = (1 - g_1)\,\mu_s \tag{44}$$

2.3.3 The diffusion approximation

In a high-albedo (predominantly scattering) medium, the time for a substantial change in flux $\boldsymbol{J}$ is much longer than the time to traverse one transport mean free path. Thus, over one transport mean free path itself, the fractional change in flux is much less than unity. The *diffusion approximation* results from making the following assumptions:

$$\frac{\partial \boldsymbol{J}(\boldsymbol{r},t)}{\partial t} = 0 \tag{45}$$

$$\boldsymbol{q_1}(\boldsymbol{r},t) = 0 \tag{46}$$

Dropping the dipole moment of the source is reasonable assuming an isotropic source. Eq. 43 then becomes *Fick's law*:

$$\boldsymbol{J}(\boldsymbol{r},t) = -\frac{1}{3\left(\mu_a + u_s'\right)}\nabla\Phi(\boldsymbol{r},t) \tag{47}$$

Usually the factor multiplying the gradient is called *diffusion coefficient*, $D = \frac{1}{3(\mu_a+\mu_s')}$. We notice that in high-albedo medium ($\mu_s' \gg \mu_a$) it doesn't depend on absorption and can be calculated as $D \approx \frac{1}{3\mu_s'}$[3].

[3] This is consistent with the similarity principle previously introduced [Martelli et al. (2010)].

Substituting into Eq. 42 we finally have the *diffusion equation* (DE):

$$\frac{1}{v}\frac{\partial\Phi(\boldsymbol{r},t)}{\partial t} = -\mu_a\Phi(\boldsymbol{r},t) + \nabla\cdot D\nabla\Phi(\boldsymbol{r},t) + q_0(\boldsymbol{r},t) \tag{48}$$

The diffusion equation models many problems in Physics and Chemistry, such as heat propagation, ion diffusion and semiconductor doping. Analytical solution to the DE in photon migration have been carried out in symmetrical geometries such as the infinite medium, the semi-infinite medium or the semi-infinite medium with a high-absorbent inclusion.

In order to solve the DE, appropriate boundary conditions have to be declared. The most general boundary condition is the *Partial Current Boundary Condition* (PCBC):

$$\Phi(\boldsymbol{r},t) + 2AD\nabla\Phi(\boldsymbol{r},t)\cdot\hat{\boldsymbol{n}} = 0 \qquad \boldsymbol{r}\in\partial V \tag{49}$$

Where A is a coefficient depending on the refractive index and is due to Fresnel reflection [Contini et al. (1997); Martelli et al. (2010)]. In practical applications, though, the most commonly applied boundary conditions are the *Extrapolated Boundary Condition* (EBC) and the *Zero Boundary Condition* (ZBC):

$$\Phi(\boldsymbol{r},t) = 0 \qquad \boldsymbol{r}\in\partial V_{ext} \tag{50}$$

$$\Phi(\boldsymbol{r},t) = 0 \qquad \boldsymbol{r}\in\partial V \tag{51}$$

Where ∂V_{ext} is a surface distant $2AD$ from the boundary (extrapolated surface).

CW, TR and FD solutions for simple geometries have been calculated [Martelli et al. (2010)].

2.3.4 FD-NIRS

Frequency Domain Near InfraRed Spectroscopy (FD-NIRS) makes use of intensity modulated laser light (typically at radio frequencies), injecting it into the sample. The remitted wave is demodulated to obtain amplitude and phase as a function of the modulation frequency. The tissue acts like a low-pass filter: the amplitude is a decreasing function of the frequency and the phase typically increases. The analytical expressions for amplitude and phase can be obtained by a Fourier transform of the TR theoretical expression. Estimation of optical properties can thus be performed using the photon migration theory (see Fig. 4).

Some commercial device using frequency domain techniques is available and measurements and basic research often used this approach to study biological tissues oxygenation [D'Arceuil et al. (2005); Fantini et al. (1995)].

2.3.5 TR-NIRS

In section 2.2 a way to measure oxygenated and deoxygenated hemoglobin concentrations has been described. Using absorption spectroscopy techniques it is possible to investigate *in vivo* the oxygenation status of the superficial tissues and in particular of the cortical areas of the brain. Thus, CW-NIRS is a useful non-invasive technique for functional neuroimaging. As previously seen, the issue underlying Near InfraRed Spectroscopy is scattering. The way CW-NIRS deals with scattering is to perform a basal measurement and then to refer all

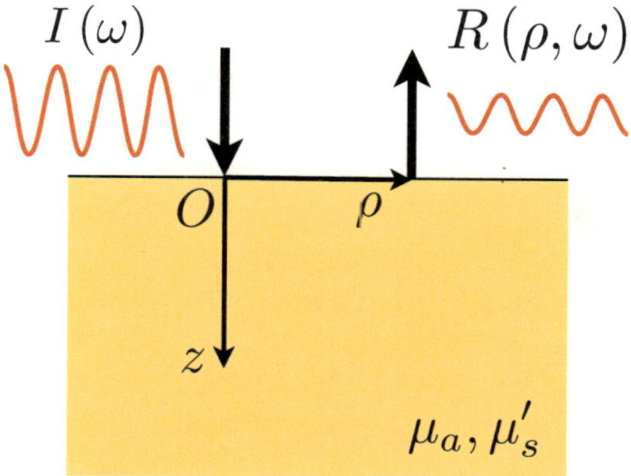

Fig. 4. Scheme of reflection geometry FD-NIRS measurement. Intensity modulated light $I(\omega)$ travels in the medium and part of it can be collected by a detector at a source-detector distance ρ. Amplitude and phase of the collected light $R(\rho,\omega)$ depend on μ_a and μ_s'.

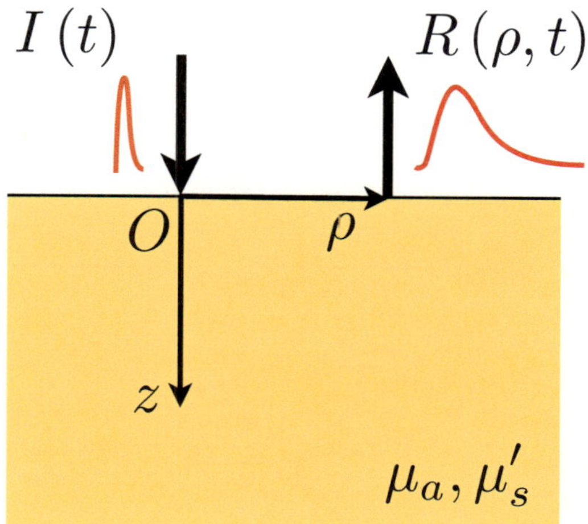

Fig. 5. Scheme of reflection geometry TD-NIRS measurement. Injected light travels in the medium and part of it can be collected by a detector at a source-detector distance ρ. Knowing the temporal shape of the injected light $I(t)$, the temporal shape of the collected light $R(\rho,t)$ depends on μ_a and μ_s'.

successive data to the baseline values, making the assumption that scattering is constant in time. This makes concentration variations the only possible obtainable data.

In section 2.3.1 the physical model for radiation propagation inside tissues has been introduced. It will be now shown how RTE gives a practically useful tool to perform a kind of measurement in which absolute hemoglobin concentrations values can be sampled.

In many biological applications the semi-infinite geometry is assumed and light intensity measurement are conducted in reflectance geometry (see Fig. 5). In this case the Green function of the Diffusion Equation with the Extrapolated Boundary Condition, expressed as the detected power per unit area (usually known as *reflectance* R), takes the form:

$$R(\rho,t) = \frac{1}{2(4\pi D v)^{3/2} t^{5/2}} e^{-\frac{\rho^2}{4Dvt}} e^{-\mu_a v t} \left[z_0 e^{-\frac{z_0^2}{4Dvt}} - z_p e^{-\frac{z_p^2}{4Dvt}} \right] \quad (52)$$

Where ρ is the source-detector distance, $z_0 = \frac{1}{\mu_s'}$, $z_p = z_0 + 2z_e$ and $z_e = 2AD$.

Looking at the the Green function of the diffusion equation it is possible to notice that absorption and scattering contributes are naturally separated in the model. Plotting these solutions for different values of the absorption coefficient and of the scattering coefficient evidence this property (see Fig. 6). This technique based on the injection of light with a known temporal shape (typical a pulse-like shape) and the estimation of the optical properties from the emitted light temporal shape is called *Time-Resolved Near InfraRed Spectroscopy* (TR-NIRS).

The light is collected by means of photomultipliers tubes (PMT) or avalanche photodiodes (APD) usually in Time Correlated Single Photon Counting (TCSPC) regime. Detailed descriptions of the way light is collected by light detectors is given in [Donati (1998)] and of TCSPC is given in [O'Connor & Phillips (1984)] and [Becker (2005)].

Estimation of the optical properties can be performed from all the analytical expressions for the TR response of a diffusive medium. Absorption and scattering coefficients can be computed by means of an inversion algorithm [Press et al. (1992)]. The instrumental response function (IRF) due to temporal dispersion in fiber, temporal jitter of detectors and finite pulse width of light sources has to be taken into account. Due to the linearity and time-invariance of the transport problem, the detected response is the convolution between the IRF and the theoretical response of the medium. Thus, a Levenberg-Marquardt non-linear minimization between experimental data and theoretical curve convoluted with the IRF is generally performed.

An estimation of the optical properties of a diffusive medium can be also performed by means of Monte Carlo simulations. A certain number of simulations are needed, then by using the scaling properties of the RTE it is possible to implement a fast search of the correct simulation [Pifferi et al. (1998)]. These two method enable an absolute estimation of optical properties.

A simple estimation of the variation of the absorption coefficient can be easily performed if only absorption changes are assumed (and usually are). If we collect at different times two reflectance curves $R_0(\rho,t)$ and $R_1(\rho,t)$, it is straightforward that:

$$\Delta\mu_a = -\frac{1}{vt} \ln\left(\frac{R_1(\rho,t)}{R_0(\rho,t)}\right) \quad (53)$$

In principle TR techniques provides a richer insight than CW to the problem of non-invasively probing of a diffusive medium. These approaches can discriminate between absorption and scattering contributions and derive absolute values for the hemodynamic parameters [Patterson et al. (1989)]. This however can be obtained only in simple geometries like the infinite or the semi-infinite homogeneous models. In a real heterogeneous medium like the human tissues and in particular the human head it is easier to derive changes with respect to a baseline or effective average parameters rather than absolute values. Advanced time-resolved perturbation models for more complicated geometries, like multi-layered media, have been derived in the last years, but they would require the use of a priori information (e.g., the

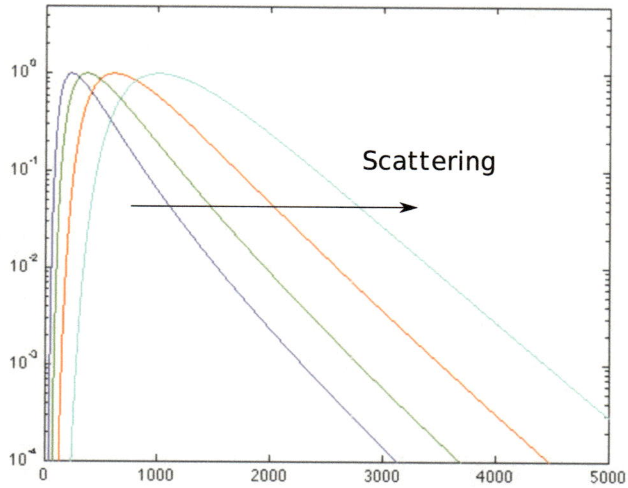

(a) Dependance from scattering ($\mu_a = 0.09$ cm^{-1}, $\mu_s' = 4, 8, 16, 32$ cm^{-1}).

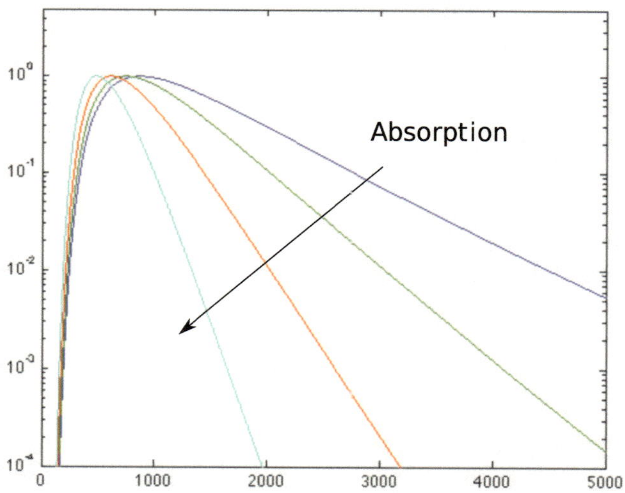

(b) Dependance from absorption ($\mu_a = 0.04, 0.08, 0.16, 0.32$ cm^{-1}, $\mu_s' = 20$ cm^{-1}).

Fig. 6. Normalized reflectance from the semi-infinite model, with source-detector distance ρ=2 cm. Reflectance vs. time is plotted in semi-logarithmic scale.

anatomy of the head as provided by a MRI scan) for their practical and effective use [Martelli et al. (2005)].

The actual potentiality of time-resolved techniques relies on an easier approach to the problem of depth sensitivity. As mentioned before, to enhance depth sensitivity, CW systems use large source-detector distance and multi-distance approaches. Conversely, depth sensitivity in TR-NIRS can be intrinsic in the measured reflectance curve having information on the time of flight of the photons in tissues.

Near InfraRed Spectroscopy applications to the brain spread from rehabilitation monitoring to neural plasticity studies, from localization of cortical activation in motor or cognitive tasks to stroke diagnosis, and more. Motor tasks such as finger tapping or hand grasping are easy to perform and hundreds of studies have been published [Torricelli et al. (2007)]. Cognitive tasks present more difficulties in activation interpretation, nevertheless a number of study is available in literature [Bandettini et al. (1997); Butti et al. (2009); Heekeren et al. (1997)]. Fig. 7 and Fig. 8 show two examples of TR-NIRS data.

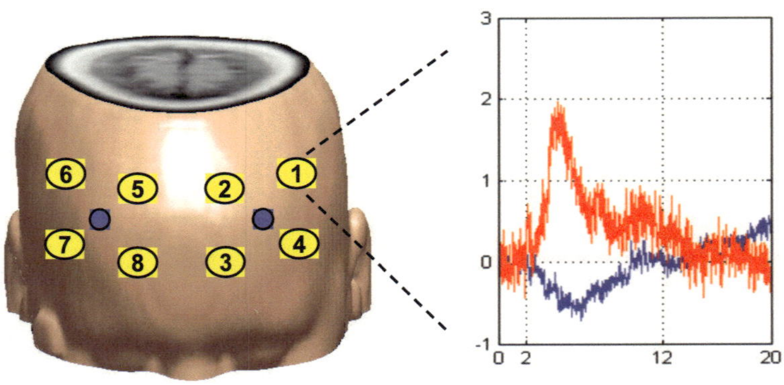

Fig. 7. Δ [Hb] (blue) and Δ [HbO_2] (red) concentrations (in arbitrary units) vs. time (in minutes) collected from the frontal area of the brain during a cognitive task of sustained attention. Vertical lines indicated the beginning and the end of the task. The average concentration value for the first two minutes block was used as baseline and then subtracted to all data.

3. Diffuse Optical Tomography (DOT)

Since the very beginning of the history of NIRS, many efforts have been made to improve space resolution and data accuracy. Near InfraRed Spectroscopy provides functional information about the oxygenation status of the explored tissues, but a single source-detector pair is only able to probe a small underlying area. In this section a way to perform functional neuroimaging starting form NIRS data will be introduced. Production of two dimensional maps, often called *topography*, by linear interpolation of NIRS data was the first application to be investigated. This imaging technique is usually called *Diffuse Optical Imaging* (DOI) and, adding depth sensitivity, is known as *Diffuse Optical Tomography* (DOT).

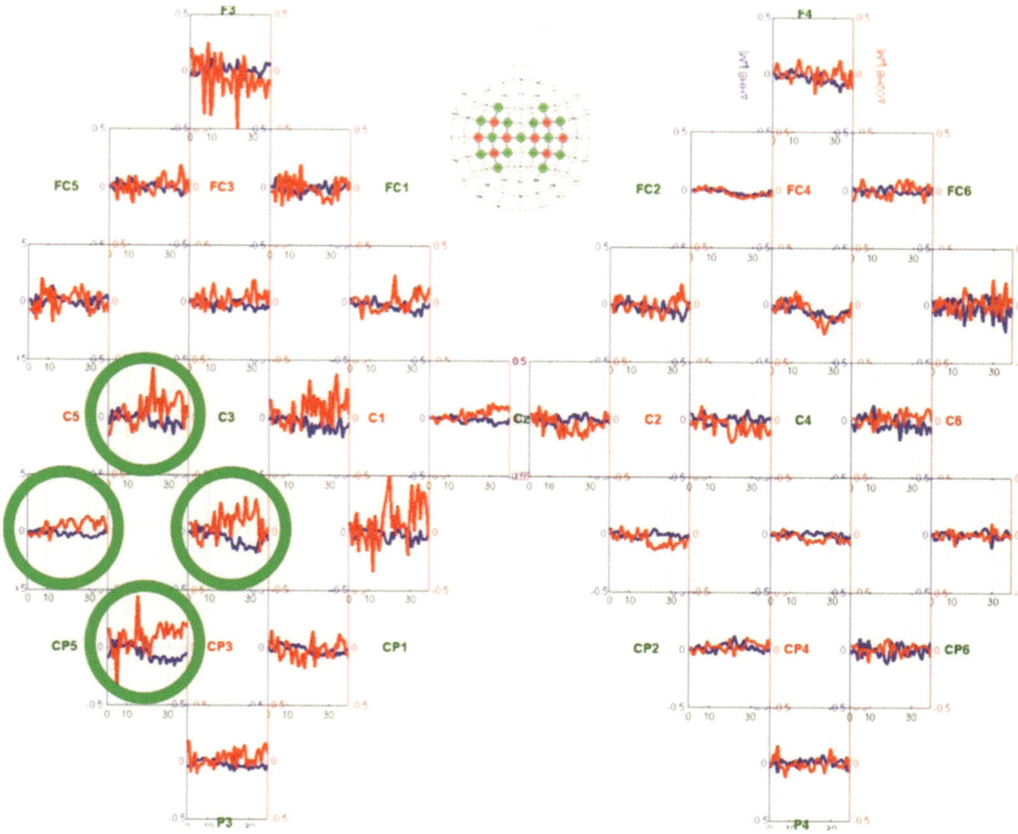

Fig. 8. Oxyhemoglobin (in red) and deoxyhemoglobin (in blue) concentrations for a hand grasping task. Single-subject, right hand movement, average of 10 repetitions, TR-NIRS device, contrast enhanced for the deep layers (see section 3.1).

To properly investigate a large area (larger than the common source-detector distance, that is 1-4 cm) a multi-channel approach is needed. The starting point is the arrangement of a number of sources and detectors to cover the area of interest and the management of the source-detector pairs. Depending on the physical dimensions of the area even a huge number could be arranged. No theoretical limitations on the number of optodes exists, however, actual technology features instrumentations with up to 32 sources and 32 detectors (CW) and 16 sources and 16 detection channels (TR). Shining NIR light on the skin and collecting the back-scattered light in a reflectance geometry from multiple points easily allows to draw a map of the hemoglobin concentrations around the area of interest. Spatial resolution is poor (depending on source-detector distances) and a little depth sensitivity (associated to the overlapping measurements in CW or intrinsic in TR) is obtained.

Concentrations time series can be plotted vs time or a spatial map can be built (see Fig. 9). A movie-like map can be obtained if each frame corresponds to a time sample. More often, especially in books and publications, averaged concentrations data over time intervals are used to obtain maps relative to a time block of seconds or minutes, just as the example in Fig 9.

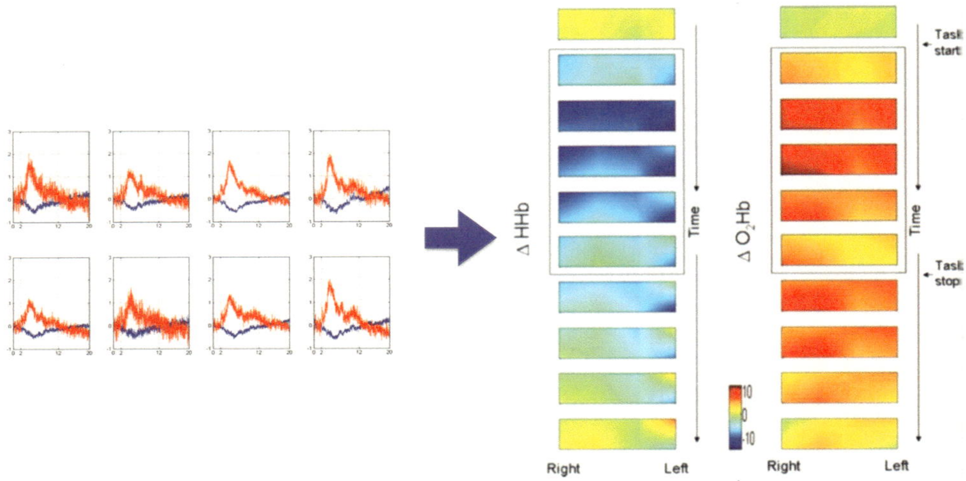

Fig. 9. The concentration time series can be visualized as spatial map. Each time sample belongs to an average position between the associated source-detector pair. The map is built by linear interpolation with the neighboring points concentration values.

More complicated ways to image optical data have been developed. Using MRI anatomical information and using suitable values for the average optical properties of the tissues a inverse problem can be established. Localized alterations of the optical properties, corresponding to a increased absorption and related to the hemodynamic responses of neural activations, can be put in correspondence with cortical features and a better localization of brain activations can be performed.

DOT systems can consist of little more than a probe with fiber-optic sources and detectors, a piece of dedicated hardware about the size of a small suitcase and a laptop computer. Systems can be much larger, depending primarily on the type of laser source and detectors employed, but the approach generally offers a degree of portability unobtainable with many other modalities. For this reason, looking into the future, DOT may be ideally suited for clinical applications such as bedside monitoring of cerebral oxygenation.

3.1 Time resolved DOT

A fundamental point in NIRS measurements, whatever technique we are using, is the ability to separate systemic hemodynamic changes occurring in the superficial tissues, such as the skin, from functional hemodynamic changes related to brain activations. In order to reach this goal is fundamental to discuss NIRS depth sensitivity. Depth sensitivity is not intrinsic in CW- and TR-NIRS measurements, but can be achieved using proper optodes configurations or using time of flight information. Multi-distance source-detector approaches, both with CW [Saager & Berger (2005)] and with TR [Liebert et al. (2004)] techniques, have been proposed to improve depth selectivity and sensitivity. Single-distance approaches have also been discussed [Selb et al. (2005); Steinbrink et al. (2001)]. Contini et al. (2007) proposed a different approach to add depth information to the tissue probing problem, based on time-domain contrast functions. Wabnitz et al. (2008) discussed a method for depth selectivity based on time windows and moments of time-of-flight distributions for TD-NIRS.

Time-resolved curves statistically contain information about tissues which light photons pass through. Photons reaching the detector at early times surely have been back-scattered from the superficial tissues and thus can bring information about the superficial layers only. Photons reaching the detector at late times have travelled inside the tissues for a longer time and statistically could have probed deeper layers and carry information about them. We usually refer to them as *early photons* and *late photons*.

A simple approach to the depth probing problem could be to develop a contrast function, considering just two domains: superficial layers and deep layers.

In order to develop models to discriminate between the variations of the absorption coefficient in the superficial layers ($\Delta\mu_a^{UP}$) and of the variation of the absorption coefficient in deep layers ($\Delta\mu_a^{DOWN}$), the quantity time-dependent photon path length, usually called Mean time-dependent Path Length (MPL) is introduced [Steinbrink et al. (2001)]. As its own name suggests, MPL is the average length of the path travelled by photons in a specific layer and can be calculated from the mean time of flight of the photons.

The reflectance curve is divided into time intervals τ, called *time gates* (TG), and the total counts (usually referred as *intensity*) are calculated for each time gate[4].

Being $I_0(t)$ the intensity for the non-absorbent medium, $L^{UP}(t)$ and $L^{DOWN}(t)$ the mean time-dependent path lengths in the superficial layers and in the deep layers, respectively, the expression for the intensity $I(t)$ in a general absorbent medium can be expressed as:

$$I(t) = I_0(t)\, e^{-\left(\Delta\mu_a^{UP} L^{UP}(t) + \Delta\mu_a^{DOWN} L^{DOWN}(t)\right)} \tag{54}$$

In the simplest case, it is possible to think that early photons carry information only about the superficial layers and that late photons are not affected by a superficial inhomogeneity, and carry information only about the deep layers. Thus, we can write for the absorption coefficient changes:

$$\Delta\mu_a^{UP} = -\frac{1}{L^{UP}(\tau_e)} \ln\left(\frac{I(\tau_e)}{I_0(\tau_e)}\right) \tag{55}$$

$$\Delta\mu_a^{DOWN} = -\frac{1}{L^{DOWN}(\tau_l)} \ln\left(\frac{I(\tau_l)}{I_0(\tau_l)}\right) \tag{56}$$

where τ_e is the mean time of flight of photons in a early time gate and τ_l is the mean time of flight for photons in a late time gate. Despite giving a general idea about how to obtain information about contributes of different layers, this model is pretty rough, indeed. The hypothesis of late photons not affected by superficial layers has to be rejected and more complicated expressions are often necessary to perform depth selection [Contini (2007)]. It can be proved that late photons carry both information about superficial and deep layers and that superficial layer absorption variations affect the deep layers absorption estimation. The subtraction of the superficial contribute is thus necessary in the estimation of $\Delta\mu_a^{DOWN}$. Such

[4] The total counts are the time integral of the reflectance curve: $I_{gate}(t) = \int_{t_{in}}^{t_{fin}} R(t)\, dt$

a subtraction can be performed as follow:

$$\Delta\mu_a^{UP} = -\frac{1}{L^{UP}(\tau_e)} \ln\left(\frac{I(\tau_e)}{I_0(\tau_e)}\right) \tag{57}$$

$$\Delta\mu_a^{DOWN} = -\frac{1}{L^{DOWN}(\tau_l)} \ln\left(1 + \frac{I(\tau_l)}{I_0(\tau_l)} - \frac{I(\tau_e)}{I_0(\tau_e)}\right) \tag{58}$$

Oxy- and deoxy-hemoglobin concentrations for the upper layer and the lower layer can be easily obtained via Lambert-Beer law, from the estimated $\Delta\mu_a$. An example of application of this stratigraphic model is shown in Fig. 10, where data where collected during a Valsalva maneuver, that forces an increase of the systemic blood volume, resulting in an increase of both oxyhemoglobin and deoxyhemoglobin concentrations in the superficial layers of the skin.

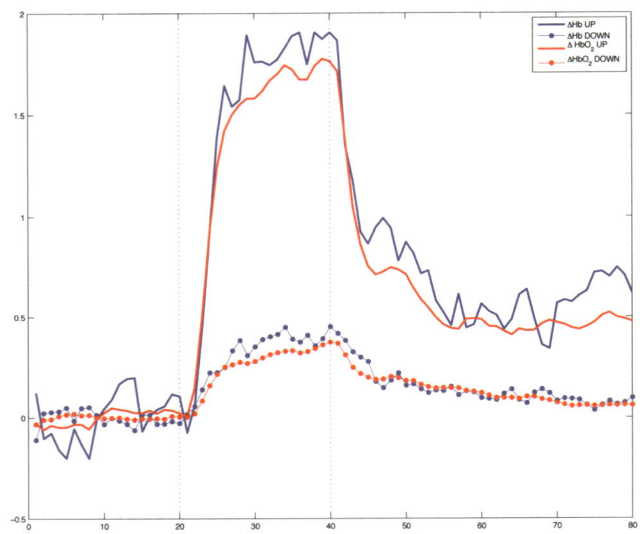

Fig. 10. Estimated ΔHbO_2 and ΔHb in the superficial layer (UP, continuous line) and in the brain (DOWN, dotted line) during the Valsalva maneuver without normalization. The two vertical dashed lines indicate the beginning and the end of the task period, respectively. During the Valsalva maneuver the sistemic blood volume dramatically increases, while the local blood volume in the brain is less affected by the maneuver effects. A proper depth selectivity remarks this differences.

3.2 Multimodality approach

Recently a great interest in multimodality approaches has grown. Merging the advantages of different imaging and functional techniques, such as co-registration of NIRS with MRI [Merritt et al. (2002)], blood flow monitors, fMRI [Torricelli et al. (2007)] and PET, gives the possibility to build anatomo-functional images and movies to largely improve information visualization.

Moreover, the comparison with standard clinical techniques such EEG or MEG can lead to a clinical standardization of the NIRS signal and push Near InfraRed Spectroscopy towards a regular clinical use [*nEUROPt Project* (2008-2012)].

Using anatomical magnetic resonance priors to perform MRI-guided optical reconstruction dramatically improves the spatial resolution of the diffuse optical tomography techniques [Boas & Dale (2005)]. Simulations of light propagation are run into the MRI head volume, using Monte Carlo statistical methods such as Fang & Boas (2009), and then the cortical activation profile is obtained solving an inverse problem. For a more detailed description of it see Caffini et al. (2011).

In the event of an unavailability of the subject-specific anatomy the efficient use of an MRI anatomical atlas has been demonstrated [Caffini et al. (2010)]. Fig. 11 reports an atlas reconstruction of a cortical activation during a visual protocol of pattern reversal checkerboard.

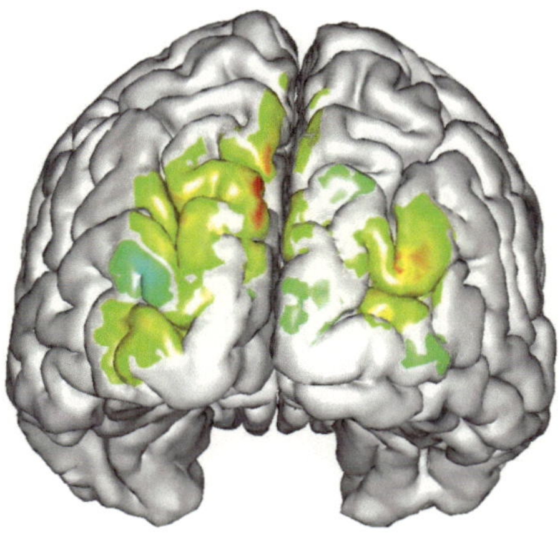

Fig. 11. Atlas map visualization of an MRI-guided optical reconstruction of the brain activation in the visual cortex (the brain is seen from the back), during a pattern reversal checkerboard protocol.

4. Conclusions

Near InfraRed Spectroscopy applied *in vivo* to cortical tissues has been widely investigated through the last two decades and big steps have been done.

From the technical point of view, the laser technology, and in particular the introduction of semiconductor laser diodes, has helped to fabricate compact and clinical instrumentations. Moreover, the improvements in light detectors has permitted to develop accurate devices, for example, in the time-resolved technology, the red-extended photocathodes well increased the quantum efficiency in the near red region.

Nevertheless, a lot more has to be done. Pulsed lasers sources are getting better and better, especially concerning time stability and output power. Photomultiplier tubes is an efficient and well established technology, but, in NIRS application, suffers the need of high voltage supplies and the necessity to work in a dark environment, to avoid background light. Single Photon Avalanche Diodes (SPAD) are the available technology that best fits the needs of Near InfraRed Spectroscopy. Actual work is to integrate SPADs into NIRS setups by means of increased light sensitive area and better quantum efficiency in the near red spectrum. For more information about SPAD detectors see [Cova et al. (2010)].

An interesting future perspective, is the so-called null-distance measurement setup, that is the possibility to collect light from the very same point of injection. Only time resolved techniques allow this possibility and a few successful efforts have been made in this direction [Pifferi et al. (2008)].

From the medical point of view, hundreds of physiological studies and psychological tasks have been carried out and a massive literature is available on the subject. For these reason, a larger clinical use of non-invasive optical imaging in the next years is expected. In particular, we expect time resolved NIRS to be the best candidate for this purpose. The four-year nEUROPt Project [*nEUROPt Project* (2008-2012)], financed by the European Union under The Seventh Framework Programme for research and technological development (FP7) for the period 2008-2011, and coordinated by the Authors, aims at the development and clinical validation of advanced non-invasive optical methodologies for in-vivo diagnosis, monitoring, and prognosis of major neurological diseases (stroke, epilepsy, ischemia), based on diffuse optical imaging by pulsed near infrared light. The consortium plans major developments in technology and data analysis that will enhance TD-NIRS with respect to spatial resolution, sensitivity, robustness of quantification as well as performance of related instruments in clinical diagnosis and monitoring. A strong clinical basis is being produced and the diagnostic value of TD-NIRS applications to brain study will be assessed, by putting using standard methodologies (such EEG) and new optical methods side by side, in a co-registration setup. The potential commercialization of TD-NIRS systems will be then evaluated by European system manufacturers.

5. Acknowledgements

We wish to acknowledge partial support from the EC's Seventh Framework Programme (FP7/ 2007 - 2013) under grant 201076.

6. References

Arridge, S. R. (1995). Photon-measurement density functions. part i: Analytical forms, *Appl. Opt.* 34(31): 7395–7409.
URL: *http://ao.osa.org/abstract.cfm?URI=ao-34-31-7395*

Arridge, S. R. (1999). Optical tomography in medical imaging, *Inverse Problems* 15(2): R41–R93.
URL: *http://stacks.iop.org/0266-5611/15/R41*

Arridge, S. R., Dehghani, H., Schweiger, M. & Okada, E. (2000). The finite element model for the propagation of light in scattering media: A direct method for domains with nonscattering regions, *Medical Physics* 27(1): 252–264.
URL: *http://link.aip.org/link/?MPH/27/252/1*

Arridge, S. R. & Hebden, J. C. (1997). Optical imaging in medicine: Ii. modelling and reconstruction, *Physics in Medicine and Biology* 42(5): 841–853.
URL: *http://stacks.iop.org/0031-9155/42/841*

Arridge, S. R. & Schweiger, M. (1995). Photon-measurement density functions. part 2: Finite-element-method calculations, *Appl. Opt.* 34(34): 8026–8037.
URL: *http://ao.osa.org/abstract.cfm?URI=ao-34-34-8026*

Arridge, S. R., Schweiger, M., Hiraoka, M. & Delpy, D. T. (1993). A finite element approach for modeling photon transport in tissue, *Medical Physics* 20(2): 299–309.
URL: *http://link.aip.org/link/?MPH/20/299/1*

Bandettini, P., Kwong, K., Davis, T., Tootell, R., Wong, E., Fox, P., Belliveau, J., Weisskoff, R. & Rosen, B. (1997). Characterization of cerebral blood oxygenation and flow changes during prolonged brain activation, *Human Brain Mapping* 5(2): 93–109.

Becker, W. (2005). *Advanced Time-Correlated Single Photon Counting Techniques*, Springer.

Boas, D. A. (1996). *Diffuse Photon Probes of Structural and Dynamical Properties of Turbid Media: Theory and Biomedical Applications*, PhD thesis, University of Pennsylvania.

Boas, D. A. & Dale, A. M. (2005). Simulation study of magnetic resonance imaging-guided cortically constrained diffuse optical tomography of human brain function, *Appl. Opt.* 44(10): 1957–1968.
URL: *http://ao.osa.org/abstract.cfm?URI=ao-44-10-1957*

Boas, D. A., Dale, A. M. & Franceschini, M. A. (2004). Diffuse optical imaging of brain activation: approaches to optimizing image sensitivity, resolution, and accuracy, *NeuroImage* 23(Supplement 1): S275 – S288. Mathematics in Brain Imaging.

Boas, D., Culver, J., Stott, J. & Dunn, A. (2002). Three dimensional monte carlo code for photon migration through complex heterogeneous media including the adult human head, *Opt. Express* 10(3): 159–170.
URL: *http://www.opticsexpress.org/abstract.cfm?URI=oe-10-3-159*

Butti, M., Contini, D., Molteni, E., Caffini, M., Spinelli, L., Baselli, G., Bianchi, A. M., Cerutti, S., Cubeddu, R. & Torricelli, A. (2009). Effect of prolonged stimulation on cerebral hemodynamic: A time-resolved fnirs study, *Medical Physics* 36(9): 4103–4114.
URL: *http://link.aip.org/link/?MPH/36/4103/1*

Caffini, M., Torricelli, A., Cubeddu, R., Custo, A., Dubb, J. & Boas, D. A. (2010). Validating an Anatomical Brain Atlas for Analyzing NIRS Measurements of Brain Activation, *Biomedical Optics*, Optical Society of America, p. JMA87.
URL: *http://www.opticsinfobase.org/abstract.cfm?URI=BIOMED-2010-JMA87*

Caffini, M., Zucchelli, L., Contini, D., Cubeddu, R., Spinelli, L., Boas, D. & Torricelli, A. (2011). Anatomical brain atlas for nirs measurements of brain activation, *Proc. SPIE* 8088(1): 808809.

Contini, D. (2007). *Time-resolved functional Near Infrared Spectroscopy for Neuroscience*, PhD thesis, Politecnico di Milano.

Contini, D., Martelli, F. & Zaccanti, G. (1997). Photon migration through a turbid slab described by a model based on diffusion approximation. i. theory, *Appl. Opt.* 36(19): 4587–4599.
URL: *http://ao.osa.org/abstract.cfm?URI=ao-36-19-4587*

Contini, D., Spinelli, L., Torricelli, A., Pifferi, A. & Cubeddu, R. (2007). Novel method for depth-resolved brain functional imaging by time-domain nirs, *Diffuse Optical Imaging of Tissue*, Optical Society of America, p. 6629.

Cova, S., Ghioni, M., Zappa, F., Gulinatti, A., Rech, I. & Tosi, A. (2010). Single photon counting detectors in action: Retrospect and prospect, *2010 23rd Annual Meeting of the IEEE Photonics Society, PHOTINICS 2010*, pp. 177–178.
URL: *www.scopus.com*

D'Arceuil, H. E., Hotakainen, M. P., Liu, C., Themelis, G., de Crespigny, A. J. & Franceschini, M. A. (2005). Near-infrared frequency-domain optical spectroscopy and magnetic resonance imaging: a combined approach to studying cerebral maturation in neonatal rabbits, *Journal of Biomedical Optics* 10(1).

Donati, S. (1998). *Fotorivelatori*, 2a edizione edn, AEI.

Fang, Q. & Boas, D. A. (2009). Monte carlo simulation of photon migration in 3d turbid media accelerated by graphics processing units, *Optics Express* 17(22): 20178–20190.
URL: *http://www.opticsexpress.org/abstract.cfm?URI=oe-17-22-20178*

Fantini, S., Franceschini, M.-A., Maier, J. S., Walker, S. A., Barbieri, B. B. & Gratton, E. (1995). Frequency-domain multichannel optical detector for noninvasive tissue spectroscopy and oximetry, *Optical Engineering* 34(1): 32–42.
URL: *http://link.aip.org/link/?JOE/34/32/1*

Feynman, R. P., Leighton, R. B. & Sands, M. (1964). *The Feynman Lectures on Physics including Feynman's Tips on Physics: The Definitive and Extended Edition*, Addison-Wesley.

Heekeren, H. R., Obrig, H., Wenzel, R., Eberle, K., Ruben, J., Villringer, K., Kurth, R. & Villringer, A. (1997). Cerebral haemoglobin oxygenation during sustained visual stimulation – a near–infrared spectroscopy study, *Philosophical Transactions of the Royal Society of London. Series B: Biological Sciences* 352(1354): 743–750.
URL: *http://rstb.royalsocietypublishing.org/content/352/1354/743.abstract*

Ishimaru, A. (1978). *Wave Propagation and Scattering in Random Media*, Academic Press.

Jackson, J. D. (1999). *Classical Electrodynamics*, 3rd edn, Wiley.

Liebert, A., Wabnitz, H., Steinbrink, J., Obrig, H., Möller, M., Macdonald, R., Villringer, A. & Rinneberg, H. (2004). Time-resolved multidistance near-infrared spectroscopy of the adult head: Intracerebral and extracerebral absorption changes from moments of distribution of times of flight of photons, *Appl. Opt.* 43(15): 3037–3047.
URL: *http://ao.osa.org/abstract.cfm?URI=ao-43-15-3037*

Martelli, F., Bianco, S. D., Ismaelli, A. & Zaccanti, G. (2010). *Photon Migration Through Diffusive Media: Theory, Solutions and Software*, SPIE Press.

Martelli, F., Bianco, S. D. & Zaccanti, G. (2005). Perturbation model for light propagation through diffusive layered media, *Physics in Medicine and Biology* 50(9): 2159–2166.
URL: *http://stacks.iop.org/0031-9155/50/2159*

Merritt, S., Bevilacqua, F., Durkin, A. J., Cuccia, D. J., Lanning, R. & Tromberg, B. J. (2002). Near-infrared spectroscopy and mri co-registration of tumor tissue physiology, *Biomedical Topical Meeting*, Optical Society of America, p. SuE1.
URL: *http://www.opticsinfobase.org/abstract.cfm?URI=BIO-2002-SuE1*

Mie, G. (1908). Beiträge zur optik trüber medien, speziell kolloidaler metallösungen, *Annalen der Physik* 330(3): 377–445.
URL: *http://dx.doi.org/10.1002/andp.19083300302*

nEUROPt Project (2008-2012).
URL: *www.neuropt.eu*

O'Connor, D. V. & Phillips, D. (1984). *Time correlated single photon counting*, Academic Press.

Patterson, M. S., Chance, B. & Wilson, B. C. (1989). Time resolved reflectance and transmittance for the non-invasive measurement of tissue optical properties, *Appl. Opt.* 28(12): 2331–2336.
URL: *http://ao.osa.org/abstract.cfm?URI=ao-28-12-2331*

Pifferi, A., Taroni, P., Valentini, G. & Andersson-Engels, S. (1998). Real-time method for fitting time-resolved reflectance and transmittance measurements with a monte carlo model, *Appl. Opt.* 37(13): 2774–2780.
URL: *http://ao.osa.org/abstract.cfm?URI=ao-37-13-2774*

Pifferi, A., Torricelli, A., Spinelli, L., Contini, D., Cubeddu, R., Martelli, F., Zaccanti, G., Tosi, A., Mora, A. D., Zappa, F. & Cova, S. (2008). Time-resolved functional near-infrared spectroscopy at null source-detector separation, *Biomedical Optics*, Optical Society of America, p. BWC6.
URL: *http://www.opticsinfobase.org/abstract.cfm?URI=BIOMED-2008-BWC6*

Press, W. H., Teukolsky, S. A., Vetterling, W. T. & Flannery, B. P. (1992). *Numerical Recipes in C - The Art of Scientific Computing*, Cambridge University Press.

Rutherford, E. (1911). The scattering of alpha and beta particles by matter and the structure of the atom, *Philosophical Magazine Series 6* 21(125): 669–688.

Saager, R. B. & Berger, A. J. (2005). Direct characterization and removal of interfering absorption trends in two-layer turbid media, *J. Opt. Soc. Am. A* 22(9): 1874–1882.
URL: *http://josaa.osa.org/abstract.cfm?URI=josaa-22-9-1874*

Sanchez, R. & McCormick, N. J. (1982). A review of neutron transport approximations, *Nuclear Science and Engineering* 80(4): 481–535.

Sassaroli, A. & Fantini, S. (2004). Comment on the modified beer-lambert law for scattering media, *Physics in Medicine and Biology* 49(14): N255–N257.
URL: *http://stacks.iop.org/0031-9155/49/N255*

Selb, J., Stott, J. J., Franceschini, M. A., Sorensen, A. G. & Boas, D. A. (2005). Improved sensitivity to cerebral hemodynamics during brain activation with a time-gated optical system: analytical model and experimental validation, *Journal of Biomedical Optics* 10(1): 011013.
URL: *http://link.aip.org/link/?JBO/10/011013/1*

Steinbrink, J., Wabnitz, H., Obrig, H., Villringer, A. & Rinneberg, H. (2001). Determining changes in nir absorption using a layered model of the human head, *Physics in Medicine and Biology* 46(3): 879–896.
URL: *http://stacks.iop.org/0031-9155/46/879*

Strangman, G., Boas, D. A. & Sutton, J. P. (2002). Non-invasive neuroimaging using near-infrared light, *Society of Biological Psychiatry* 52: 679–693.

Torricelli, A., Contini, D., Pifferi, A., Spinelli, L., Cubeddu, R., Nocetti, L., Manginelli, A.-A. & Baraldi, P. (2007). Simultaneous acquisition of time-domain fnirs and fmri during motor activity, *Proc. SPIE* 6631(1): 66310A.
URL: *http://dx.doi.org/doi/10.1117/12.727699*

Tsuchiya, Y. (2001). Photon path distribution and optical responses of turbid media: theoretical analysis based on the microscopic beer-lambert law, *Physics in Medicine and Biology* 46(8): 2067–2084.
URL: *http://stacks.iop.org/0031-9155/46/2067*

Wabnitz, H., Liebert, A., Contini, D., Spinelli, L. & Torricelli, A. (2008). Depth selectivity in time-domain optical brain imaging based on time windows and moments of time-of-flight distributions, *Biomedical Optics*, Optical Society of America, p. BMD9. URL: *http://www.opticsinfobase.org/abstract.cfm?URI=BIOMED-2008-BMD9*

Wolf, M., Ferrari, M. & Quaresima, V. (2007). Progress of near-infrared spectroscopy and topography for brain and muscle clinical applications, *Journal of Biomedical Optics* 12(6): 062104.
URL: *http://link.aip.org/link/?JBO/12/062104/1*

Zege, E. P., Ivanov, A. I. & Katsev, I. L. (1991). *Image Transfer through a Scattering Medium*, Springer-Verlag.

5

Intraoperative Human Functional Brain Mapping Using Optical Intrinsic Signal Imaging

Sameer A. Sheth, Vijay Yanamadala and Emad N. Eskandar
Department of Neurosurgery, Massachusetts General Hospital, Harvard Medical School, Boston, USA

1. Introduction

Functional brain mapping strives to describe the brain's organization as a mosaic of distinct regions, each of which subserves a particular function. Advances in our understanding of functional brain organization over the past decades have been propelled by the availability of increasingly sophisticated methods for assessing various aspects of neuronal activity *in vivo*. These methods can be broadly categorized as "direct" or "indirect" measures of neuronal activity (Figure 1). Direct techniques measure changes in electromagnetic fields resulting from neuronal action potentials and synaptic activity. Indirect techniques measure changes in other tissue properties that are related to neural activity. This distinction does not imply the superiority of direct over indirect techniques. Certain disadvantages of direct measures were the very motivation for the development of indirect measures. Indeed, the most widely used functional brain imaging modality currently is functional magnetic resonance imaging (fMRI), an indirect technique. A subset of indirect techniques are based on changes in blood flow subsequent to and produced by neural activity. These perfusion-dependent functional brain imaging techniques include fMRI, positron emission tomography (PET), and others. Although they are among the most commonly used methods for investigating brain function, they rely on vascular responses that are not completely understood. In this chapter, we will focus on indirect measures of brain activity, emphasizing the technique of optical intrinsic signal imaging (OISI). We discuss the physical basis of perfusion imaging and OISI, animal and human studies of OISI to date, and its potential as a powerful intraoperative functional brain mapping tool.

2. Perfusion-based functional brain imaging

In framing OISI, we first discuss the broad category of perfusion-based imaging techniques to which it belongs. Perfusion-based brain imaging techniques measure physiological events linked to neuronal activity, such as changes in metabolism or blood flow, and include positron emission tomography (PET), functional magnetic resonance imaging (fMRI), and OISI. These techniques do not measure neuronal activity *per se*; rather, they measure surrogate metabolic and vascular markers of activity. In essence, hemodynamic responses provide a map of neuronal activity spatially and temporally broadened by passage through a vascular filter. Despite their indirect nature, however, perfusion-based brain imaging techniques are among the most commonly used, and have provided numerous important clinical and basic research insights.

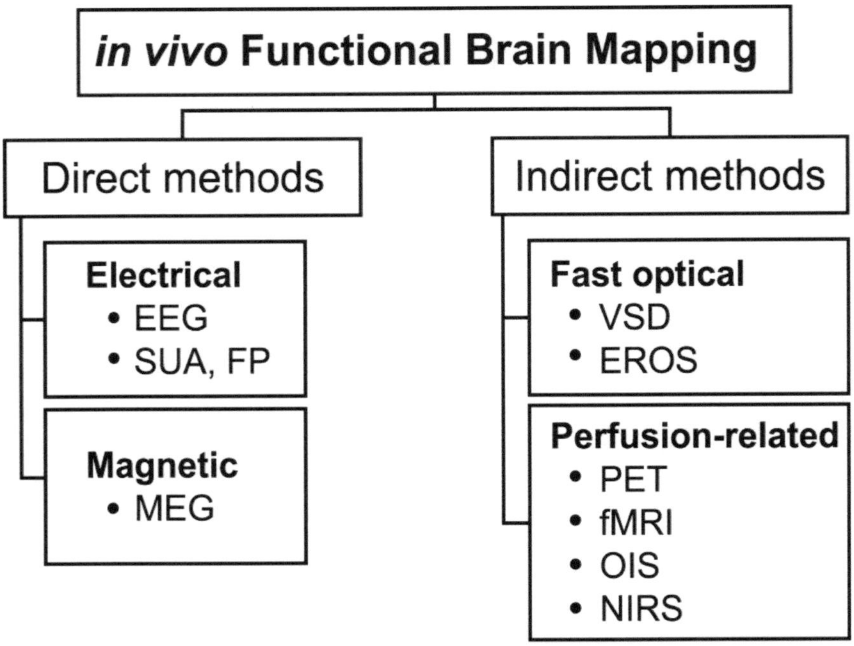

Fig. 1. Categorical division of *in vivo* functional brain mapping techniques. Direct methods measure electrical and magnetic field changes produced by neuronal action potentials and synaptic potentials. Electrical measures include both non-invasive techniques such as electroencephalography (EEG) and invasive techniques such as single unit activity (SUA) and field potential (FP) recording. The most common magnetic measure is magnetoencephalography (MEG). Indirect methods, on the other hand, are sensitive to other tissue changes that accompany neural activation. Structural changes produce variations in optical properties that follow the millisecond timecourse of neural events. Techniques taking advantage of these processes include voltage sensitive dye (VSD) imaging, which measures transmembrane voltage changes, and event-related optical signal (EROS) imaging, which measures optical scattering changes putatively produced by ionic movement. Indirect assessment is also possible using changes in blood flow elicited by neural activity. Hemodynamic events follow a much slower time course (several seconds), but are the most commonly used signals for functional imaging. A full appreciation of their importance for basic neurophysiology and functional imaging requires a detailed understanding of neurovascular coupling, or the relationship between neuronal activity and perfusion. PET, positron emission tomography; fMRI, functional magnetic resonance imaging; OISI, optical intrinsic signal imaging; NIRS, near-infrared spectroscopy.

3. Neurovascular coupling

Understanding the capacities and limitations of perfusion-based techniques requires an appreciation of the relationship between changes in neuronal activity and blood flow. In brief, the concept of "neurovascular coupling" describes the observation that increases in neuronal activity trigger local increases in blood flow. Whether the perfusion response is necessary to supply an increased metabolic demand is under debate. This physiological blood flow response has several measurable properties that form the basis for the techniques described below.

The idea of neurovascular coupling dates to the late 19th century. In his tome *Principles of Psychology*, William James states,

The fluctuations of the blood-supply to the brain ... followed the quickening of mental activity almost immediately. We must suppose a very delicate adjustment whereby the circulation follows the needs of the cerebral activity. Blood very likely may rush to each region of the cortex according as it is most active, but of this we know nothing. I need hardly say that the activity of the nervous matter is the primary phenomenon, and the afflux of blood its secondary consequence.

William James (1890)

James draws these conclusions from the observations of the Italian scientist Mosso, who found that cerebral blood flow was redistributed based on emotional or intellectual activity. In the same year, Roy and Sherrington published their landmark study, "On the regulation of the blood supply of the brain", in which they hypothesized a connection between neuronal activity and blood flow. Decades later in 1928, Fulton (then a neurosurgical resident under Harvey Cushing, the "father" of neurosurgery) described a clinical case involving a patient with an occipital arteriovenous malformation that produced an audible bruit when the patient engaged in visual activity [1]. This finding further strengthened the case for a causal connection between brain activity and vascular responses. Important developments occurred in the 1950s, when Kety and Sokoloff pioneered methods for measuring metabolism and blood flow changes in the whole brain using radioactive tracers [2]. Ingvar and Lassen furthered these techniques by demonstrating regional blood flow changes in response to neuronal activity in humans [3]. These methods were combined with reconstruction algorithms developed for X-ray computed tomography to give rise to PET, the first of the modern perfusion-based brain imaging techniques.

4. The hemodynamic response

Although it took over half a century to appreciate the significance of the coupling between brain activity and cerebral blood flow, the last few decades have seen a considerable advancement in our understanding of its spatiotemporal dynamics. The "hemodynamic response" refers to changes in blood flow, volume, and oxygenation generated by neuronal activation. Because perfusion-based imaging modalities are based on various aspects of the hemodynamic response, their proper interpretation requires an understanding of the characteristics of the response and its relationship to neuronal activity.

Because neurons are thought to rely on oxidative metabolism for energy production, an increase in neuronal activity leads to increased oxygen consumption, which results in extraction of oxygen from the surrounding tissue and capillaries. These events take place within the first 100-300 milliseconds following activation onset. Local oxygen extraction produces a transient increase in the relative concentration of deoxyhemoglobin (Hbr) that peaks at 0.75 - 2 seconds, depending on cortex, species, and physiological condition. Neuronal activity also triggers an increase in local cerebral blood flow (CBF), via a host of possible mediators and incompletely understood mechanisms. The CBF response begins near the site of neural activity in small arterioles, the primary resistance vessels, and propagates retrograde to larger vessels, peaking at 2-4 seconds. The influx of oxygenated arterial blood rapidly reverses local tissue oxygenation, decreasing Hbr and increasing oxyhemoglobin (HbO_2). This oxygenation change greatly overshoots baseline, resulting in relative hyperoxygenation, peaking at 3-6 seconds. As the inflowing blood drains into the venous system, these later oxygenation changes occur in medium to large veins. If neuronal activation lasts fewer than ~4 seconds, the oxygenation changes gradually return to baseline over 10-20 seconds. If activation lasts longer, blood volume and oxygenation remain elevated for the duration of stimulation at a lower "plateau" level, and then return to baseline over several seconds after stimulus offset.

The reliance of neurons on oxidative metabolism mentioned above is a recently developed hypothesis. In the late 1980s Fox and Raichle found that relative increases in CBF were six times greater than increases in oxygen utilization [5-6]. The authors suggested that this mismatch represented uncoupling between CBF and oxygen metabolism, which they interpreted as suggesting neurons use means other than oxygen metabolism to support their energy demand. For several years, a glycoltyic mechanism for ATP production was thought to support neuronal activity. In the late 1990s, however, Buxton and Frank proposed a biophysical model of the hemodynamic response that accounted for these measurements [7-9]. They suggested that the capacity for oxygen diffusion from capillary red blood cells to neurons was reduced during the CBF response due to a decrease in capillary transit time. Blood flowing more quickly had less time to exchange oxygen with the tissue. According to this "oxygen limitation" model, a relatively larger increase in CBF was necessary to compensate for the reduced oxygen extraction, and that Fox and Raichle's data actually supported tight coupling between CBF and oxygen metabolism. This model supported the notion that oxidative metabolism accounted for the bulk of neuronal energy production. Studies using MR spectroscopy [10] and fMRI [11] provided experimental validation of this theory. In the last few years, a number of additional studies have demonstrated focal decreases in tissue oxygenation and increases in oxygen metabolism rate [12-15].

The debate over the physiology of energy metabolism has occurred almost in parallel with the debate over its implication for perfusion-based functional imaging. Some have suggested that a local increase in Hbr due to decreased tissue oxygenation would generate a transient drop in blood oxygen-level dependent (BOLD) signal ("initial dip" in fMRI parlance) [16-17]. Its close relationship to neuronal metabolism would putatively allow the initial dip to serve as a spatially accurate mapping signal for functional imaging. Although several studies have observed the dip with BOLD fMRI [18-27] and OIS spectroscopy [13, 28-31], others have not [32-36], and its existence remains somewhat controversial. Some have suggested that slightly different spatiotemporal dynamics between cerebral blood flow (CBF) and volume (CBV) could create an initial dip in BOLD signal without an increase in oxygen metabolism [9, 37]. The observation that CBV increases at least 0.5 seconds after tissue pO_2 begins to drop [15], however, makes that possibility unlikely. There now seems to be general agreement that the dip exists and is related to increased oxygen consumption. Its small size [38] and susceptibility to baseline physiological conditions [7, 32] however, jeopardize its usefulness as a mapping signal.

Although general aspects of the hemodynamic response have been fairly well characterized, relatively little is known about the mediators of the response [39]. Hypotheses explaining the molecular communication between neural activity and blood flow fall roughly into four groups [40]. According to one, byproducts of neuronal activity such as adenosine and K^+ released extracellularly cause vasodilatation in nearby blood vessels [41]. A second hypothesis promotes the role of nitric oxide (NO). In this scenario, glutamate, the predominant excitatory neurotransmitter, also acts as a mediator of neurovascular coupling. Glutamate released into the synapse binds to postsynaptic NMDA receptors and activates guanylyl cyclase to produce NO, which diffuses to neighboring blood vessels and causes vasodilatation [42]. According to a third line of thought, neuronal processes directly innervate local blood vessels and transmit vasodilatory signals through acetylcholine [43], dopamine [44], or serotonin [45]. The final and most recent argument also implicates glutamate, but highlights the role of astrocytes. Astrocytic processes ensheathing the synapse sense glutamate levels through metabotropic receptors that produce graded intracellular Ca^{2+} increases. The Ca^{2+} wave propagates to the astrocyte endfeet, which are in intimate contact with blood vessels, and triggers vasodilatation through release of various molecules including prostanoids [46].

Historically, the most commonly used perfusion-based functional brain mapping techniques have been positron emission tomography (PET) and functional magnetic resonance imaging (fMRI). The latter has experienced tremendous growth over the last ten years, eclipsing all other brain imaging techniques [47]. The demand for high-resolution imaging has also brought OISI to the forefront, along with its lower resolution but noninvasive cousin, near-infrared spectroscopy (NIRS).

Each of these imaging modalities is based on one or more aspects of the hemodynamic response. The following discussion introduces the development, basic methodology, and relative advantages and disadvantages of these techniques, with particular emphasis given to OISI and related optical techniques.

4.1 Positron emission tomography (PET)

Throughout the 1950s and 1960s, radionuclide scans were a popular tool for neurodiagnostics. The application of tomographic reconstruction techniques developed for X-ray computerized tomography (CT) to nuclear medicine heralded the rise of positron emission tomography (PET) and single photon emission computed tomography (SPECT). Introduced in 1975 by Michael Phelps [48], PET imaging was the first non-invasive (or at least minimally invasive) perfusion-based functional brain imaging modality. This technological breakthrough allowed autoradiographic measurement of metabolism [49] and blood flow [2], previously restricted to animals, to be performed in humans in the form of *in vivo* autoradiograms. The development of several biologically useful positron-emitting molecules rapidly increased the utility of PET through the late 1970s and 1980s.

PET imaging relies on the use of radioactive atoms decaying by emitting positrons, which have the same mass as electrons but a positive charge. These positron-emitting atoms are generated either through the decay of another generating element (e.g., ^{68}Ga through the decay of ^{68}Ge), or by direct production in a cyclotron (e.g., ^{15}O). Molecules containing these radioactive elements are chemically synthesized, and trace amounts injected into the subject.

The labeled molecules circulate according to their biological properties, all the while emitting positrons. The emitted positrons travel a short distance (on the order of a few mm), until they encounter their anti-particles, electrons, with which they annihilate. The annihilation produces a characteristic release of so-called synchrotron energy in the form of two 511 keV gamma rays, which travel in opposite directions, close to 180° apart.

Because of the gamma rays' high energy, PET system detectors employ elements with high atomic number and therefore high stopping power. The original detectors used thallium-doped sodium iodide (NaI[Tl]) crystals, but modern scanners use either bismuth germinate (BGO; $Bi_4Ge_3O_{12}$) or lutetium oxyorthosilicate (LSO). The detector electronics use a coincidence detection system that reduces background radiation and scatter by rejecting events that are not recorded almost simultaneously (within the preset coincidence time window) on both sides of the head. The source is assumed to exist on a line connecting the two detectors that recorded the events, and its position is determined based on the coincidence time difference. Events are recorded in this manner, and the source distribution within the brain is then calculated by solving the inverse problem using filtered back-projection or iterative approaches.

One of the advantages of PET imaging is the diversity of metabolic, hemodynamic, and biochemical processes that can be assessed using different tracers. Those that are most relevant for hemodynamic functional brain mapping are ^{15}O-labelled water ($H_2{}^{15}O$) and ^{18}F-labelled 2-fluoro-2-deoxy-D-glucose (^{18}FDG). $H_2{}^{15}O$ distributes within the circulation and collects proportionally to the regional blood flow. $H_2{}^{15}O$ PET is therefore the most common method for non-invasive cerebral blood flow (CBF) measurement. ^{18}FDG is actively transported into cells via glucose transporters, where it is phosphorylated in the cytoplasm and thereby sequestered intracellularly. Its 2-fluoro group prevents it from undergoing further glycolysis, so the amount accumulated within the cell indicates the rate of glucose metabolism.

More than 25 years since its introduction, PET imaging is still an important and widely used technique for clinical diagnosis and basic science research. PET offers versatility for measuring a range of physiological processes and the ability to quantify them in absolute terms. Its reliance on radiopharmaceuticals, however, limits the potential subject population and number of studies that can be performed in the same subject. In addition, PET affords rather poor spatial (several millimeters) and temporal (10s of seconds to minutes) resolution.

SPECT imaging is similar to PET in its reliance on exogenous radioisotope contrast agents. SPECT radioisotopes undergo gamma decay by emitting a single high-energy photon, as its name implies, as opposed to the two gamma rays produced by positron-electron annihilation in PET. As in PET, the contrast agents can be chosen to measure physiological responses such as CBF (e.g., ^{99m}Tc-hexamethylpropyleneamineoxime [HMPAO]). Many of the radiopharmaceuticals are commonly used in nuclear medicine and therefore do not require a cyclotron for their production. Factors such as these make SPECT imaging significantly cheaper than PET, although it suffers from even lower spatial resolution.

4.2 Functional magnetic resonance imaging (fMRI)

In 2001, fMRI surpassed EEG as the most widely used brain imaging technique, in terms of the number of published papers. Whereas EEG required 72 years to reach this level, fMRI required only 11. This surge in popularity is a consequence of the technique's noninvasiveness and balance between sensitivity and resolution. In addition, many types of studies can be performed in clinical MRI magnets, which are increasingly available in modern health care facilities. Over the past decade, great progress has been made in improving the versatility, spatial and temporal resolution, and clinical utility of fMRI.

The phenomenon of nuclear magnetic resonance (NMR) was observed independently by Bloch and Purcell in 1945, a finding for which they were jointly awarded the Nobel Prize in Physics in 1952. NMR describes the behavior of atomic nuclei in magnetic fields. Because nuclei possess both charge and spin, they also possess an intrinsic magnetic moment. When placed in an external magnetic field ($\vec{B}_o$), nuclei align their magnetic moments parallel or anti-parallel to the field and precess about the field like a gyroscope precessing in the Earth's gravitational field. If molar quantities of spinning atoms are considered, a small fraction more tend to align parallel to $\vec{B}_o$, resulting in a net magnetization vector $\vec{M}$ parallel to $\vec{B}_o$.

Precession occurs at a characteristic frequency (the Larmor frequency, $\vec{\omega}$), which is a function of $\vec{B}_o$ and the atom's inherent properties (called its gryomagnetic constant, γ): $\vec{\omega} = \gamma \cdot \vec{B}_o$. The resonance phenomenon dictates that externally applied energy at this frequency will be transferred to the spinning atoms. Because the Larmor frequency is in the radio wave spectrum, the applied energy is called the radiofrequency (RF) pulse. The RF energy exerts a torque on $\vec{M}$, rotating it towards the transverse plane. Because the spins are still precessing, the time varying magnetic field they produce in the transverse plane induces current in a coil of wire oriented perpendicular to it. Thus transverse magnetization produces a detectable signal.

This signal decays by two processes: longitudinal (spin-lattice) and transverse (spin-spin) relaxation. The first describes the relaxation of $\vec{M}$ back to its equilibrium position, parallel to $\vec{B}_o$, and occurs with a characteristic time constant T_1. The second describes dephasing of spins due to precession at different rates, and occurs with a time constant T_2. This difference arises from spins experiencing slightly different magnetic field strengths, caused either by interactions with other spins (pure T_2 effects) or by small field inhomogeneities (T_2* effects). Variations in the latter provide contrast for the most commonly used form of fMRI.

Imaging based on NMR involves spatially encoding the position of different spins using magnetic field gradients. Whereas NMR can be performed with any atom possessing non zero spin, imaging applications prefer spin ½ nuclei because they have only two possible energy levels. Several spin ½ atoms have been used for imaging and spectroscopy applications, including ^{3}He [50], ^{13}C [51], ^{31}P [52], and ^{129}Xe [53], but by far the most common is ^{1}H because of its abundance in the form of H_2O in biological material.

Biological imaging using NMR was developed in the late 1970s, with the first human images appearing in 1977 [54]. The word "nuclear" was dropped in the mid 1980s to avoid the associated negative connotation, in favor of the term magnetic resonance imaging (MRI). In the early 1990s, Belliveau, Rosen, and colleagues performed the first functional studies using an injected paramagnetic contrast agent [55-57]. Contrast agents with high magnetic susceptibility produce large magnetic field gradients in the local environment, decreasing T_2* in proportion to the amount present. Using tracer kinetic models, they compared the decrease in T_2* weighted signal during visual activity and rest and generated a CBV weighted functional image of visual cortex [55].

At the same time, Ogawa and colleagues showed in animals that functional images could be generated without an exogenous contrast agent [58]. They took advantage of the natural difference in magnetic properties between oxy- (HbO_2) and deoxyhemoglobin (Hbr). Whereas the former is weakly diamagnetic and has little effect on magnetic fields, the latter is paramagnetic and causes local field disturbances. Hbr therefore acts as an endogenous contrast agent. The CBF response produced by functional activity reduces local Hbr content and therefore increases signal strength.

These lines of research converged in 1992, when these two groups and a third almost simultaneously demonstrated that this intrinsic oxygenation-based contrast could be used to map brain activity [59-61]. This so-called blood oxygenation level dependent (BOLD) contrast is by far the most common in fMRI studies. BOLD fMRI has spearheaded the surge in functional brain imaging over the last decade, surpassing PET due to its superior spatial and temporal resolution and avoidance of exogenous radioactive tracers.

Because it is based on blood Hbr content, BOLD fMRI temporal characteristics closely follow those of oxygenation changes, starting within 1-2 seconds of stimulation onset and peaking at 4-6 seconds. Spatially, it emphasizes venous structures because oxygenation changes are most prominent in medium to large veins. This bias tends to decrease the spatial specificity of conventional T_2* BOLD fMRI somewhat, as veins are often millimeters away from the neuronal areas they drain. Spatial precision of a few millimeters may be sufficient for many types of cognitive studies investigating the entire brain with moderate resolution (and is certainly superior to that of PET, EEG, or MEG), but it is not sufficient for high resolution studies of columnar functional architecture.

In 1996, Malonek and Grinvald observed a small increase in Hbr before the CBF-induced hyperoxygenation [17]. They attributed this transient deoxygenation to an increase in oxidative metabolism that decreased local tissue oxygen tension before the onset of the CBF response. They suggested that imaging based on the dip could improve spatial specificity, since it was restricted to metabolically active areas.

A transient increase in Hbr would appear as a brief decrease in BOLD signal prior to the conventional positive BOLD response. Over the next several years, many investigators looked for this "initial dip" in a variety of cortices and species. It has been successfully identified in the visual cortex of cat [22-23], monkey [21], and human [18-20, 24-27], and human motor cortex [25, 27]. Although these studies identified the dip in the BOLD signal timecourse, only one study has been able to generate a map using this signal [23]. Other groups have tried, but found that the maps were not reproducible [62]. Indeed, several fMRI studies in rat somatosensory cortex have been unable to detect the dip altogether [34-36]. These discrepancies may be due to anesthesia, differences in cortical architecture, or other effects.

Alternatives to BOLD fMRI include CBF- (or perfusion-) weighted fMRI and CBV-weighted fMRI. In CBF fMRI, ^1H spins in arterial blood water are used as endogenous flow tracers [63-

64]. Spins outside the region of interest are labeled with an RF pulse. Labeled spins are allowed to enter the imaging region after a suitable time delay (0.5 – 2 s), where they exchange with tissue water. The amount of signal detected in the imaging slice is proportional to the flow rate into the slice. Advantages of CBF fMRI include better spatial specificity than BOLD, with less emphasis on large draining veins. In addition, whereas BOLD signals include a complex mixture of CBV, CBF, and oxygenation contributions, CBF fMRI can isolate and quantify the CBF component. This technique suffers, however, from relatively poor temporal resolution (several seconds) and lower sensitivity than BOLD [65].

The original reports of functional imaging using MRI used CBV contrast [55-57]. Current CBV fMRI studies use exogenous paramagnetic contrast agents with a long blood half-life, avoiding the need for kinetic tracer models and allowing repeated imaging. The large magnetic field disruptions introduced by the contrast agents lead to decreased T_2*-weighted signals in proportion to CBV. The temporal resolution of CBV fMRI is similar to that of BOLD fMRI, and its contrast-to-noise ratio (CNR) is much higher. The major drawback is the requirement for contrast injection, which also precludes human studies, although clinical trials are underway [66].

5. Optical intrinsic signal imaging (OISI)

Intraoperative OISI maps the brain by measuring activity-related changes in cortical light reflectance. Activity related reflectance changes were first demonstrated in nervous tissue in vitro more than 50 years ago [67] and have since been observed in vivo in rodents, cats, nonhuman primates, and humans. It is a particularly attractive brain-mapping modality because it can rapidly assess the functional activity of large cortical areas with very high spatial resolution (50–100 μm). Because of its versatility, OISI has been used to characterize numerous physiological phenomena, including neurovascular coupling [67-69], hemodynamic refractory periods [70], vasomotion [71], the organization of the visual cortex [71-73], cortical plasticity [71-76], cortical spreading depression [77], seizure [78-79], and language organization in the human brain [80]. Haglund and colleagues [81] were the first to observe optical signals in humans during seizure and cognitive tasks. Since then, the authors of studies on intraoperative OISI have described optical signal evolution in human cortex [82], the mapping of primary sensory and motor cortices [70], and the delineation of language cortices within [83] and across languages [80].

5.1 Intrinsic optical signals

OISI detects perfusion-related and metabolic signals that are coupled to neuronal activity, including hemoglobin concentration and oxygenation changes, cytochrome oxidation changes, and light scattering caused by altered blood volume, blood flow, and cell swelling [15, 17, 30, 84-86], which in turn create a functional map of the brain. Each of these different phenomena is observed and best quantified at different imaging wavelengths [30, 87]. For example, imaging at 610 nm best detects deoxyhemoglobin concentration changes because the absorbance of oxyhemoglobin is much less than that of deoxyhemoglobin at 610 nm [30]. Thus, OISI at 610 nm is analagous to BOLD fMRI [20], which capitalizes on local magnetic susceptibility changes due to differences between deoxyhemoglobin and oxyhemoglobin concentration.

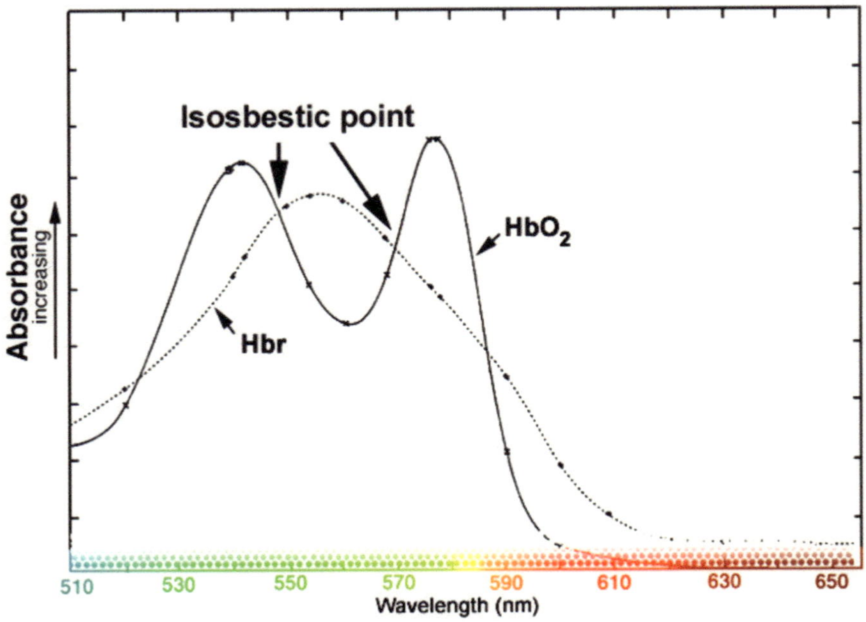

Fig. 2. Hemoglobin absorption spectrum. Optical intrinsic signal imaging (OISI) relies on changes in cortical light reflectance produced by the hemodynamic response. The most important absorber in the visible spectrum is hemoglobin (Hb). Because oxy- (HbO_2) and deoxyhemoglobin (Hbr) absorb light differentially, OISI is wavelength dependent. By selecting different imaging wavelengths, different aspects of the hemodynamic response can be assessed. Both Hb species absorb equally at isosbestic points (549, 569 nm; green light), so reflectance changes at these wavelengths emphasize changes in total Hb, a measure of blood volume. The increased absorbance of Hbr in the 605-630 nm range (red light) permits estimation of oxygenation changes by imaging in this range.

5.2 OISI mapping

Optical maps are integrated comparisons between the cortex at rest and during prescribed activity. OISI can only be performed intraoperatively in humans because it must be performed following craniotomy and dural reflection. A CCD camera is used to detect small optical changes (0.5–5%) and is mounted onto an operating microscope (Figure 3) or other support structure for imaging. The cortex is then epi-illuminated with white light, and the CCD camera captures the reflected light after it passes through a band-pass filter. Maps of functional change are calculated by comparing images during activation to images at rest [70, 80, 82-83, 89-91]. Multiple trials are averaged to increase the SNR.

Respirophasic and cardiophasic movements of the brain are significant sources of noise during imaging. Using a glass plate to immobilize the cortex [81], synchronizing image acquisition with respiration and heart rate [82] and using image registration [80-81, 83] allow for a reduction in this noise. Vascular artifacts from blood vessels are another major source of noise. Focusing 1-2 mm below the cortical surface [87] and imaging only immediately after stimulus onset [92] can minimize this artifact when the area being imaged is close to large vessels [13, 71, 93].

Commercial systems for clinical intraoperative OISI imaging are not yet available. Investigational systems can be developed from an existing operating microscope with the addition of a camera, camera controller, personal computer, and software to control image acquisition and analysis.

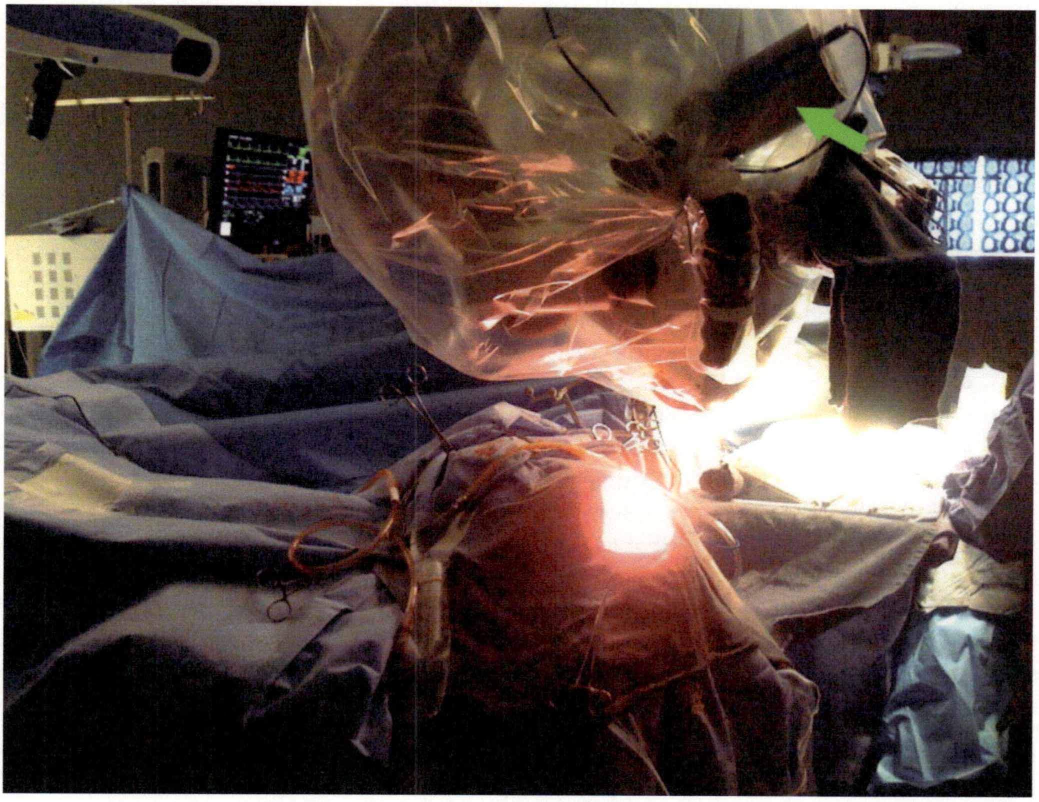

Fig. 3. Intraoperative photograph showing CCD camera mounted on operating microscope. The cortex is illuminated with white light, and the reflected light is filtered at a particular wavelength of interest. Images are captured by a very sensitive CCD camera (shown with green arrow), and reflectance changes between rest and stimulation are measured. These changes correspond to evolving aspects of the hemodynamic response generated as a consequence of underlying cortical activity.

5.3 OISI in animal models

OISI has been extensively used in animals to date and has paved the way for major breakthroughs in our understanding of the functional organization, physiology and pathophysiology of the brain [30, 68-69, 72, 74-78, 84-85, 92, 94-97]. OISI studies in animals have defined the functional topography of visual [72] and other cortices, helped elucidate the coupling between electrophysiology and perfusion-related signals, characterized the robustness of neurovascular response capacities, and described perfusion-related changes induced by pathophysiological processes such as cortical spreading depression and seizure. These studies have repeatedly demonstrated the versatility of this modality and its numerous potential applications. The specificity of optical maps generated through OISI has been consistently confirmed in these various studies when compared to other established invasive methodologies, including single unit activity measurement [87, 95], maximum field potential measurement [96-97], and cytochrome oxidase-staining [68, 95]. OISI has also been used for mapping seizure propagation in the cortex [78] and for identifying epileptogenic foci [79].

5.4 OISI in humans

The first OISI maps of human function were created by asking the patient to engage in simple motor tasks such as tongue movement and simple language task such as visual object-naming exercises. Motor tasks demonstrated clear optical signals in the motor cortex, and language tasks demonstrated activity in both Broca and Wernicke areas [81]. Optical responses in humans typically appear within 1 second, peak between 3 and 4 seconds, and disappear by 9 seconds, similar to those observed in animal models [82, 89]. Indeed, this similar timing of optical signals across species suggests that we are indeed imaging similar phenomena, and because we have clearer physiological correlates in animals obtained through invasive methodologies, we can extrapolate that we are imaging the same neural activity. In line with this assertion, hemodynamic refractory periods originally observed in rodents were also observable in humans during OISI mapping [70]. In further corroboration, all human OISI studies to date indicate that the observed reflectance changes are spatially correlated with somatosensory evoked potential (SSEP) data. Median and ulnar nerve stimulation leads to a decrease in optical signal obtained at 610 nm in an area that colocalizes with the largest SSEPs in both somatosensory and motor cortices [82]. More importantly, OISI maps similarly colocalize with intraoperative electrocortical stimulation mapping (ESM), the current gold standard of cortical mapping [80-81, 83]. Areas that are identified by ESM as essential for a specific task consistently demonstrate optical activity [80-81, 83].

A notable phenomenon with optical signals is "vascular spread." OISI maps demonstrate signal in some surrounding areas (approximately 25%) that are not identified as essential on ESM. This has been demonstrated in both rodent models [98-100] and human intraoperative imaging. Spread may occur in part because intraoperative OISI is detecting both essential and secondary cortices whereas ESM is only detecting essential areas. Spread may also be related to imprecise physiological coupling of neuronal activity, metabolism, and perfusion. The sensitivity, specificity, positive predictive value, and negative predictive value of intraoperative OISI relative to ESM as a gold standard have not been fully quantified [101-102], and such quantification will be essential to the broadening of intraoperative OISI as a fundamental clinical tool.

OISI has also begun to provide a finer resolution of cortical mapping with regards to task specific activity. For example, OISI demonstrates differentially activated gyri during tongue movement and naming tasks, activities which require similar movements but which are otherwise distinct [81]. Median and ulnar nerve stimulation produces distinct maps within the same gyrus, possibly providing a fine resolution of somatosensory and motor activity in the cortex [82]. Distinct maps of face, thumb, and index and middle fingers have also been obtained within the same gyrus [70], and although there is some overlap between these areas, the areas of maximum optical signal are distinct for each task. Such specificity has also been observed in language areas (Broca and Wernicke areas) [83].

5.5 Advantages of intraoperative OISI mapping

The ultimate goal of intraoperative mapping is to predict when resection of a cortical area will cause functional deficits. As such, ESM is the current gold standard for intraoperative mapping because it produces reversible lesions such as would occur permanently with resection. However, ESM interpretation is complicated by the fact that cortical stimulation may disrupt remote areas via stimulation of neuronal projections [103-104], and this may lead to imprecise maps [105]. Thus, direct activation-based techniques such as OISI that rely on the detection of local neuronal activity may create a clearer picture when used in conjunction with established methods like ESM.

The spatial resolution of ESM is also one of its important drawbacks. Resection within 1 cm of essential areas identified by ESM increases the likelihood of postoperative neurological deficits [106-107]. Because of this local current spread, the resolution of this techique is relatively coarse. On the other hand, OISI offers a resolution as high as 50 to 100 μm as demonstrated by numerous studies, potentially allowing for a much finer delineation of eloquence.

Rapidity of assessment is another consideration. ESM requires the testing of several sites, at different current levels, during numerous tasks. The process requires several repetitions and is relatively quite time-consuming. Intraoperative OISI provides a faster assessment of the cortical surface, as the entire field of view can be imaged at once. This advantage is particularly important when mapping multiple tasks in an area that covers several possible functional representations.

Another advantage of OISI is its non-tactile nature, as it relies solely on light reflection. ESM requires direct contact with the brain, and the application of current to its surface. This process can precipitate abnormal electrical propagation known as after-discharge activity, which can escalate into a clinical seizure. Intraoperative seizures are not only dangerous, but also often preclude further mapping, as the brain is relatively depressed afterwards.

Furthermore, essential areas identified by ESM are consistently demonstrated by intraoperative OISI maps, suggesting that they do indeed offer a relatively high sensitivity. Thus, cortical regions not demonstrating task-related OISI activity can probably be resected without functional consequence. However, vascular spread, as previously described, may produce false-positive results in OISI maps by highlighting secondary and/or non-essential cortical areas, thus hindering our ability to produce a maximal resection. Thus, OISI may not completely replace ESM but may be used in conjunction as a complementary modality to improve the accuracy of cortical maps.

OISI can also be used in conjunction with fluorescent dyes that allow for more precise physical localization of pathological tissues such as tumors. Dyes were first used in animal studies [15, 96, 107-108] for this purpose. For example, optical imaging of an intravenously injected dye in rodents demonstrates intracranial tumors with high accuracy [107], and this has correlated well with human studies as well. Preoperative injection of 5-aminolevulinic acid, a precursor of fluorescent porphyrin, could be used to identify malignant gliomas with 85% sensitivity and 100% specificity [108]. The 5-aminolevulinic acid accumulates within the malignant tissue, where it is converted to its fluorescent derivative, which is then imaged intraoperatively using optical imaging with special optics. This is a powerful adjunctive application to optical imaging that can provide spatial information of the relationship between pathological tissue and essential cortical areas.

Importantly, like all intraoperative imaging modalities, OISI presents a distinct advantage over preoperative functional mapping (as provided by fMRI or PET) because it can correct for "brain shift" following craniotomy and dural reflection [109]. This is a non-trivial problem that confounds our ability to rely on preoperative functional mapping alone. Intraoperative OISI requires only minimal modification of the neurosurgical equipment already found in the operating room and does not impact the surgery or affect normal brain tissue as it relies solely on measuring reflected light from the brain.

5.6 Limitations of intraoperative OISI mapping

While neurovascular and neurometabolic coupling to neuronal activity appear to be consistent in numerous studies to date [15, 80, 82-83, 86-87, 95-97], the major limitation of intraoperative OISI continues to be the fact that the signal does not directly arise from neuronal activity. This becomes particularly relevant when dealing with pathological cortex, as is frequently the case during neurosurgical interventions, where the coupling may not be as tight as in normal cortex. This is a major question that remains to be elucidated and arguably can only be investigated with high-resolution intraoperative measures such as OISI.

Vascular lesions such as arteriovenous malformations (AVMs) present perhaps the most important challenge. Abnormal vascular networks may provide altered and unreliable signal in cortical areas adjacent to AVMs. While several studies have found that perfusion-related mapping signals can be detected directly adjacent to AVMs and can therefore be used reliably to predict essential language sites identified by ESM [110-112], the interpretation of results in these patients should still be approached cautiously.

Vascular spread in OISI maps is another confounder in the use of intraoperative OISI as a single modality. Indeed, using it as a lone modality may produce significant false-positive results that would prevent maximum resection of pathological and non-eloquent tissue. Until we understand this spread phenomenon better and are able to control for it, intraoperative OISI cannot replace ESM. However, it may provide an important complementary modality - for example, intraoperative OISI can be used to rapidly map cortical areas of interest with high spatial resolution, and those areas found to demonstrate optical activity can then be verified by ESM.

Another potential drawback of OISI is its limited signal-to-noise ratio (SNR). In language mapping trials, SNR values range from 5:1 to 9:1 when averaging four trials. This limited SNR can be attributed to patient head motion as well as respirophasic and cardiophasic cortical movements. While SNR can be improved by increasing the number trials that are averaged, reducing cortical movements by using a glass plate [81], or synchronizing image acquisition with respiration and pulse [82], this is still a challenge that remains to be addressed. Furthermore, increasing the number of trials elongates the time required for the procedure, a distinct disadvantage. Furthermore, unlike fMRI and PET, which afford three-dimensional maps, intraoperative OISI produces surface maps, usually to a maximum depth of 1 mm. This represents a further limitation.

As the utilization of OISI increases, we will begin to understand its strengths and weaknesses to a greater extent, potentially enabling the development of auxiliary technologies that augment these strengths or overcome these weaknesses. On the whole, however, OISI presents important new advances that can potentially improve clinical outcomes when used in conjunction with other established modalities.

6. OIS spectroscopy

One potential shortcoming of OISI, alluded to above, is its ambiguous etiology. Studies using OISI usually report "activity" as a certain fractional change in reflectance from baseline. These reflectance changes incorporate changes in absorbance and scattering related to a number of physiological processes. Specific hemodynamic processes can be isolated to some degree by choosing appropriate wavelengths, but other contributions certainly exist.

This drawback was addressed in the late 1990s by Malonek and Grinvald [16-17]. They disambiguated the various contributions of absorbance and scattering by developing a variant of OISI known as OIS spectroscopy. In its most common form, broadband light reflected from the cortex is focused on a primary image plane containing a spectrographic slit instead of a detector. The one-dimensional column of light is then incident upon a diffraction grating that disperses the light into its constituent wavelengths along a second orthogonal axis. This two-dimensional "spatio-spectral" image is then refocused on a second image plane and captured by a camera. The x-dimension of the image represents the wavelength of light at a particular point along the slit, and the y-dimension represents vertical position. Spatio-spectral images are taken over time to capture the hemodynamic response, as in other techniques.

This approach essentially sacrifices one dimension of spatial information for an extra dimension of spectral information. The advantage gained is the ability to fit the spectra acquired over time to a model containing physiological parameters that are known to change during the hemodynamic response and affect light reflectance. Models are usually based on the Beer-Lambert law, which describes light attenuation in the presence of absorbers: $Abs = \sum_i \varepsilon_i c_i l$, where ε_i is the extinction coefficient of the ith absorber, c is the absorber concentration, and l is the pathlength through the tissue. In living tissue under normal physiological circumstances, Hbr and HbO_2 are the most important absorbers in visible wavelengths. Cytochrome oxidase also absorbs in the visible range, but its oxidation state only changes in cases of extremely low oxygen saturation. Because its absorbance is also an order of magnitude smaller than hemoglobin, it is generally not considered an important model component [71]. Early models incorporated scattering as an additive linear term: $Abs = \sum_i (\varepsilon_i c_i l) + S$, which would also capture residual errors.

Spectral data are fit to the model to extract the timecourses of the model parameters, i.e., Hbr and HbO_2. OIS spectroscopy therefore provides changes in physiological variables rather than (somewhat arbitrary) reflectance changes. This advantage allows for more direct comparison between OIS data and other modalities such as fMRI.

The results derived from OIS spectroscopy are only as valid as the model. The most important model refinements have been better consideration of wavelength dependency. The fact that different wavelengths of light penetrate biological tissue to different depths has been recognized for several years [113]. Longer wavelengths penetrate deeper into tissue and therefore travel through a longer pathlength (l in the above equations), another way of saying that they experience more scattering. To properly account for the optical pathlength and scattering, therefore, this dependency must be taken into account.

Mayhew and colleagues performed Monte Carlo simulations to calculate the distribution of differential pathlength factors in the visible spectrum [71]. Since then, several studies have incorporated wavelength dependency into the Beer-Lambert model to more accurately simulate the behavior of light transport through highly scattering biological tissue [28, 33, 114-115]. Their results have shown that accounting for wavelength dependency is critical, especially when assessing small transients in the response such as the initial dip.

6.1 Near-infrared spectroscopy (NIRS)

In 1977 Jobsis showed that the intact human skull was not necessarily a barrier for light [116]. He found that wavelengths of light beyond the visible spectrum in the near-infrared range (~670-900 nm) can penetrate through several centimeters of skin and skull. This range is ideally situated between the strong absorption spectra of hemoglobin (<~630 nm) and water (>~950 nm), and has therefore been dubbed the "biological window" for noninvasive optical imaging [117-118].

NIRS is based on the same principles as visible range spectroscopy described above. Changes in light attenuation are fit to a modified Beer-Lambert law incorporating scattering and absorption by hemoglobin. The wavelength dependency of the pathlength must be taken into account. Differential pathlength factors can also be calculated using a Monte Carlo simulation, but another method exists in the case of NIRS. Pathlengths can be directly measured using time-resolved spectroscopy systems [113, 119]. These instruments have very fast (picosecond) detectors that are capable of measuring the time of flight of photons traveling through the head, which is directly related to the distance traveled. Alternatively, frequency domain systems can measure the phase difference between incident and remitted light [120-121].

The main difference between NIRS and visible spectroscopy is the way in which light is emitted and collected. Because the cortex is not exposed, light cannot illuminate the entire area. Instead, light is directed into the head through fiber optic guides and diffuses through the skin, skull, and cortex. A detector fiber guide is positioned a few centimeters from the emitter, and captures photons that have scattered through the head in an arc-shaped path from emitter to detector. The greater the distance between emitter and detector, the more likely it is that photons will travel through a deeper arc. On the other hand, a greater separation reduces the number of photons detected. Studies have theoretically and experimentally determined the optimal spacing (2.5-4 cm) to allow the photons to "sample" the top layers of cortex [122-123]. Because functional activation is not expected to produce changes in the skull or scalp, any differences in measured light intensity are attributed to cortical hemodynamic processes, i.e., changes in oxygenation or volume.

NIRS can be performed using broadband or laser illumination. The former situation is directly analogous to visible spectroscopy: remitted light is spectrally decomposed and captured by a camera. This approach affords excellent spectral resolution, but the emitted power per wavelength band is low. In contrast, laser diodes produce more power in a narrow wavelength band, but the number of wavelengths is limited to a few (2-4 in conventional systems), decreasing spectral resolution. Detectors for laser illumination are usually photodiodes, which are much more sensitive than CCDs.

The principle advantage of NIRS over other optical techniques is its noninvasive nature. NIRS provides information about functional oxygenation and volume changes that are directly comparable to fMRI, but the apparatus is much less costly and confining. NIRS can be performed in pediatric populations much more easily than fMRI [124], and it can be transported to the bedside for clinical evaluations [125-128]. Because NIRS signals are detected several centimeters from the cortex, however, the spatial resolution of the technique is low (~1-2 cm). Spatial coverage can be increased by using arrays of emitters and detectors, but the emitter-detector spacing must be at least 2-3 cm to allow the light to sample cortex.

Modifications to the acquisition and analysis methods allow images to be created from NIRS data [129]. In this variant, a grid of emitters and detectors is placed on the head, providing several emitter-detectors pairs. NIRS imaging, or diffuse optical tomography (DOT), is the optical analog of PET, EEG, or MEG, in that it requires measurement of surface signals and calculation of the source distribution that could have produced them. It therefore also involves solving an inverse problem, which is again poorly constrained. Recent work has shown, however, that analyzing multi-channel NIRS data with this imaging approach provides better estimates of functional changes than single-channel NIRS [129].

7. Multi-modality approaches

The brain mapping techniques described above, both direct and indirect, can be combined, such that the information gained by their combination surpasses their advantages individually. The most beneficial combinations usually involve compensating for limitations of one technique with another, or concurrently measuring different aspects of the same response to better understand its physiological basis. For example, combined OISI-fMRI studies have also contributed to our knowledge of the etiology of these signals [101, 130-131]. The recent development of a system that allows simultaneous fMRI and OIS spectroscopy [132] promises to further this endeavor. This combination has also been used to test the clinical utility of intraoperative human OISI for neurosurgical guidance by comparing intraoperative OISI maps with pre-surgical fMRI maps [101, 130-131].

8. Conclusions

A central tenet in neurosurgery is avoidance of new postoperative neurological deficit. This goal is especially challenging when operating in or near "eloquent cortex", or regions subserving known specific functions, such as sensation, motor control, or language. Given individual neuroanatomical variations, eloquent regions must be delineated at the time of surgery, within the individual patient. The conventional method for identifying eloquent cortex intraoperatively is electrical stimulation mapping (ESM), during which regions of cortex are directly stimulated with a small electrical current using a hand-held probe. However, ESM has several limitations including limited spatial resolution, lengthy protocol time which places the patient at increased anesthesia and infection risk and increases costs, and a higher risk of seizure due to direct electrical stimulation of the cortex. Intraoperative OISI can provide maps of cortical function rapidly and without contacting the brain, therefore reducing operative time and seizure likelihood. These maps will be complementary to ESM for the localization of eloquent cortex. Furthermore, these maps can also be used for basic research, including the fine-scale determination of the functional organization of the brain. Optical imaging thus presents a powerful new avenue for the advancement of clinical neurosurgery and neuroscience research.

Although intraoperative OISI has only been used for research purposes, it has significant potential as a clinical mapping tool as well. Although it is unlikely to replace ESM, it may, if used in conjunction with conventional intraoperative mapping techniques, decrease mapping time, provide high spatial resolution cortical maps, and allow mapping of multiple tasks.

9. References

[1] Fulton, J.F., *Vasomotor and Reflex Sequelae of Unilateral Cervical and Lumbar Ramisectomy in a Case of Raynaud's Disease, with Observations on Tonus*. Ann Surg, 1928. 88(5): p. 827-41.
[2] Landau, W.M., et al., *The local circulation of the living brain; values in the unanesthetized and anesthetized cat*. Trans Am Neurol Assoc, 1955(80th Meeting): p. 125-9.
[3] Lassen, N.A., et al., *Regional Cerebral Blood Flow in Man Determined by Krypton*. Neurology, 1963. 13: p. 719-27.
[4] Bonvento, G., N. Sibson, and L. Pellerin, *Does glutamate image your thoughts?* Trends Neurosci, 2002. 25(7): p. 359-64.
[5] Fox, P.T. and M.E. Raichle, *Focal physiological uncoupling of cerebral blood flow and oxidative metabolism during somatosensory stimulation in human subjects*. Proc Natl Acad Sci U S A, 1986. 83(4): p. 1140-4.
[6] Fox, P.T., et al., *Nonoxidative glucose consumption during focal physiologic neural activity*. Science, 1988. 241(4864): p. 462-4.
[7] Buxton, R.B., *The elusive initial dip*. Neuroimage, 2001. 13(6 Pt 1): p. 953-8.
[8] Buxton, R.B. and L.R. Frank, *A model for the coupling between cerebral blood flow and oxygen metabolism during neural stimulation*. J Cereb Blood Flow Metab, 1997. 17(1): p. 64-72.
[9] Buxton, R.B., E.C. Wong, and L.R. Frank, *Dynamics of blood flow and oxygenation changes during brain activation: the balloon model*. Magn Reson Med, 1998. 39(6): p. 855-64.
[10] Hyder, F., et al., *Oxidative glucose metabolism in rat brain during single forepaw stimulation: a spatially localized 1H[13C] nuclear magnetic resonance study*. J Cereb Blood Flow Metab, 1997. 17(10): p. 1040-7.
[11] Hoge, R.D., et al., *Linear coupling between cerebral blood flow and oxygen consumption in activated human cortex*. Proc Natl Acad Sci U S A, 1999. 96(16): p. 9403-8.
[12] Ances, B.M., et al., *Dynamic changes in cerebral blood flow, O2 tension, and calculated cerebral metabolic rate of O2 during functional activation using oxygen phosphorescence quenching*. J Cereb Blood Flow Metab, 2001. 21(5): p. 511-6.
[13] Mayhew, J., et al., *Spectroscopic analysis of neural activity in brain: increased oxygen consumption following activation of barrel cortex*. Neuroimage, 2000. 12(6): p. 664-75.
[14] Thompson, J.K., M.R. Peterson, and R.D. Freeman, *Single-neuron activity and tissue oxygenation in the cerebral cortex*. Science, 2003. 299(5609): p. 1070-2.
[15] Vanzetta, I. and A. Grinvald, *Increased cortical oxidative metabolism due to sensory stimulation: implications for functional brain imaging*. Science, 1999. 286(5444): p. 1555-8.

[16] Malonek, D., et al., *Vascular imprints of neuronal activity: relationships between the dynamics of cortical blood flow, oxygenation, and volume changes following sensory stimulation.* Proc Natl Acad Sci U S A, 1997. 94(26): p. 14826-31.

[17] Malonek, D. and A. Grinvald, *Interactions between electrical activity and cortical microcirculation revealed by imaging spectroscopy: implications for functional brain mapping.* Science, 1996. 272(5261): p. 551-4.

[18] Ernst, T. and J. Hennig, *Observation of a fast response in functional MR.* Magn Reson Med, 1994. 32(1): p. 146-9.

[19] Menon, R.S., et al., *BOLD based functional MRI at 4 Tesla includes a capillary bed contribution: echo-planar imaging correlates with previous optical imaging using intrinsic signals.* Magn Reson Med, 1995. 33(3): p. 453-9.

[20] Hu, X., T.H. Le, and K. Ugurbil, *Evaluation of the early response in fMRI in individual subjects using short stimulus duration.* Magn Reson Med, 1997. 37(6): p. 877-84.

[21] Logothetis, N.K., et al., *Functional imaging of the monkey brain.* Nat Neurosci, 1999. 2(6): p. 555-62.

[22] Duong, T.Q., et al., *Spatiotemporal dynamics of the BOLD fMRI signals: toward mapping submillimeter cortical columns using the early negative response.* Magn Reson Med, 2000. 44(2): p. 231-42.

[23] Kim, D.S., T.Q. Duong, and S.G. Kim, *High-resolution mapping of iso-orientation columns by fMRI.* Nat Neurosci, 2000. 3(2): p. 164-9.

[24] Yacoub, E. and X. Hu, *Detection of the early negative response in fMRI at 1.5 Tesla.* Magn Reson Med, 1999. 41(6): p. 1088-92.

[25] Yacoub, E. and X. Hu, *Detection of the early decrease in fMRI signal in the motor area.* Magn Reson Med, 2001. 45(2): p. 184-90.

[26] Yacoub, E., et al., *Further evaluation of the initial negative response in functional magnetic resonance imaging.* Magn Reson Med, 1999. 41(3): p. 436-41.

[27] Yacoub, E., et al., *Investigation of the initial dip in fMRI at 7 Tesla.* NMR Biomed, 2001. 14(7-8): p. 408-12.

[28] Jones, M., et al., *Concurrent optical imaging spectroscopy and laser-Doppler flowmetry: the relationship between blood flow, oxygenation, and volume in rodent barrel cortex.* Neuroimage, 2001. 13(6 Pt 1): p. 1002-15.

[29] Jones, M., J. Berwick, and J. Mayhew, *Changes in blood flow, oxygenation, and volume following extended stimulation of rodent barrel cortex.* Neuroimage, 2002. 15(3): p. 474-87.

[30] Nemoto, M., et al., *Analysis of optical signals evoked by peripheral nerve stimulation in rat somatosensory cortex: dynamic changes in hemoglobin concentration and oxygenation.* J Cereb Blood Flow Metab, 1999. 19(3): p. 246-59.

[31] Shtoyerman, E., et al., *Long-term optical imaging and spectroscopy reveal mechanisms underlying the intrinsic signal and stability of cortical maps in V1 of behaving monkeys.* J Neurosci, 2000. 20(21): p. 8111-21.

[32] Lindauer, U., et al., *Neuronal activity-induced changes of local cerebral microvascular blood oxygenation in the rat: effect of systemic hyperoxia or hypoxia.* Brain Res, 2003. 975(1-2): p. 135-40.

[33] Lindauer, U., et al., *No evidence for early decrease in blood oxygenation in rat whisker cortex in response to functional activation.* Neuroimage, 2001. 13(6 Pt 1): p. 988-1001.

[34] Mandeville, J.B., et al., *Dynamic functional imaging of relative cerebral blood volume during rat forepaw stimulation.* Magn Reson Med, 1998. 39(4): p. 615-24.

[35] Marota, J.J., et al., *Investigation of the early response to rat forepaw stimulation.* Magn Reson Med, 1999. 41(2): p. 247-52.
[36] Silva, A.C., et al., *Early temporal characteristics of cerebral blood flow and deoxyhemoglobin changes during somatosensory stimulation.* J Cereb Blood Flow Metab, 2000. 20(1): p. 201-6.
[37] Hathout, G.M., B. Varjavand, and R.K. Gopi, *The early response in fMRI: a modeling approach.* Magn Reson Med, 1999. 41(3): p. 550-4.
[38] Ugurbil, K., L. Toth, and D.S. Kim, *How accurate is magnetic resonance imaging of brain function?* Trends Neurosci, 2003. 26(2): p. 108-14.
[39] Villringer, A. and U. Dirnagl, *Coupling of brain activity and cerebral blood flow: basis of functional neuroimaging.* Cerebrovasc Brain Metab Rev, 1995. 7(3): p. 240-76.
[40] Parri, R. and V. Crunelli, *An astrocyte bridge from synapse to blood flow.* Nat Neurosci, 2003. 6(1): p. 5-6.
[41] Faraci, F.M., *Regulation of the cerebral circulation by endothelium.* Pharmacol Ther, 1992. 56(1): p. 1-22.
[42] Iadecola, C., *Regulation of the cerebral microcirculation during neural activity: is nitric oxide the missing link?* Trends Neurosci, 1993. 16(6): p. 206-14.
[43] Vaucher, E. and E. Hamel, *Cholinergic basal forebrain neurons project to cortical microvessels in the rat: electron microscopic study with anterogradely transported Phaseolus vulgaris leucoagglutinin and choline acetyltransferase immunocytochemistry.* J Neurosci, 1995. 15(11): p. 7427-41.
[44] Krimer, L.S., et al., *Dopaminergic regulation of cerebral cortical microcirculation.* Nat Neurosci, 1998. 1(4): p. 286-9.
[45] Reinhard, J.F., Jr., et al., *Serotonin neurons project to small blood vessels in the brain.* Science, 1979. 206(4414): p. 85-7.
[46] Zonta, M., et al., *Neuron-to-astrocyte signaling is central to the dynamic control of brain microcirculation.* Nat Neurosci, 2003. 6(1): p. 43-50.
[47] Illes, J., M.P. Kirschen, and J.D. Gabrieli, *From neuroimaging to neuroethics.* Nat Neurosci, 2003. 6(3): p. 205.
[48] Phelps, M.E., et al., *Application of annihilation coincidence detection to transaxial reconstruction tomography.* J Nucl Med, 1975. 16(3): p. 210-24.
[49] Sokoloff, L., et al., *The [14C]deoxyglucose method for the measurement of local cerebral glucose utilization: theory, procedure, and normal values in the conscious and anesthetized albino rat.* J Neurochem, 1977. 28(5): p. 897-916.
[50] Middleton, H., et al., *MR imaging with hyperpolarized 3He gas.* Magn Reson Med, 1995. 33(2): p. 271-5.
[51] Shulman, R.G., F. Hyder, and D.L. Rothman, *Biophysical basis of brain activity: implications for neuroimaging.* Q Rev Biophys, 2002. 35(3): p. 287-325.
[52] Constantinidis, I., *MRS methodology.* Adv Neurol, 2000. 83: p. 235-46.
[53] Mair, R.W., et al., *Reduced xenon diffusion for quantitative lung study--the role of SF(6).* NMR Biomed, 2000. 13(4): p. 229-33.
[54] Damadian, R., M. Goldsmith, and L. Minkoff, *NMR in cancer: XVI. FONAR image of the live human body.* Physiol Chem Phys, 1977. 9(1): p. 97-100, 108.
[55] Belliveau, J.W., et al., *Functional mapping of the human visual cortex by magnetic resonance imaging.* Science, 1991. 254(5032): p. 716-9.

[56] Belliveau, J.W., et al., *Functional cerebral imaging by susceptibility-contrast NMR.* Magn Reson Med, 1990. 14(3): p. 538-46.
[57] Rosen, B.R., et al., *Contrast agents and cerebral hemodynamics.* Magn Reson Med, 1991. 19(2): p. 285-92.
[58] Ogawa, S., et al., *Brain magnetic resonance imaging with contrast dependent on blood oxygenation.* Proc Natl Acad Sci U S A, 1990. 87(24): p. 9868-72.
[59] Bandettini, P.A., et al., *Time course EPI of human brain function during task activation.* Magn Reson Med, 1992. 25(2): p. 390-7.
[60] Kwong, K.K., et al., *Dynamic magnetic resonance imaging of human brain activity during primary sensory stimulation.* Proc Natl Acad Sci U S A, 1992. 89(12): p. 5675-9.
[61] Ogawa, S., et al., *Intrinsic signal changes accompanying sensory stimulation: functional brain mapping with magnetic resonance imaging.* Proc Natl Acad Sci U S A, 1992. 89(13): p. 5951-5.
[62] Logothetis, N., *Can current fMRI techniques reveal the micro-architecture of cortex?* Nat Neurosci, 2000. 3(5): p. 413-4.
[63] Duong, T.Q., et al., *Localized cerebral blood flow response at submillimeter columnar resolution.* Proc Natl Acad Sci U S A, 2001. 98(19): p. 10904-9.
[64] Kim, S.G., *Quantification of relative cerebral blood flow change by flow-sensitive alternating inversion recovery (FAIR) technique: application to functional mapping.* Magn Reson Med, 1995. 34(3): p. 293-301.
[65] Kim, S.G. and K. Ugurbil, *Functional magnetic resonance imaging of the human brain.* J Neurosci Methods, 1997. 74(2): p. 229-43.
[66] Sharma, R., et al., *Safety profile of ultrasmall superparamagnetic iron oxide ferumoxtran-10: phase II clinical trial data.* J Magn Reson Imaging, 1999. 9(2): p. 291-4.
[67] Hill, D.K. and R.D. Keynes, *Opacity changes in stimulated nerve.* J Physiol, 1949. 108(3): p. 278-81.
[68] Blood, A.J., S.M. Narayan, and A.W. Toga, *Stimulus parameters influence characteristics of optical intrinsic signal responses in somatosensory cortex.* J Cereb Blood Flow Metab, 1995. 15(6): p. 1109-21.
[69] Blood, A.J. and A.W. Toga, *Optical intrinsic signal imaging responses are modulated in rodent somatosensory cortex during simultaneous whisker and forelimb stimulation.* J Cereb Blood Flow Metab, 1998. 18(9): p. 968-77.
[70] Cannestra, A.F., et al., *Topographical and temporal specificity of human intraoperative optical intrinsic signals.* Neuroreport, 1998. 9(11): p. 2557-63.
[71] Mayhew, J., et al., *Spectroscopic analysis of changes in remitted illumination: the response to increased neural activity in brain.* Neuroimage, 1999. 10(3 Pt 1): p. 304-26.
[72] Bonhoeffer, T. and A. Grinvald, *Iso-orientation domains in cat visual cortex are arranged in pinwheel-like patterns.* Nature, 1991. 353(6343): p. 429-31.
[73] Shmuel, A. and A. Grinvald, *Coexistence of linear zones and pinwheels within orientation maps in cat visual cortex.* Proc Natl Acad Sci U S A, 2000. 97(10): p. 5568-73.
[74] Dinse, H.R., et al., *Optical imaging of cat auditory cortex cochleotopic selectivity evoked by acute electrical stimulation of a multi-channel cochlear implant.* Eur J Neurosci, 1997. 9(1): p. 113-9.
[75] Dinse, H.R., et al., *Optical imaging of cat auditory cortical organization after electrical stimulation of a multichannel cochlear implant: differential effects of acute and chronic stimulation.* Am J Otol, 1997. 18(6 Suppl): p. S17-8.

[76] Polley, D.B., C.H. Chen-Bee, and R.D. Frostig, *Two directions of plasticity in the sensory-deprived adult cortex.* Neuron, 1999. 24(3): p. 623-37.

[77] O'Farrell, A.M., et al., *Characterization of optical intrinsic signals and blood volume during cortical spreading depression.* Neuroreport, 2000. 11(10): p. 2121-5.

[78] Chen, J.W., A.M. O'Farrell, and A.W. Toga, *Optical intrinsic signal imaging in a rodent seizure model.* Neurology, 2000. 55(2): p. 312-5.

[79] Schwartz, T.H. and T. Bonhoeffer, *In vivo optical mapping of epileptic foci and surround inhibition in ferret cerebral cortex.* Nat Med, 2001. 7(9): p. 1063-7.

[80] Pouratian, N., et al., *Optical imaging of bilingual cortical representations. Case report.* J Neurosurg, 2000. 93(4): p. 676-81.

[81] Haglund, M.M., G.A. Ojemann, and D.W. Hochman, *Optical imaging of epileptiform and functional activity in human cerebral cortex.* Nature, 1992. 358(6388): p. 668-71.

[82] Toga, A.W., A.F. Cannestra, and K.L. Black, *The temporal/spatial evolution of optical signals in human cortex.* Cereb Cortex, 1995. 5(6): p. 561-5.

[83] Cannestra, A.F., et al., *Temporal and topographical characterization of language cortices using intraoperative optical intrinsic signals.* Neuroimage, 2000. 12(1): p. 41-54.

[84] Frostig, R.D., et al., *Cortical functional architecture and local coupling between neuronal activity and the microcirculation revealed by in vivo high-resolution optical imaging of intrinsic signals.* Proc Natl Acad Sci U S A, 1990. 87(16): p. 6082-6.

[85] Grinvald, A., *Optical imaging of architecture and function in the living brain sheds new light on cortical mechanisms underlying visual perception.* Brain Topogr, 1992. 5(2): p. 71-5.

[86] Narayan, S.M., et al., *Functional increases in cerebral blood volume over somatosensory cortex.* J Cereb Blood Flow Metab, 1995. 15(5): p. 754-65.

[87] Hodge, C.J., Jr., et al., *Identification of functioning cortex using cortical optical imaging.* Neurosurgery, 1997. 41(5): p. 1137-44; discussion 1144-5.

[88] Grinvald, A., et al., *High-resolution optical imaging of functional brain architecture in the awake monkey.* Proc Natl Acad Sci U S A, 1991. 88(24): p. 11559-63.

[89] Cannestra, A.F., et al., *The evolution of optical signals in human and rodent cortex.* Neuroimage, 1996. 3(3 Pt 1): p. 202-8.

[90] Cannestra, A.F., et al., *Temporal spatial differences observed by functional MRI and human intraoperative optical imaging.* Cereb Cortex, 2001. 11(8): p. 773-82.

[91] Cannestra, A.F., et al., *Refractory periods observed by intrinsic signal and fluorescent dye imaging.* J Neurophysiol, 1998. 80(3): p. 1522-32.

[92] Chen-Bee, C.H., et al., *Visualizing and quantifying evoked cortical activity assessed with intrinsic signal imaging.* J Neurosci Methods, 2000. 97(2): p. 157-73.

[93] Chen-Bee, C.H., et al., *Areal extent quantification of functional representations using intrinsic signal optical imaging.* J Neurosci Methods, 1996. 68(1): p. 27-37.

[94] Fukunishi, K. and N. Murai, *Temporal coding in the guinea-pig auditory cortex as revealed by optical imaging and its pattern-time-series analysis.* Biol Cybern, 1995. 72(6): p. 463-73.

[95] Masino, S.A., et al., *Characterization of functional organization within rat barrel cortex using intrinsic signal optical imaging through a thinned skull.* Proc Natl Acad Sci U S A, 1993. 90(21): p. 9998-10002.

[96] Narayan, S.M., et al., *Imaging optical reflectance in rodent barrel and forelimb sensory cortex.* Neuroimage, 1994. 1(3): p. 181-90.

[97] Narayan, S.M., E.M. Santori, and A.W. Toga, *Mapping functional activity in rodent cortex using optical intrinsic signals.* Cereb Cortex, 1994. 4(2): p. 195-204.

[98] Chen-Bee, C.H. and R.D. Frostig, *Variability and interhemispheric asymmetry of single-whisker functional representations in rat barrel cortex.* J Neurophysiol, 1996. 76(2): p. 884-94.
[99] Godde, B., et al., *Optical imaging of rat somatosensory cortex reveals representational overlap as topographic principle.* Neuroreport, 1995. 7(1): p. 24-8.
[100] Masino, S.A. and R.D. Frostig, *Quantitative long-term imaging of the functional representation of a whisker in rat barrel cortex.* Proc Natl Acad Sci U S A, 1996. 93(10): p. 4942-7.
[101] Pouratian, N., et al., *Intraoperative optical intrinsic signal imaging: a clinical tool for functional brain mapping.* Neurosurg Focus, 2002. 13(4): p. e1.
[102] Pouratian, N., et al., *Shedding light on brain mapping: advances in human optical imaging.* Trends Neurosci, 2003. 26(5): p. 277-82.
[103] Penfield, W. and K. Welch, *The supplementary motor area of the cerebral cortex; a clinical and experimental study.* AMA Arch Neurol Psychiatry, 1951. 66(3): p. 289-317.
[104] Wilson, C.L. and J. Engel, Jr., *Electrical stimulation of the human epileptic limbic cortex.* Adv Neurol, 1993. 63: p. 103-13.
[105] Ojemann, G.A., *Functional mapping of cortical language areas in adults. Intraoperative approaches.* Adv Neurol, 1993. 63: p. 155-63.
[106] Haglund, M.M., et al., *Cortical localization of temporal lobe language sites in patients with gliomas.* Neurosurgery, 1994. 34(4): p. 567-76; discussion 576.
[107] Haglund, M.M., et al., *Enhanced optical imaging of rat gliomas and tumor margins.* Neurosurgery, 1994. 35(5): p. 930-40; discussion 940-1.
[108] Stummer, W., et al., *Intraoperative detection of malignant gliomas by 5-aminolevulinic acid-induced porphyrin fluorescence.* Neurosurgery, 1998. 42(3): p. 518-25; discussion 525-6.
[109] Maurer, C.R., Jr., et al., *Investigation of intraoperative brain deformation using a 1.5-T interventional MR system: preliminary results.* IEEE Trans Med Imaging, 1998. 17(5): p. 817-25.
[110] Baumann, S.B., et al., *Comparison of functional magnetic resonance imaging with positron emission tomography and magnetoencephalography to identify the motor cortex in a patient with an arteriovenous malformation.* J Image Guid Surg, 1995. 1(4): p. 191-7.
[111] Leblanc, R. and E. Meyer, *Functional PET scanning in the assessment of cerebral arteriovenous malformations. Case report.* J Neurosurg, 1990. 73(4): p. 615-9.
[112] Maldjian, J., et al., *Functional magnetic resonance imaging of regional brain activity in patients with intracerebral arteriovenous malformations before surgical or endovascular therapy.* J Neurosurg, 1996. 84(3): p. 477-83.
[113] Delpy, D.T., et al., *Estimation of optical pathlength through tissue from direct time of flight measurement.* Phys Med Biol, 1988. 33(12): p. 1433-42.
[114] Sato, C., M. Nemoto, and M. Tamura, *Reassessment of activity-related optical signals in somatosensory cortex by an algorithm with wavelength-dependent path length.* Jpn J Physiol, 2002. 52(3): p. 301-12.
[115] Sato, K., et al., *Intraoperative intrinsic optical imaging of neuronal activity from subdivisions of the human primary somatosensory cortex.* Cereb Cortex, 2002. 12(3): p. 269-80.
[116] Jobsis, F.F., *Noninvasive, infrared monitoring of cerebral and myocardial oxygen sufficiency and circulatory parameters.* Science, 1977. 198(4323): p. 1264-7.

[117] Cope, M. and D.T. Delpy, *System for long-term measurement of cerebral blood and tissue oxygenation on newborn infants by near infra-red transillumination.* Med Biol Eng Comput, 1988. 26(3): p. 289-94.

[118] Obrig, H. and A. Villringer, *Beyond the visible--imaging the human brain with light.* J Cereb Blood Flow Metab, 2003. 23(1): p. 1-18.

[119] Chance, B., et al., *Comparison of time-resolved and -unresolved measurements of deoxyhemoglobin in brain.* Proc Natl Acad Sci U S A, 1988. 85(14): p. 4971-5.

[120] Fantini, S., et al., *Non-invasive optical monitoring of the newborn piglet brain using continuous-wave and frequency-domain spectroscopy.* Phys Med Biol, 1999. 44(6): p. 1543-63.

[121] Tsuchiya, Y., *Photon path distribution and optical responses of turbid media: theoretical analysis based on the microscopic Beer-Lambert law.* Phys Med Biol, 2001. 46(8): p. 2067-84.

[122] Firbank, M., et al., *Experimental and theoretical comparison of NIR spectroscopy measurements of cerebral hemoglobin changes.* J Appl Physiol, 1998. 85(5): p. 1915-21.

[123] van der Zee, P., et al., *Experimentally measured optical pathlengths for the adult head, calf and forearm and the head of the newborn infant as a function of inter optode spacing.* Adv Exp Med Biol, 1992. 316: p. 143-53.

[124] Hoshi, Y. and S.J. Chen, *Regional cerebral blood flow changes associated with emotions in children.* Pediatr Neurol, 2002. 27(4): p. 275-81.

[125] Adcock, L.M., et al., *Neonatal intensive care applications of near-infrared spectroscopy.* Clin Perinatol, 1999. 26(4): p. 893-903, ix.

[126] Hopton, P., T.S. Walsh, and A. Lee, *CBF in adults using near infrared spectroscopy (NIRS): potential for bedside measurement?* Br J Anaesth, 1996. 77(1): p. 131.

[127] Sokol, D.K., et al., *Near infrared spectroscopy (NIRS) distinguishes seizure types.* Seizure, 2000. 9(5): p. 323-7.

[128] Soul, J.S. and A.J. du Plessis, *New technologies in pediatric neurology. Near-infrared spectroscopy.* Semin Pediatr Neurol, 1999. 6(2): p. 101-10.

[129] Boas, D.A., et al., *The accuracy of near infrared spectroscopy and imaging during focal changes in cerebral hemodynamics.* Neuroimage, 2001. 13(1): p. 76-90.

[130] Hess, A., et al., *New insights into the hemodynamic blood oxygenation level-dependent response through combination of functional magnetic resonance imaging and optical recording in gerbil barrel cortex.* J Neurosci, 2000. 20(9): p. 3328-38.

[131] Pouratian, N., et al., *Spatial/temporal correlation of BOLD and optical intrinsic signals in humans.* Magn Reson Med, 2002. 47(4): p. 766-76.

[132] Paley, M., et al., *Design and initial evaluation of a low-cost 3-Tesla research system for combined optical and functional MR imaging with interventional capability.* J Magn Reson Imaging, 2001. 13(1): p. 87-92.

6

Functional Holography and Cliques in Brain Activation Patterns

Yael Jacob[1,2,3], David Papo[1,4], Talma Hendler[1,2] and Eshel Ben-Jacob[3,5]
[1]*The Sackler School of Medicine, Tel Aviv University, Tel Aviv,*
[2]*Functional Brain Imaging Unit, Wohl Institute for Advanced Imaging, Tel Aviv Sourasky Medical Center, Tel Aviv ,*
[3]*School of Physics and Astronomy, Tel Aviv University, Tel Aviv,*
[4]*Center for Biomedical Technology, Universidad Politécnica de Madrid, Pozuelo de Alarcón, Madrid,*
[5]*The Center for Theoretical and Biological Physics, University of California San Diego, La Jolla, California*
[1,2,3]*Israel*
[4]*Spain*
[5]*USA*

1. Introduction

The brain is a complex spatially extended biological system, where a great number of neurons (~10^{11}) interact to carry out extremely sophisticated tasks. Alongside a well-established tradition of studies of single neuron activity, a wealth of neuroimaging techniques has been developed where brain activity at various spatial scales is observed in terms of multichannel recordings of the dynamics of its components.

Early neuroimaging studies of brain activity mainly focused on the functional specialization of segregated brain modules. The main concern of these studies was that of finding which brain areas change their activity as subjects carry out well-controlled tasks. A robust statistical underpinning for the quantitative analysis of results was offered by the general linear model and Gaussian field theory (Worsley & Friston, 1995), which allowed delineating a collection of significant cortical *activations* and *deactivations* associated with the execution of these tasks. From a computational point of view, this general univariate framework treated the brain as a collection of independent brain regions.

While the brain developed largely segregated modules, communication between and within these modules is essential to the transfer and processing of information. Accordingly, neuroimaging studies started incorporating the idea that the neural activity associated with the execution of given cognitive tasks is indeed diffuse, and that the influence that one brain region exerts over the others cannot be neglected. As a consequence, over the past few years, the neuroimaging literature has seen a shift towards a focus on measures of functional integration of brain activity. Many methods were developed to estimate functional and effective connectivity (Friston, 1994). These methods were designed to investigate how a generally rather small set of brain areas interact, and how different experimental manipulations may affect their mutual relationships (Friston et al., 1997). More or less coarse-grained brain regions are identified with the nodes of a network, while some metric of brain coupling between these regions is identified with an edge between these nodes. Prominent among these methods are *data-driven* methods such as Independent component analysis (ICA) (McKeown et al., 1998), Fuzzy Clustering Analysis (FCA) (Windischberger et al., 2003), Temporal Clustering Analysis (TCA) (Zhao et al., 2007), and autoregressive models such as the Granger Causal Mapping (GCM) (Goebel et al., 2003) and *model-driven* dynamical models expressed in dynamic causal modeling (DCM) (Friston et al., 2003). The former set of methods started exploiting the inherent multivariate and stochastic nature of fMRI data. Model-driven approaches, on the other hand, used causal influences among neural sources to produce an explicit computational model generating the observed signal. This method improved on early methods by incorporating an explicit temporal component into effective connectivity estimation (Penny et al., 2004). The main merits of these methods were that of making explicit the spatially non-local nature of task-related brain activity, and of adding to it a (rather coarse) temporal dimension. However, these methods are typically limited in the number of regions they can incorporate. Furthermore, while these methods incorporate the idea that correlations among neuronal assemblies play an important role in brain activity (Segev et al., 2004), no clear distinction between information processing and information transfer is made, and the output is essentially a flow-chart of communication between nodes. As a consequence, the meaningfulness of the networks that are delineated boils down to the combined functional properties attributed to the segregated brain regions that are identified with the network nodes, but it is unrelated to some general property of the network *per se*. This in turn implies, among other things, that no clear relationship exists between brain anatomy, the structure of functional networks of brain activity and the dynamics taking place on them.

While single region activity can be characterized in a straightforward way through time-varying profiles of amplitudes of some aspect of brain activity, network activity needs appropriate non-trivial observables to be defined. Graph theory (Boccaletti et al., 2006) offers a convenient and flexible way to analyze topological properties of systems with a network organization (Bullmore et al., 2009). Most importantly for neuroscientists, graph theory can be used to understand the complex relationship between structure, dynamics and function in the brain. Graph theory shows that the topology of structural networks influences the dynamical processes (namely synchronization) taking place on them (Boccaletti et al., 2006). For instance, small-world properties of dense or clustered local connectivity with relatively few long-range connections confer distinctive dynamical and functional properties: in addition to optimizing information processing (Strogatz, 2001), facilitating synchronization (Bucolo et al., 2003), ensuring rapid response and emergence of coherent oscillations (Lago-Fernández et al., 2000), and conferring resilience against pathological attack, small-world architecture has been shown to provide an optimum trade-off between efficiency and wiring costs, conferring high local and global efficiencies for relatively low connection costs (Latora & Marchiori, 2001).

Recently, an increasing number of neuroimaging studies using graph theoretical tools have started showing that the brain developed in such a way that a clear correspondence exists between anatomical network topology and dynamical processes taking place on it. It has been convincingly shown that brain anatomical networks have characteristically small-world properties of dense or clustered local connectivity with relatively few long-range connections (Sporns et al., 2004). Similarly, human brain functional networks associated with the execution of cognitive tasks have also been associated with fractal small-world architecture (Achard et al., 2006; Bassett et al., 2006; Eguíluz et al., 2005; Salvador et al., 2005), which support efficient parallel information transfer at relatively low costs and is differently impaired by normal aging and pharmacological manipulations (Achard & Bullmore, 2007; Bassett et al., 2009). Furthermore, specific neuroanatomical connectivity patterns are univocally associated with given functional complexity levels, and networks capable of producing highly complex functional dynamics share common structural motifs (see e.g. (Sporns et al., 2000, 2002)). Finally, simulations showed that brain dynamics exhibits a modular hierarchical organization, where clusters coincide with the topological community structure of anatomical networks (Zhou et al., 2006).

Arguably graph theory's greatest strengths is that it has made possible to address a whole range of new research questions, far exceeding the original main one addressed by neuroimaging, of localizing brain activity, particularly issues related to *how* the brain organizes its activity as it carries out tasks of arbitrary complexity. A relative limitation of graph theoretical applications, in their current form, to neuroimaging is that both computations and visualization of functional brain networks are performed based on the Euclidean coordinates of observed activity. However, it has long been known that there is no straightforward correspondence between spatial and functional proximity between brain regions, so that regions that are contiguous to each other can in fact be involved in the execution of completely different tasks. It is then of great interest to be able to represent the topology of the functional space, and ultimately to delineate the correspondence between anatomical and functional spaces.

Here we propose a new method, Functional Holography (FH), designed to describe the information content of a network as it functions as a whole unit. The term used for the familiar holograms indicates that the photographic plates can capture the whole information about the 3D image. The FH method can overcome the main limitations of previous methods by visualizing networks of correlated activity in an auxiliary space of correlations and linking the components according to similarities between them.

The main objectives of the FH method are:

1. To overcome the limitations of existing methods taking into account only a fraction of the network components.
2. To identify underlying functional motives embedded in complex spatio-temporal behavior.
3. To identify functional subgroups functional clusters and to reveal the causal relations between them.
4. To relate the observed temporal ordering activity propagation to underlying causal motives propagation of information and causal connectivity.
5. To be able to compare the activity of two different networks or different modes of behavior of the same network.

In the remainder of this chapter, we will first illustrate the mathematical procedure of the method; we will then show some applications of the method to various neurophysiological signals, and will finally conclude by discussing the scope of the FH method in the context of brain imaging data analysis.

2. Methods and applications

2.1 FH analysis

The FH method was developed from the perspective of cultured networks (Segev et al., 2004). Yet it can be applied to essentially any type of neural signal from the analysis of slices, to cortex-recorded activities, ranging from electro- or magneto-encephalographic (EEG and MEG respectively) to functional magnetic resonance imaging (fMRI) signals. Moreover, it makes it possible to place the recordings from all of these levels within the same presentation schema for comparative studies.

The FH approach allows identifying additional motifs embedded in the inter-neuron correlation matrices— analogous to the inter-location coherence matrices evaluated for ECoG recordings of brain activity (Milton & Jung, 2002; Towle et al., 1999) that are not transparent in the real space connectivity networks. The correlation matrix is represented in a higher dimensional space of functional correlations, or correlation affinities.

The FH method involves the following steps:

1. Evaluation of the similarity matrix between components.
2. Clustering by sorting or reordering of the similarity matrix.
3. Construction of a matrix of functional correlations.
4. Dimension reduction.
5. Retrieval from the correlation matrix of the information lost in the dimension reduction.
6. Inclusion of temporal causal information describing the activity propagation in the network.
7. Holographic zooming and comparison.

2.1.1 Correlation matrices

The first stage in the FH analysis is computation of the signals correlation matrices - the matrices of correlations between the dynamical responses of all pairs of signals. We used the Pearson formula (Pearson, 1901) to calculate the correlation $C(i,j)$ between signals (i) and (j):

$$C(i,j)=\frac{\sum_{k=1}^{T}\left(X(i,k)-\mu(i)\right)\left(X(j,k)-\mu(j)\right)}{\sigma(i)\sigma(j)} \tag{1}$$

where $X(i)$ and $X(j)$ are the recorded time signals (i) and (j), with corresponding means $\mu(i)$, $\mu(j)$ and standard deviations $\sigma(i)$, $\sigma(j)$.

For N signals, the pair-wise correlations define a symmetric NxN correlation matrix. In order to reveal subgroups in the correlation matrix, we make use of the commonly used dendrogram clustering algorithm (Dubes & Jain, 1980). This algorithm reorders the correlation matrix such that highly correlated signals are closely located. This is performed using the correlation distance D(i,j) between signals (i) and (j), which is the Euclidean distance between the rows i and j in the correlation matrix (the vectors of correlations of each one of the signals with all other ones)

$$D(i,j) = \left\| \vec{C}(i) - \vec{C}(j) \right\| = \sqrt{\sum_{k=1}^{N} \left(C(i,k) - C(j,k) \right)^2} \tag{2}$$

where $\vec{C}(i)$ is the correlation vector between signal (i) and all other signals. Next, the algorithm reorders the correlation matrix by sorting it according to the hierarchical tree of correlation distances. In such a way we produce a real metric that satisfies the triangle inequality. In Fig. 1 we illustrate the analysis with a simple example. We generate 25 signals to imitate a multichannel recording of the activity of a network of 25 components. The signals (Fig. 1a) include two subgroups of periodic signals with higher correlations and a group of random signals. In Fig. 1b we show the corresponding correlation matrix computed using the Pearson correlations. Applying the dendrogram clustering algorithm (Fig. 1c) on the correlation matrix, the subgroups are delineated in the resulting sorted (reordered) matrix (Fig. 1d). The correlation matrix can be associated with the *correlation space*, i.e. the N-1 dimensional space of correlations (Baruchi et al., 2006; Baruchi et al., 2004). We note that the correlation space does not represent a real space in the sense that the eigenvectors do not create an orthogonal mathematical space.

2.1.2 Collective normalization

The next step of the analysis is designed to capture mutual or relative effects between several signals. A collective normalization of the correlations (cross-correlation) is performed and an affinity matrix is computed. The affinity transformation represents a collective property of all channels, and can help capturing hidden collective motifs related to functional connectivity in the network behaviors (Baruchi et al., 2006; Baruchi et al., 2004). The affinity matrix is calculated using the meta-correlation matrix *MC(i,j)*, which is the Pearson's correlation between the rows of the reordered correlation matrix of any two components *(i)* and *(j)* as described in Eq.3. The affinity collective normalized matrix is the product of the correlation matrix and the meta-correlation matrix as defined in Eq. 4.

$$MC(i,j) = \frac{\sum_{k \neq i,j}^{N} \left(C(i,k) - \mu c(i) \right)\left(C(j,k) - \mu c(j) \right)}{\sqrt{\left\langle \hat{C}(i)^2 \right\rangle \cdot \left\langle \hat{C}(j)^2 \right\rangle}} \tag{3}$$

$$A(i,j) = \sqrt{C(i,j) \cdot MC(i,j)} \tag{4}$$

This MC matrix is calculated on the reshuffled rows of the matrix in such a way that all the elements between the signals (i) and (j) themselves are not included in the calculation. We note that the affinity transformation is performed after rescaling the range of the correlations to [0,1].

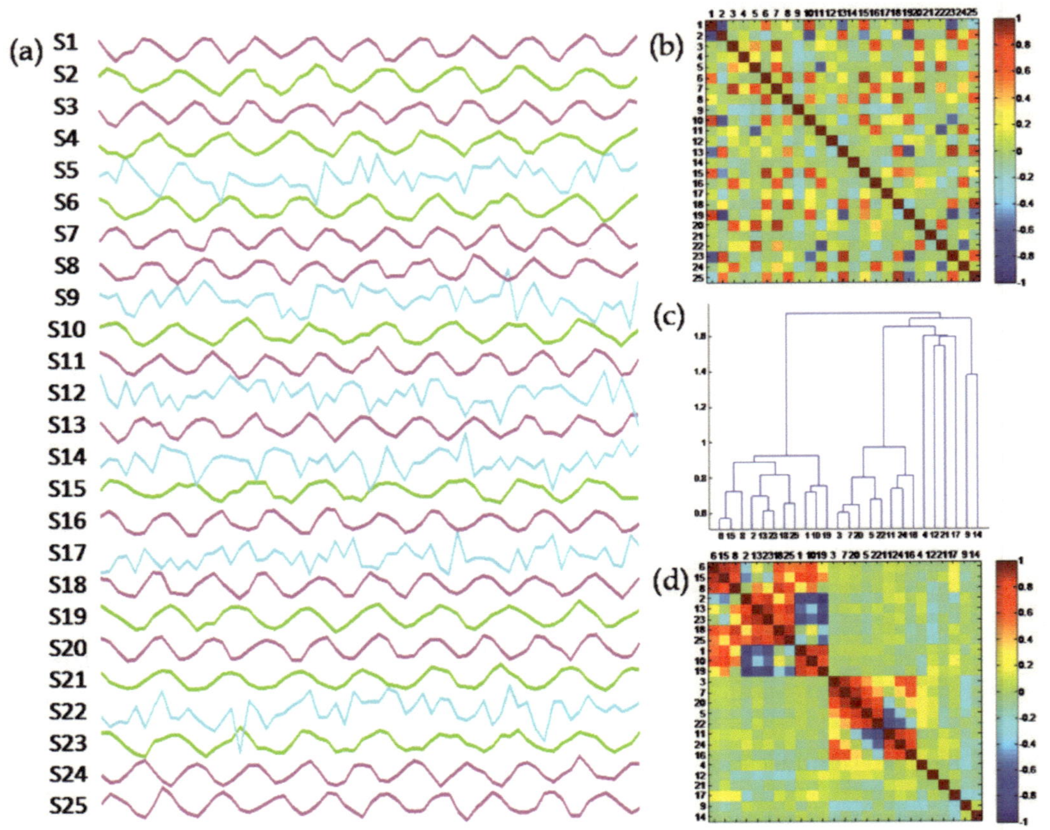

Fig. 1. Correlation matrix of synthetically produced signals. (a) Synthetic signals that include three groups—the first subgroup of nine signals (color coded in magenta) was generated by harmonic signals with the same periodicity, a phase shift of about 2π/10 and added noise. The second subgroup signals (color coded in green), is another set of harmonic signals, with a different frequency. The other signals just have pure noise with no correlations. (b) The corresponding correlation matrix that was computed using the Pearson's correlations. (c) The dendrogram tree. The vertical axis is the correlation distance between the signals (the Euclidian distance between the vectors of correlations of each signal with all the others, or the row in the correlation matrix that corresponds to the signal). Longer/shorter distances correspond to lower/higher correlations. (d) The sorted correlation matrix using the dendrogramed clustering algorithm. In this matrix the two subgroups form distinct clusters.

2.1.3 Dimension reduction and construction of the holographic networks

To search for hidden functional motifs of brain activity induced by the execution of a given task, dimension reduction of the correlation matrices is performed. Principal component analysis (PCA) a standard dimension reduction algorithm can be used to extract the maximal relevant information embedded in the signal correlation matrices. The relevant information can then be presented in a 3-dimensional principal component space (Baruchi et al., 2006; Baruchi et al., 2004) the axes of which are the three leading PCA principal vectors.

Each node is placed in this space according to its three eigenvalues for the three leading principal vectors. Reduction to three dimensions (projection on the three leading principal components) typically extracts most of the relevant information (above 85%), (Baruchi et al., 2006; Madi et al., 2008). To retrieve the information lost as a result of dimension reduction, we link each pair of nodes by lines color coded according to the correlations between them (Baruchi et al., 2006; Baruchi et al., 2004; Madi et al., 2008). The result is a holographic representation (Fig. 2) of a network (or manifold) of linked nodes in the PCA space.

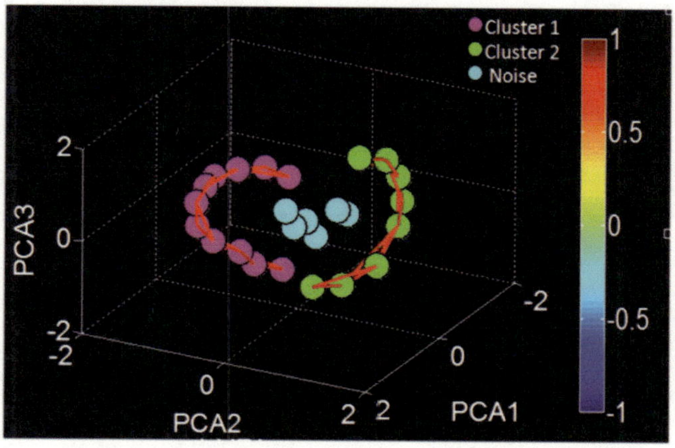

Fig. 2. Holographic representation of the synthetically produced signals from Fig.1 in the 3D space. The axes are the three leading principal PCA vectors of the correlation matrix. Each node is located in this space according to its eigenvalues corresponding to the leading principal vectors. All the nodes with correlations above 0.8 are linked by lines color coded according to the correlations (represented in the colorbar), creating the holographic manifold.

2.1.4 Holographic zooming

Often, one is interested in more details about a part of the manifold. Details cannot be extracted simply by rescaling of the axes as done, for example, when a part of a picture is magnified. The idea of the *holographic zooming* is to take advantage of the collective normalization in the following way: 1) Identifying the part of the manifold to be magnified; 2) isolating the *subsimilarity* matrix for the cluster; 3) performing a second iteration on this matrix, i.e., the affinity transformation, dimension reduction and construction of a manifold (see Fig. 3).

2.1.5 Inclusion of temporal information

An essential, though often neglected aspect of brain activity is represented by its temporal dimension. The similarity matrices, the cornerstone of the FH method exposed so far, do not include essential information about the temporal propagation of activity across the components. When available, this information can be presented in temporal ordering matrices the generic $T_{i,j}$ element of which describes the relative timing or phase difference between the activity of components i and j. Various methods can be used to evaluate the temporal ordering matrices. Recently, a new notion—the *temporal center of mass*, or temporal location was introduced in the context of cultured networks (Segev et al., 2004), but works equally well for other fast continuous neurophysiological signals, ECoG and EEG, and though with minor modifications even for relatively slow signals, viz. fMRI.

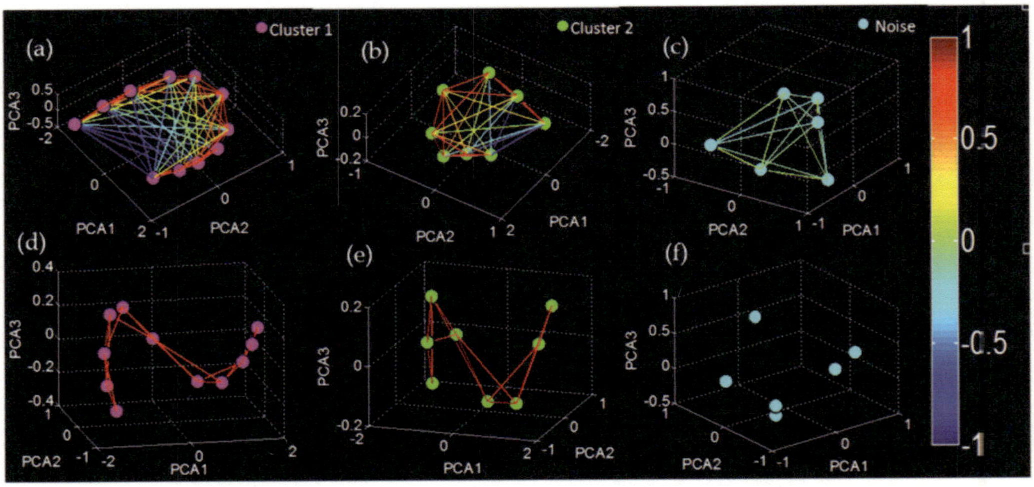

Fig. 3. Holographic zooming. The FH algorithm conducted for each cluster separately; (a) cluster 1 (b) cluster 2 (c) noise signals nodes. All the nodes are linked by lines color coded according to the correlations (represented in the colorbar), creating the holographic manifold. Note that the two clusters are highly correlated whereas the noise group has no high or low correlations between them. The FH diagrams in (d,e and f) represent the same diagrams as in (a,b and c) from a different point of view while all nodes with correlations above 0.8 are linked.

The idea is to regard the activity density of each node i as a temporal weight function so that it's temporal center of mass, T_{in}, during a synchronized bursting event (SBEs), i.e. a time segment in which most of the recorded neurons exhibit rapid firing is given by T_i

$$T_i^n = \frac{\int (t-T_n) D_t^n (t-T_n) dt}{D_t^n (t-T_n) dt} \tag{5}$$

where the integral is over the time window of the SBE, and T_n marks the temporal location of the n_{th} SBE, which is the combined "center of mass" of all the neurons. The temporal center of mass of each neuron can vary between the different SBEs. Therefore we define the relative timing of a neuron i to be $T_i = \langle T_i^n \rangle_n$ the average of the sequence of SBEs. Similarly, we define the temporal ordering matrix as follows:

$$T_{i,j} = \langle T_i^n - T_j^n \rangle \tag{6}$$

Interestingly, when the temporal information is superimposed on the 3-D space of leading PCA eigenvectors, the activity propagates along the manifold in an orderly fashion from one end to the other (Fig. 4). For this reason, it is proposed to view the resulted manifold, which includes the temporal information as a causal manifold.

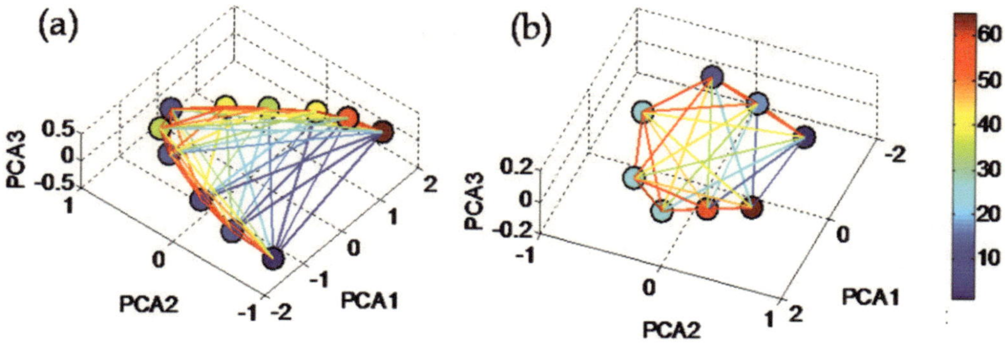

Fig. 4. Inclusion of temporal information. (a) and (b) show the inclusion of the causal information for the holographic network shown in Fig. 3a,b respectively. The activity propagation is added by coloring the nodes location according to the relative phases or time lag between them. Blue is for early time (negative phases) and red for late times (positive phases). Note that adding this information helps to reveal the phase shifts imposed in the generation of the signals.

2.1.6 Holographic comparison and superposition of networks activity

A versatile method of data analysis should also come with the ability to quantitatively assess difference between experimental conditions. Clustering algorithms are often used for comparison between the activities of different networks, e.g., gene expression in different groups of patients, or between two modes of behavior of the same network, e.g., during and between epileptic seizures of the same patient. We propose the following holographic comparison between networks: 1) Compute the PCA leading eigenvectors of the affinity matrix for each network. 2) Project the affinity matrix of each network on the leading eigenvectors of the other one. Clearly, this approach can also be used for comparison between different modes of activity of the same networks, like the above-mentioned case of brain activity in between and during seizure, or different clusters identified in a given matrix. Once the clusters are identified, the similarity matrix for each is isolated from the combined matrix and the above two stages are applied. The holographic superposition is designed as additional method for comparison between different modes of activity of the same network. The idea is similar to the holographic comparison; however, the projection is on the mutual PCA leading eigenvectors, i.e. the leading eigenvectors of a combined matrix that includes the different modes.

2.1.7 Quantifying cluster information: Cluster entropy

Once clusters of functional brain activity are singled out, it is often useful to describe them in a quantitative fashion. This in particular enables to compare different clusters within and across subjects.

Entropy has been used in statistics and information theory to develop measures of the information content of signals (Shannon, 1948). However, entropy can also be used to measure the amount of information or variance embedded in a cluster, and to quantify the deviation of the cluster's eigenvalue distribution from a uniform one (Alter et al., 2000). This idea has been used in the context of biological systems (Varshavsky et al., 2007; Varshavsky et al., 2006) and economic systems (Shapira et al., 2009). The eigenvalue entropy is defined as

$$S = -\frac{1}{\log(N)}\sum_{i=1}^{N}\Omega(i)\log\left[\Omega(i)\right] \tag{7}$$

where Ω is given by,

$$\Omega(i) = \frac{\lambda(i)^2}{\sum_{i=1}^{N}\lambda(i)^2} \tag{8}$$

N the number of signals, and $\lambda(i)$ denotes the matrix eigenvalues. S ranges from 0 to 1. Note that $1/\log(N)$ is a normalization factor ensuring that S reaches its maximum (S=1) for a uniform eigenvalue distribution (i.e. random correlations matrix).

2.1.8 Extracting topological information: MST analysis

The correlation matrix of the system creates a topological network structure, where the links between nodes are the pair-wise correlations, and the correlation coefficients as the weights of these links. Valuable information can be extracted from the topological properties of the network, over and above the mere localization in the brain volume. To extract this information, graph theoretical techniques can be applied to the data.

The graph induced by the correlation matrix is complete and therefore difficult to interpret per se. Extracting meaningful information from this complete graph involves providing a more compact description of the graph and analyzing its topological properties (e.g. (Newman, 2003; Tumminello et al., 2007). A graph and its connectivity can be synthetically described by its minimum spanning tree (MST) (West, 2001), i.e. a connected, undirected graph composed of subgroups of edges with the following two properties: I) The tree spans the graph, i.e. connects all the nodes of the graph. The number of links retained is (n − 1) for a network of (n) nodes. II) The sum of the edges' weights is minimal out of all possible spanning trees. The MST creates a subgraph without loops, maintains the connection of all nodes, using only the links with minimal weight.

The topological structure of the constructed tree creates a new visualization of the complex system, which allows visually tracking clusters of nodes, as well as structural similarities and differences of the system under different conditions. Other graph properties, such as node degree, node centrality and betweenness can be used to extract information from the tree (Newman, 2003; Tumminello et al., 2007; West, 2001).

The MST can be constructed based of the correlation matrix (i.e. the correlation based system) obtained by the FH algorithm. Plotting the MST upon the PCA affinity space and on the anatomical slice image enables us to monitor the dynamical changes of the selected voxels and the tree they create (their connections) over the entire time course of the experiment.

The MST method requires assigning weights to the links between the nodes. The weights are assigned according to the affinity matrix. A commonly used distance transformation is the ultrametric distance, suggested by Rammal et al. (1986) (Rammal et al., 1986) and Mantegna et al. (2000) (Mantegna & Stanley, 2000). Using this distance, the pairwise correlation coefficient for each pair of nodes is translated into the distance between those two nodes. The ultrametric distance is *UD(i,j)* given by

$$UD(i,j) = \sqrt{2\cdot(1 - C(i,j))} \tag{9}$$

where *C(i,j)* is the correlation coefficient between nodes *i* and *j*. This distance metric satisfies the ultrametric inequality, (I) $UD(i,j) = 0$ if and only if $i = j$, (II) $UD(i,j) = UD(j,i)$, (III) $UD(i,j) \leq \text{Max}\{UD(i,k), UD(k,j)\}$.

The result of the ultrametric transformation is that strong positive correlations are translated into short distances, and strong negative correlations are translated into long distances. For the case of perfect positive correlation, i.e. $C(i,j) = 1$, the distance is 0; for the case of no correlation, i.e. $C(i,j) = 0.5$, the distance is 1; and for the case of perfect negative correlation, i.e. $C(i,j) = 0$, the distance is $\sqrt{2}$. The ultrametric distance matrix describes the complete network´s topological structure that yields no significant information (West, 2001). To construct the MST, the Kruskal algorithm (Kruskal, 1956) can be applied. This algorithm is considered greedy, as it runs in polynomial time (this problem however is not particularly severe if the networks have about 300 nodes, which renders the problem computable), and in each phase some local optimum is chosen. Fig. 5 demonstrates the use of the Kruskal algorithm to find the MST for a complete graph.

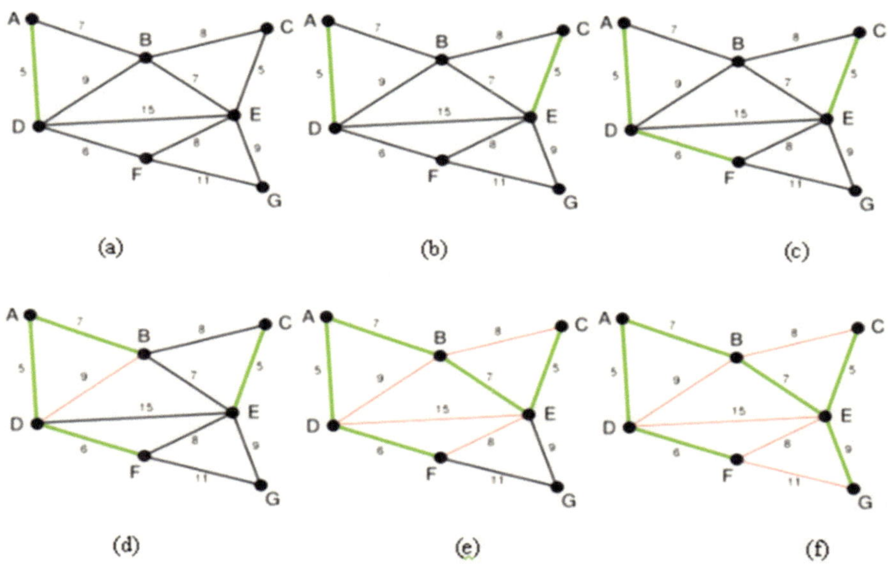

Fig. 5. An example of how the Kruskal algorithm can be used in order to find the minimal spanning tree from the complete graph. (a) Original graph. The numbers near the links indicate their weight. AD and CE are the shortest links, with length 5, and AD highlighted to indicate that it has been arbitrarily chosen. (b) CE is now the shortest link with length 5, which does not form a cycle, so it is highlighted as the second link. (c) The next

link, DF with length 6, is highlighted using the same method. (d) The next-shortest links are AB and BE, both with length 7. AB is chosen arbitrarily, and is highlighted. The link BD cannot be chosen as it would form a cycle (ABD) and has therefore been marked in red. (e) The process continues to highlight the next-smallest link, BE with length 7. Many more links are highlighted in red at this stage: BC because it would form the loop BCE, DE because it would form the loop DEBA, and FE because it would form FEBAD. (f) Finally, the process finishes with the link EG, of length 9, and the minimum spanning tree is found.

The MST analysis can be used in combination with FH analysis. The FH analysis performs the aforementioned PCA dimension reduction algorithm creating a visualization of this complex network. The nodes in the reduced 3D space are then linked according to the MST connections, with lines color coded according to their original correlations. These lines create a topological MST manifold upon the 3D correlations space (see figs. 11 and 14 in section 2.2.2). This MST manifold is displayed on the brain slice image in the same way as that of the FH, thus providing information about connectivity on the real space (see figs. 12 and 15 in section 2.2.2).

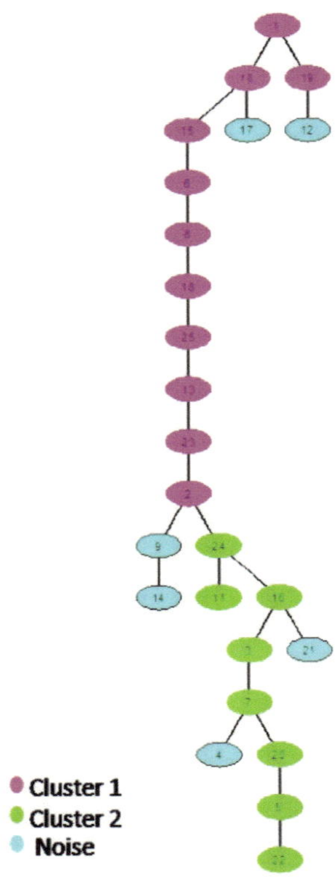

Fig. 6. The MST representation of the synthetically produced signals from Fig.1. The magenta and green colors represent clusters 1 and 2 respectively, and the cyan color represents the noise signals.

2.1.9 Dissimilarity measure for MSTs

The MST can conveniently be used to quantify similarities between different networks of brain activity. This can be done by resorting to the divergence rate measure developed by

Lee et al. (Lee et al., 2006). This measure is based on the information metric d(X,Y), which quantifies the conditional entropies (or the difference) between two information sources,

$$d(X,Y) = H(X\,|\,Y) + H(Y\,|\,X)\,, \tag{10}$$

where H(X|Y) and H(Y|X) are the conditional entropies between sources X and Y. This metric satisfies the triangle inequality. The conditional entropy H(X|Y) denotes the amount of information that is obtained by measuring an information source Y with the knowledge of a different source X. The information gain can be approximated by the information change between two different sources. The source X is transformed into the Y source space by the transformation Y=f(X). The average information change by the transformation is defined as

$$\overline{\Delta H} = \frac{1}{N}\sum_{i=1}^{N} \ln\left|\frac{\Delta f(x_i)}{\Delta x_i}\right|, \tag{11}$$

where N is the number of elements of an information source.

The divergence rate can be defined as an approximation of the average information change in order to apply it between two MSTs,

$$D(Y\,|\,X) = \frac{1}{N}\sum_{i=1}^{N} \log_{10}\left|\frac{D(Y\,|\,X)_{(i)}}{D(X)_{(i)}}\right|. \tag{12}$$

Where $D(X)_{(i)}$ is the sum of all distances taken from a reference node i to the neighboring nodes in the XMST, and $D(X\,|\,Y)_{(i)}$ is the sum of all distances taken from the node i to the nodes in the YMST. Given the distances between node i to its neighbors in the XMST, $D(Y\,|\,X)_{(i)}$ evaluates how much the distance changed in the YMST. Note that the number of neighboring nodes for every reference node is different. This measure evaluates how much information is needed on average to explain YMST, given XMST. Then, to quantify the dissimilarity between two MSTs the metric distance is given by,

$$D(X,Y) = D(Y\,|\,X) + D(X\,|\,Y) \tag{13}$$

If the MSTs are identical, $D(X,Y) = 0$, otherwise $D(X,Y) > 0$. Subgroups in the metric distance can then be delineated using the dendrogram clustering algorithm.

2.2 Applications

2.2.1 Analyzing ECoG recorded human brain activity

The occurrence of epilepsy is rising and is estimated to affect, at some level, 1% - 2% of the world population (Towle et al., 2002). Due to availability of many antiepileptic drugs, approximately 80% of all epileptic patients can be kept seizure free. But for the remaining 20%, the only cure is surgical resection of the seizure focus (Chkhenkeli et al., 1998; Doyle & Spencer, 1998). One of the most challenging tasks facing epileptologists is precise identification of brain areas to be removed so that the problem can be cured with minimal damage and side effects. Often, the precise location of the epileptogenic region remains uncertain after obtaining conventional, noninvasive measurements such as electroencephalogram (EEG) and magnetoencephalogram (MEG) cannot provide sufficient information because of the relatively low spatial resolution of these methods. In these cases, the activity is directly recorded by the electrocorticography (ECoG) procedure in which the recording electrodes are placed directly on the brain surface.

Here we illustrate how the FH method can be applied to reveal the existence of hidden causal manifolds in the electrical brain activity of epileptic patients with implanted electrodes. We note that the method can also be applied to experimental seizure studies that have gained much attention (Ben-Jacob et al., 2007). Typical results are presented in Fig. 7.

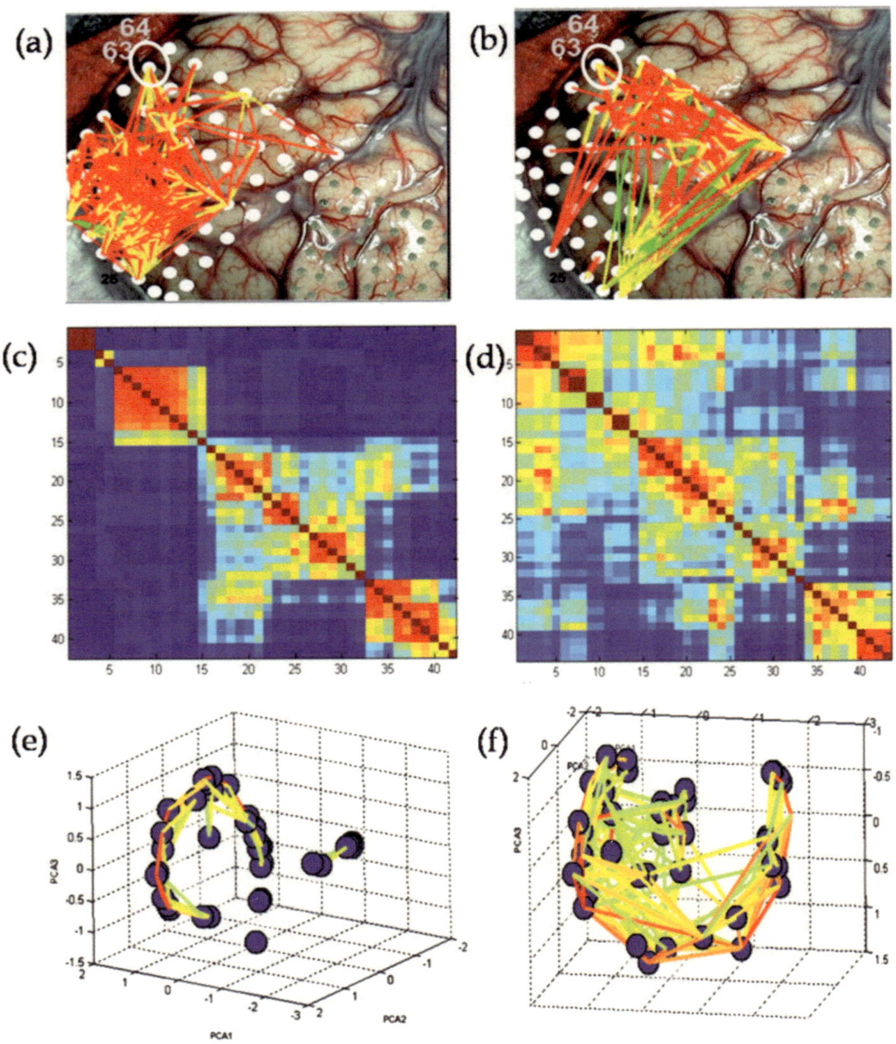

Fig. 7. Holographic networks of recorded brain activity. The holographic networks are for the ECoG recorded human brain activity for the inter-Ictal and Ictal activities. (a) and (b) show the connectivity diagram for the inter-Ictal and Ictal respectively, constructed upon the set of electrodes placed on the surface of the brain (the frontal lobe in this case). (c) and

(d) show the corresponding dendrogram correlation matrices. (e) and (f) show the corresponding FH manifolds in the PCA affinity space. In the analysis we included only electrodes whose correlations with the other electrodes are above noise level. Note, that the locations change their functional role during seizure (Ictal) relative to those during the inter-Ictal durations.

Notably, the manifold of the inter-ictal activity has a very simple topology of almost circular horseshoe like part and another subgroup perpendicular to its plane and position at the center of the horseshoe. Although the new manifold has as expected a more complex topology, it retains some of the features of the one associated with inter-Ictal activity, when viewed from specific angle. Preliminary analyses also indicate that causal features are captured when the temporal (i.e., phase coherences) information is imposed on the manifolds. These results bear the promise that functional holography might become a valuable diagnostic procedure in the treatment of intractable epilepsy.

2.2.2 Analyzing fMRI recorded human brain activity

When applied to fMRI data, FH is an effective clustering method, capable of capturing system level networks using voxel-voxel correlation matrices (Jacob et al., 2010). Here we show how the algorithm using a dendrogram clustering method combined with a standard deviation (STD) filter can effectively be used to identify and extract voxel clusters. Subjects were instructed to clench and open either their left or right hand, according to an auditory cue. The paradigm consisted of 11 blocks of 114 volumes. Each consisted of a resting period with cross fixation (6–15 s), an auditory instruction period regarding hand movement (right or left; 3 s), and a period of hand movement execution (15 s). The blocks were presented in a constant order across subjects with regard to which hand to move. Two types of sequences were examined: *repetitive* (two consecutive movements of the same hand) and *alternating* hand movements.

Even for this simple hand clenching motor task, the FH analysis conducted for a single block revealed interesting motifs. For example, unilateral hand movement yielded two clusters, one located in the contralateral primary motor cortex showing increased signal (i.e. activation), and the other one in the ipsilateral homologue region, showing reduced signal (i.e. deactivation) (Fig. 8). Inspection of repetitive vs. alternating hand movements suggested that this pattern could be indicative of an inhibition mechanism of the ipsilateral hemisphere. In addition, a single-block level analysis, using only 12 time points corresponding to a 36 second recording session, was enough to determine which hand was moved by the subject, while other methods required the entire experiment time course. Moreover, cluster quantification based on eigenvalue entropy showed lower entropy for the motor-dominant hemisphere clusters. This lower entropy demonstrates less variability in the cluster's correlations, suggesting a higher modular organization in specific motor dominant hemisphere.

The MST was extracted for each subject and each block. The divergence rate measure was used for quantification of the structural similarities and differences of the system under the two different conditions of right or left hand movement. Fig. 9 displays examples of the dendrograms constructed from the divergence rate measure. Each dendrogram represents the distance, i.e. the divergence rate measure or similarity between all pairwise MSTs of the experiment's different blocks. Half of the subjects exhibited good separation between right and left hand movement MSTs (e.g. Fig. 9a), displaying clusters of 3-4 same hand movement trees. The other half of the subjects did not yield such good separation (e.g. Fig. 9b). Fig. 10 depicts the MSTs for a single subject that showed good separation. To elucidate the functional and structural meaning of the MST, the tree's nodes were colored according to their location in the brain; the red and blue colors represent voxels in the right and left hemisphere respectively, while yellow represents the midline SMA region. All the resulting MSTs showed two distinct clusters, one dominated by the right (red) and one by the left hemisphere (blue). The interesting result is that this representation highlights for all blocks a few red voxels in the blue cluster and blue ones in the red cluster, these voxels are the same in every block.

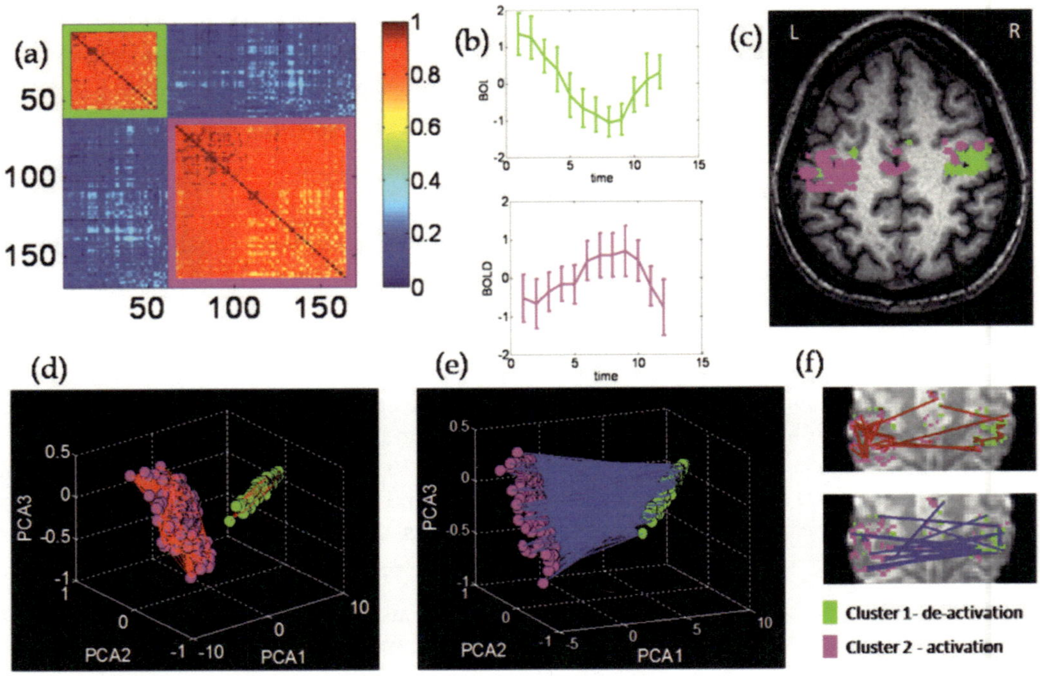

Fig. 8. FH applied on fMRI data. Presented here is an example of the results of a right-handed single subject, for a right hand movement block (12 TRs). (a) The correlation matrix shows a pattern of two dominant distinguished clusters. (b) The magenta cluster averaged BOLD signal demonstrated clear activation, whereas the green cluster showed deactivation. (c) The magenta activation cluster was located at the left hemisphere in the M1 region and, as expected. The second green cluster was located in the M1 region of the ipsihemisphere. (d) and (e) show the holographic presentations of the voxels or the holographic networks while the voxels with correlations above 0.8 are linked in (d) and voxels with correlations below -0.4 are linked in (e). (f) Displays the corresponding holographic networks on the brain slice image for correlations with a specific range of 0.98-0.99 and (-0.9)–(-1.0).

To further investigate whether the two groups of subjects as obtained by the divergence rate measure, differed in terms of topological structure of their functional networks of correlated activity, the MST was used in combination with the FH visualization. The MST constructed for every single block shows a good separation between the hemispheres. For half of the subjects, the divergence rate measure allowed to partition the MSTs into two clusters of right and left hand movements. Figs.11-15 depicts the MSTs on the FH correlation PCA space, and on the anatomical brain slice image of a single subject that showed a good separation between right and left hand movements (Figs.11-12). A single subject who did not yield a good separation is also shown (Figs.13-15). Looking at the dynamic changes of the MSTs along the experiment time course in the anatomical slice image it becomes visible that blocks of sequences of repetitive hand movements resulted in numerous connections between the clusters as opposed to the alternating hand movements' blocks. The graph in Fig. 16 displays the average Z score of the number of connections between the clusters for each block across subjects (N=15). This demonstrates that these two kinds of sequences can also be differentiated by the MST visualization.

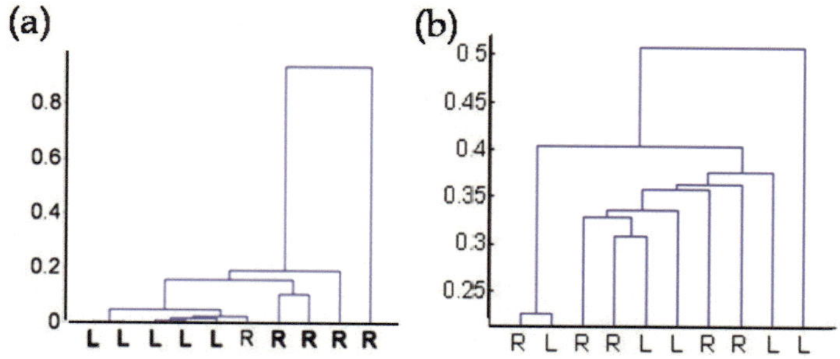

Fig. 9. Dendrograms constructed from the divergence rate measure for two different subjects. Each dendrogram represents the distances i.e. the divergence rate measure between all pair wise MSTs. The dendrogram clusters all the MSTs that show similar structure. The subjects were divided into two groups; (a) An example of a subject who's MSTs had much similarity showing clusters separating between right and left hand movement MSTs. (b) An example of a subject that showed no distinct clusters for MSTs associated with right and left hand movements.

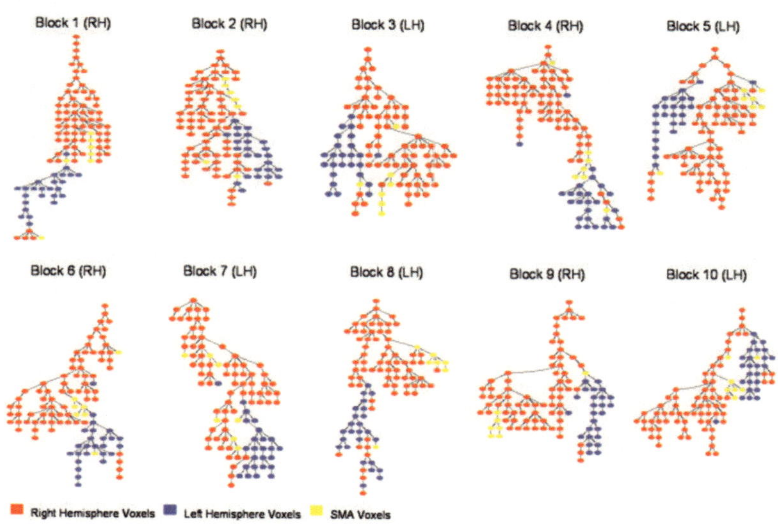

Fig. 10. Example of the MSTs constructed for a single left-handed male subject that shows a good separation in the divergence rate dendrogram. Displaying the MSTs for all the experiment's ten blocks i.e. right hand (RH) and left hand (LH) movements. The MST color

coded according to the brain anatomic structure. The red and blue colors represent the right and left hemisphere voxels respectively, and the yellow color represents the SMA area. The MSTs give a good separation between the right and left hemisphere. Note that in every MST there are few red voxles in the blue cluster and one blue voxle in the red cluster, since all the voxles are labeled a closer inspection shows that these outlier voxels are the exact same voxles in every MST.

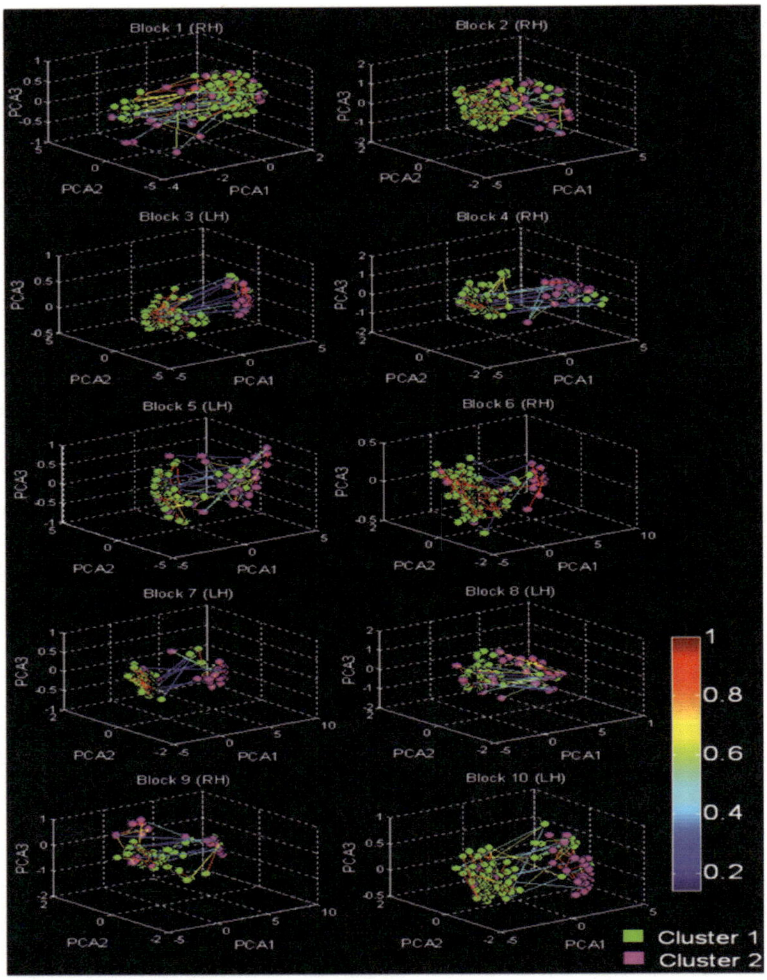

Fig. 11. The MSTs from fig. 10 constructed on the FH affinity PCA space. Displaying the MSTs of a subject that resulted in a good separation between right and left hand MSTs, showing high similarity between right hand block MSTs, and between left hand block MSTs. Each 3D graph represent the same voxels (color coded according to their original cluster with magenta and green), for each experiment block. These voxels are presented in their new location in the correlation space and connected according to the block's MST with lines color coded according to their correlation coefficient. In this visualization it is hard to detect the similarities and dissimilarities between the tree's structures. However it becomes visible in this case, that right hand movement's MSTs yielded a better separation of the clusters as opposed to left hand movements.

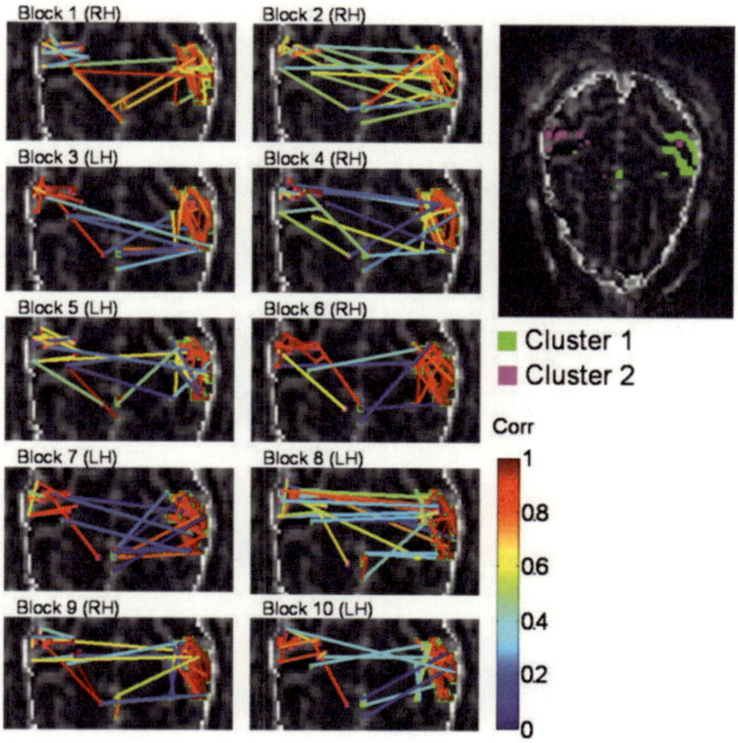

Fig. 12. The same MSTs from figs. 10 and 11 constructed upon the brain slice EPI image. This presentation shows that according to the MSTs the two hemispheres are highly coupled (with positive correlation and with negative correlation) in the motor task.

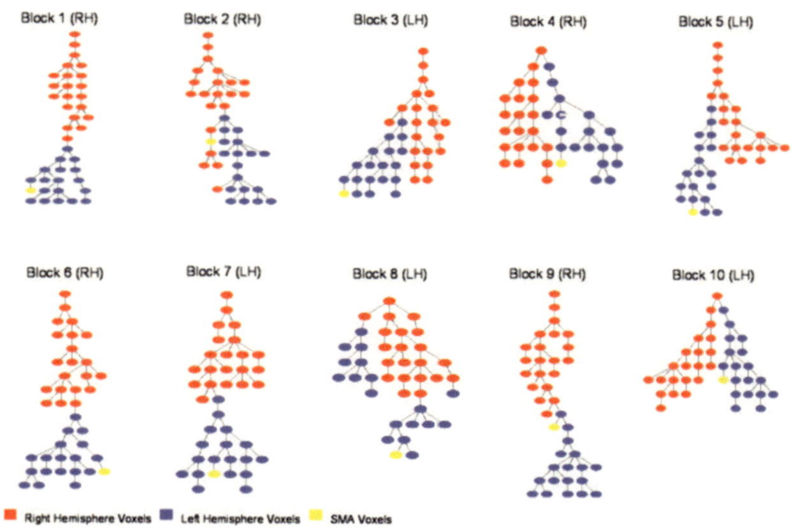

Fig. 13. Example of the MSTs constructed for a single left-handed subject that does not show a good separation in the divergence rate dendrogram. Displaying the MSTs for all ten blocks i.e. right hand (RH) and left hand (LH) movements. The red and blue colors represent the

right and left hemisphere voxels respectively, and the yellow color represents the SMA area. Although this subject does not yield a good separation between the right and left hand MSTs his MSTs do show a good separation between the right and left hemispheres.

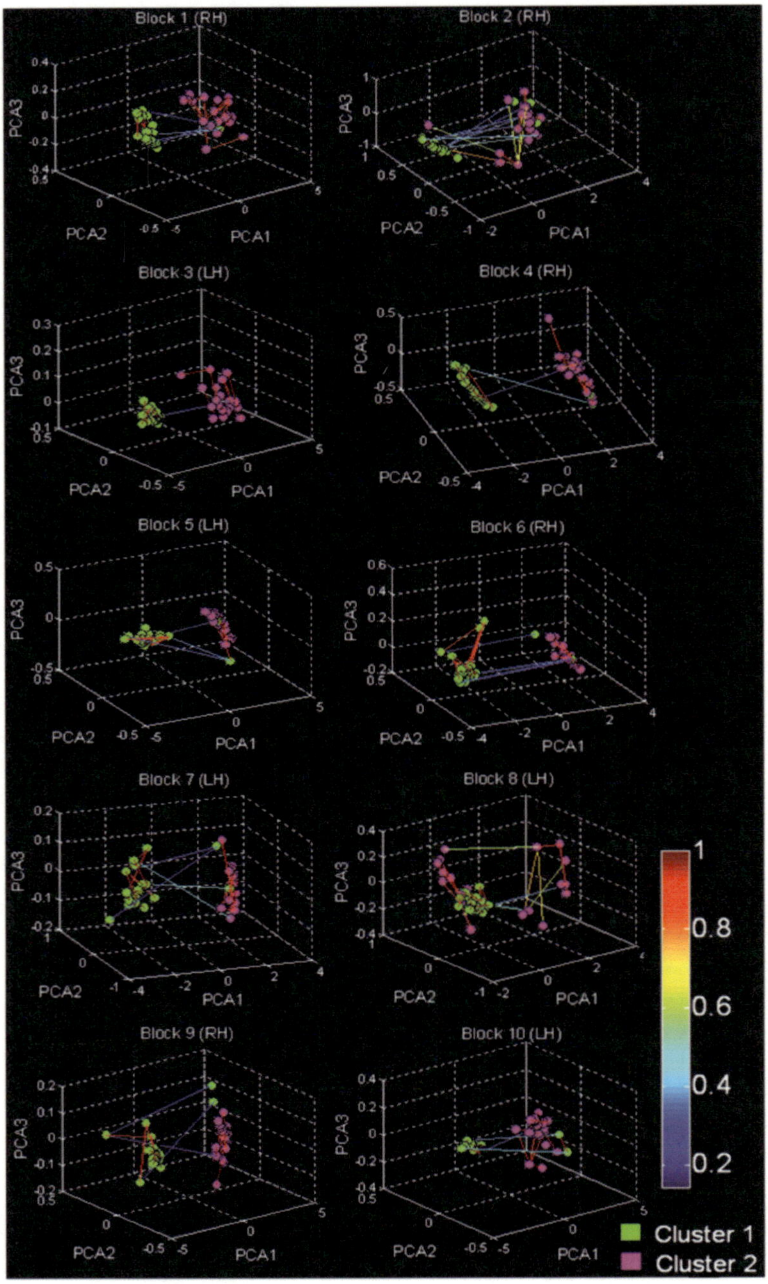

Fig. 14. The MSTs from fig. 13 constructed on the FH affinity PCA space. Demonstrating the MSTs of a subject who displayed no similarities or dissimilarities between right and left hand block MSTs in the divergence rate dendrogram tree.

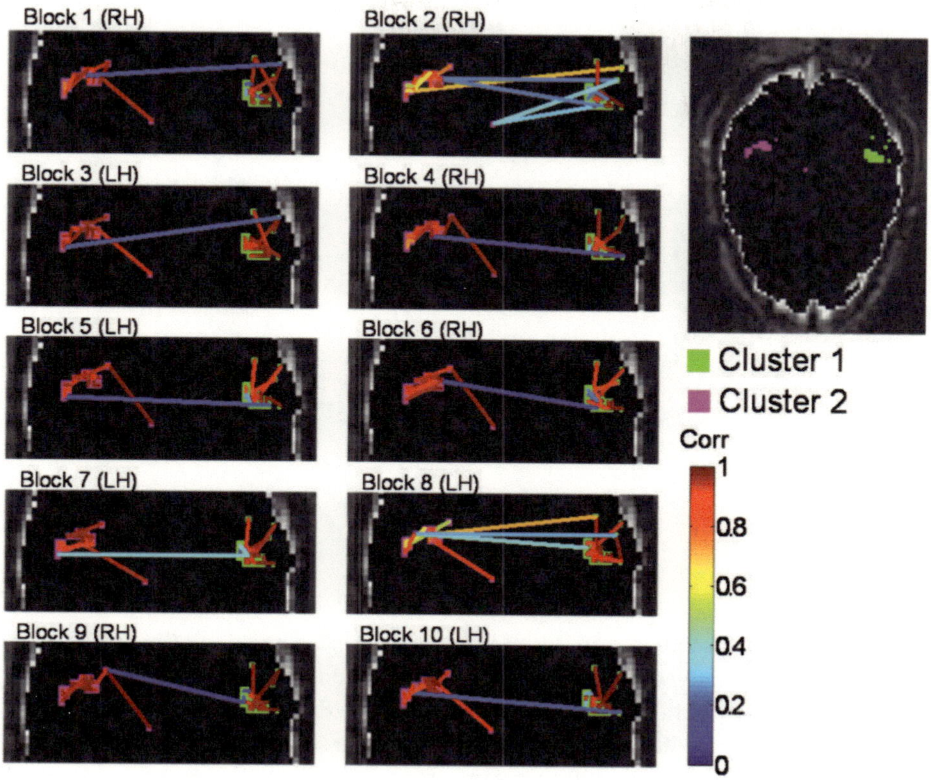

Fig. 15. The same MSTs from figs. 13 and 14 constructed upon the brain slice image. In this presentation, the two hemispheres seem to be highly negatively connected within the motor task blocks.

The topological structure of the constructed tree allows visual tracking clusters of nodes, and the variations undergone by the system as it faces different experimental conditions. This visualization is of paramount importance when dealing with highly complex systems, and is particularly helpful in the identification of clusters and their hierarchies. Thus two different clusters, each dominated by one hemisphere (figs. 10 and 13) or "outlier" voxels, which may have an important part in inter-hemispheric communication, could be highlighted.

Finally we point out one drawback of the MST method. When applied on a correlation-based system the MST uses the shortest distances. This induces a bias to positive correlations, while anti-correlations are overlooked. Further analysis of the data treating positive and the negative correlations on a par level (e.g. using the absolute values of the correlation matrix) may be recommended.

Overall, with this extremely simple example, we have illustrated how analyzing a very basic topological network property of networks of correlated activity associated with different cognitive conditions can reveal, in a rather parsimonious way, it's most important connections, suggesting the potential of this type of analysis in dealing with more challenging and rich data.

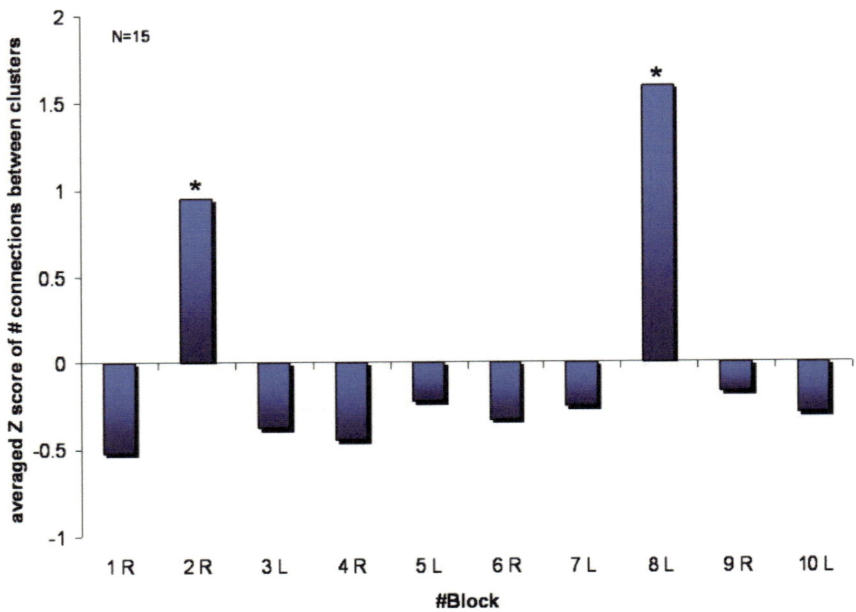

Fig. 16. The averaged Z score of number of links in the MST connecting the two clusters across subjects (N=15) for each experiment block. The two repetitive hand movements (i.e. blocks 2 and 8) resulted in higher average than the rest of the blocks. A statistical Z-test was calculated for each block with the null hypothesis that the scores in each block are a random sample from a normal distribution with mean zero. According to this test the two repetitive hand movements were found significant ($p=2x10^{-4}$ and $p=6.9x10^{-10}$ for blocks 2 and 8 respectively).

3. Conclusion

Over the past two decades, the development of new neuroimaging techniques has produced spectacular improvements in the amount of detail with which brain activity can be monitored. As precision has rapidly been gained, though, so has the typical data set size grown steadily. The range of questions that researchers and clinicians alike have started finding an answer for with neuroimaging techniques has also dramatically expanded. All this, in turn, has created a demand for new methods of data analysis, These new methods were developed on the one hand to provide new ways to represent brain activity, and on the other hand, to make quantitative sense of the rich information embedded in very high dimensional data and to visualize them in a way that can be read and understood in a sufficiently straightforward way by researchers first and, ultimately, by clinicians.

In this chapter, we presented FH a method which effectively tackles these issues. The FH algorithm deals with the multivariate and multiscale nature of brain imaging data sets and simplifies their complexity by representing patterns in a low-dimensional space which preserves the higher dimensional information of the original pattern of connectivity. In this sense, the FH analysis may be regarded as a system-level analysis that produces a complete, holographic, representation of brain activation.

The method also provides an effective visualization of the system, of critical importance when dealing with highly complex systems, and is particularly helpful in the identification of clusters and their hierarchies. Even more important though is the ability of the FH analysis to reveal subtle, system-level dynamical features that are hard to detect through other methods, even at the single subject level. And that might be overlooked due to prior assumptions by hypothesis-driven methods. In fact, the FH method can capture sensitive hemodynamic variations at the single block level, without further need for averaging or for contrasts between experimental conditions. In addition the method requires far less time point to localize activations than other clustering methods, viz. ICA (Bell & Sejnowski, 1995), FCA (Windischberger et al., 2003) or TCA (Zhao et al., 2007), suggesting that the FH method may play a prominent role in the development of classification algorithms for blind identification of different conditions in extremely short time series.

It is important to portray the FH method not only as an alternative but also as a valuable complement to existing methods. For instance, its dimension reduction step could be carried out using a variety of clustering techniques. Perhaps even more cogently, there is a clear complementarily between network theory and the FH method. The application of the former that we presented, i.e. the MST, clearly represents but one out of the many possible applications. To the extremely vast field of issues that network theory allows to address in a versatile but quantitatively rigorous and qualitatively explicit way, the FH method adds a compact representation in an auxiliary field that makes functional networks more explicit, as it divorces them from the anatomical space in which they live.

A distinctive quality of the FH method is represented by its versatility. While originally developed for cultured neural networks, the method can be applied to the analysis of essentially any type of signal, including the main tools for system-level neuroimaging, viz. EEG/MEG and fMRI. Although fewer examples of application to the latter are and further investigation of the method on different (viz. event-related) designs is needed, the proposed method shows great potential even for fMRI data in differentiating experimental conditions particularly when the corresponding signals are separated (Jacob et al., 2010). Since the outcome of the analysis is a holographic presentation in an abstract reduced space, it represents an ideal tool for multi-modal analysis of data from experiments combining EEG´s temporal precision with fMRI´s spatial one. Finally, the principles and implementation of the FH analysis are relatively simple and straightforward; taken together with the methods efficiency in delineating and tracking the time-varying unfolding of fine details of clustered activity at different spatial scales, it may represent a tool of election for brain scientists and for clinical neurologists alike.

4. Acknowledgment

We are most thankful to Asaf Madi, Dror Kenett, Amir Rapson, Michal Kafri and Keren Rosenberg for fruitful discussions. This research has been supported in part by the Israel-US Binational Science Foundation - 2005385 (EBJ, TH), the Maguy-Glass chair in physics of complex systems (EBJ), the Tauber Family Funds and the Italy-Israel program in System Level Network Neuroscience at Tel Aviv University (EBJ), the National Science Foundation Grants PHY- 0216576 and 0225630 at UCSD (EBJ), the Israel Science Foundation - 1747/07 (TH) and by the U.S Department Of Defense W81XWH-11-2-0008 (TH).

5. References

Achard, S. & Bullmore, E. Efficiency and Cost of Economical Brain Functional Networks. PLoS Comput Biol, 2007; 3: e17.

Achard, S., Salvador, R., Whitcher, B., Suckling, J. & Bullmore, E. A Resilient, Low-Frequency, Small-World Human Brain Functional Network with Highly Connected Association Cortical Hubs. The Journal of Neuroscience, 2006; 26: 63-72.

Alter, O., Brown, P.O. & Botstein, D. Singular value decomposition for genome-wide expression data processing and modeling. Proceedings of the National Academy of Sciences of the United States of America, 2000; 97: 10101-6.

Baruchi, I. & Ben-Jacob, E. Functional holography of recorded neuronal networks activity. Neuroinformatics, 2004; 2: 333-52.

Baruchi, I., Grossman, D., Volman, V., Shein, M., Hunter, J., Towle, V.L. & Ben-Jacob, E. Functional holography analysis: simplifying the complexity of dynamical networks. Chaos, 2006; 16: 015112.

Baruchi , I., Towle , V.L. & Ben-Jacob , E. Functional holography of Complex Networks Activity—From Cultures to the Human Brain. Complexity, 2004; 10: 38–51.

Bassett, D.S., Bullmore, E.T., Meyer-Lindenberg, A., Apud, J.A., Weinberger, D.R. & Coppola, R. Cognitive fitness of cost-efficient brain functional networks. Proceedings of the National Academy of Sciences, 2009; 106: 11747-52.

Bassett, D.S., Meyer-Lindenberg, A., Achard, S., Duke, T. & Bullmore, E. Adaptive reconfiguration of fractal small-world human brain functional networks. Proceedings of the National Academy of Sciences, 2006; 103: 19518-23.

Bell, A.J. & Sejnowski, T.J. An Information-Maximization Approach to Blind Separation and Blind Deconvolution. Neural Computation, 1995; 7: 1129-59.

Ben-Jacob, E., Boccaletti, S., Pomyalov, A., Procaccia, I. & Towle, V.L. Detecting and localizing the foci in human epileptic seizures. Chaos, 2007 17: 043113.

Boccaletti, S., Latora, V., Moreno, Y., Chavez, M. & Hwang, D.U. Complex networks: Structure and dynamics. Physics Reports, 2006; 424: 175-308.

Bucolo, M., Fazzino, S., La Rosa, M. & Fortuna, L. Small-world networks of fuzzy chaotic oscillators. Chaos, Solitons & Fractals, 2003; 17: 557-65.

Bullmore, E., Barnes, A., Bassett, D.S., Fornito, A., Kitzbichler, M., Meunier, D. & Suckling, J. Generic aspects of complexity in brain imaging data and other biological systems. Neuroimage, 2009; 47: 1125-34.

Chkhenkeli, S.A., Towle, V.L., Milton, J.G. & Spire, J.P. Multitarget stereotactic surgery of intractable epilepsy. Abstracts of the XIII Congress of ESSFN. Freiburg: Germany, 1998: 21.

Doyle, W.K. & Spencer, D.D. Anterior temporal resections. In Engel, J.J., Pedley, T.A., editors. Epilepsy: A Comprehensive Textbook. Lippincott-Raven, 1998: 1807–17.

Dubes, R. & Jain, A. Clustering methodologies in exploratory data analysis. Advances in Computers, 1980; 19: 113-228.

Eguíluz, V.M., Chialvo, D.R., Cecchi, G.A., Baliki, M. & Apkarian, A.V. Scale-Free Brain Functional Networks. Physical Review Letters, 2005; 94: 018102.

Friston, K.J. Functional and effective connectivity in neuroimaging: A synthesis. Hum Brain Mapp, 1994; 2: 56–78.

Friston, K.J., Buechel, C., Fink, G.R., Morris, J., Rolls, E. & Dolan, R.J. Psychophysiological and Modulatory Interactions in Neuroimaging. NeuroImage, 1997; 6: 218.

Friston, K.J., Harrison, L. & Penny, W. Dynamic causal modelling. Neuroimage, 2003; 19: 1273-302.

Goebel, R., Roebroeck, A., Kim, D.-S. & Formisano, E. Investigating directed cortical interactions in time-resolved fMRI data using vector autoregressive modeling and Granger causality mapping. Magnetic Resonance Imaging, 2003; 21: 1251-61.

Jacob, Y., Rapson, A., Kafri, M., Baruchi, I., Hendler, T. & Ben Jacob, E. Revealing voxel correlation cliques by functional holography analysis of fMRI. Journal of Neuroscience Methods, 2010; 191: 126.

Kruskal, J.B. On the Shortest Spanning Subtree of a Graph and the Traveling Salesman Problem. Proceedings of the American Mathematical Society, 1956; 7: 48-50.

Lago-Fernández, L.F., Huerta, R., Corbacho, F. & Sigüenza, J.A. Fast Response and Temporal Coherent Oscillations in Small-World Networks. Physical Review Letters, 2000; 84: 2758.

Latora, V. & Marchiori, M. Efficient Behavior of Small-World Networks. Physical Review Letters, 2001; 87: 198701.

Lee, U., Kim, S. & Jung, K.-Y. Classification of epilepsy types through global network analysis of scalp electroencephalograms. Physical Review E, 2006; 73: 041920.

Madi, A., Friedman, Y., Roth, D., Regev, T., Bransburg-Zabary, S. & Ben Jacob, E. Genome holography: deciphering function-form motifs from gene expression data. PLoS ONE, 2008; 3: e2708.

Mantegna, R.N. & Stanley, H.E. An Introduction to Econophysics: Correlations and Complexity in Finance. Cambridge University Press: Cambridge UK, 2000.

McKeown, M.J., Makeig, S., Brown, G.G., Jung, T.P., Kindermann, S.S., Bell, A.J. & Sejnowski, T.J. Analysis of fMRI data by blind separation into independent spatial components. Hum Brain Mapp, 1998; 6: 160-88.

Milton, J. & Jung, P., editors. Epilepsy as a Dynamic Disease. Springer Verlag: Berlin, 2002.

Newman, M.E.J. The Structure and Function of Complex Networks. SIAM Review, 2003; 45: 256.

Pearson, K. On lines and planes of closest fit to systems of points in space. Phil. Mag, 1901.

Rammal, R., Toulouse, G. & Virasoro, M.A. Ultrametricity for physicists. Reviews of Modern Physics, 1986; 58: 765.

Salvador, R., Suckling, J., Coleman, M.R., Pickard, J.D., Menon, D. & Bullmore, E. Neurophysiological Architecture of Functional Magnetic Resonance Images of Human Brain. Cerebral Cortex, 2005; 15: 1332-42.

Segev, R., Baruchi, I., Hulata, E. & Ben-Jacob, E. Hidden neuronal correlations in cultured networks. Phys Rev Lett, 2004; 92: 118102.

Shannon, C.E. A mathematical theory of communication Part I. Bell System Technical Journal, 1948; 27: 379–423.

Shapira, Y., Kenett, D.Y. & Ben-Jacob, E. The Index cohesive effect on stock market correlations. European Physical Journal B, 2009; 72: 657-69.

Sporns, O., Chialvo, D.R., Kaiser, M. & Hilgetag, C.C. Organization, development and function of complex brain networks. Trends in Cognitive Sciences, 2004; 8: 418-25.

Sporns, O., Tononi, G. & Edelman, G.M. Connectivity and complexity: the relationship between neuroanatomy and brain dynamics. Neural Networks, 2000; 13: 909-22.

Sporns, O., Tononi, G. & Edelman, G.M. Theoretical neuroanatomy and the connectivity of the cerebral cortex. Behavioural Brain Research, 2002; 135: 69-74.

Strogatz, S.H. Exploring complex networks. Nature, 2001; 410: 268-76.

Towle, V.L., Ahmad, F., Kohrman, M., Hecox, K. & Chkhenkeli, S. Electrocorticographic Coherence Patterns of Epileptic Seizures. In P. Jung, P., Milton, J., editors. Epilepsy as a Dynamic Disease. Springer: Berlin, 2002.

Towle, V.L., Carder, R.K., Khorasani, L. & Lindberg, D. Electrocorticographic Coherence Patterns. Journal of Clinical Neurophysiology, 1999; 16: 528.

Tumminello, M., Coronnello, C., Lillo, F., Micciche, S. & Mantegna, R.N. Spanning Trees and bootstrap reliability estimation in correlation based networks. INTERNATIONAL JOURNAL OF BIFURCATION AND CHAOS IN APPLIED SCIENCES AND ENGINEERING, 2007; 17 (7): 2319 - 29.

Varshavsky, R., Gottlieb, A., Horn, D. & Linial, M. Unsupervised feature selection under perturbations: meeting the challenges of biological data. Bioinformatics, 2007; 23: 3343-9.

Varshavsky, R., Gottlieb, A., Linial, M. & Horn, D. Novel Unsupervised Feature Filtering of Biological Data. Bioinformatics, 2006; 22: e507-13.

West, D.B. An Introduction to Graph Theory. Prentice-Hall: Englewood Cliffs, NJ, 2001.

Windischberger, C., Barth, M., Lamm, C., Schroeder, L., Bauer, H., Gur, R.C. & Moser, E. Fuzzy cluster analysis of high-field functional MRI data. Artificial Intelligence In Medicine, 2003; 29: 203-23.

Worsley, K.J. & Friston, K.J. Analysis of fMRI Time-Series Revisited--Again. Neuroimage, 1995; 2: 173-81.

Zhao, X., Li, G., Glahn, D.C., Fox, P.T. & Gao, H.H. Derivative temporal clustering analysis: detecting prolonged neuronal activity. Magnetic Resonance Imaging, 2007; 25: 183-7.

Zhou, C., Zemanová, L., Zamora, G., Hilgetag, C.C. & Kurths, J. Hierarchical Organization Unveiled by Functional Connectivity in Complex Brain Networks. Physical Review Letters, 2006; 97: 238103.

7

Hyperpolarized Xenon Brain MRI

Xin Zhou
Wuhan Center for Magnetic Resonance,
State Key Laboratory of Magnetic Resonance and Atomic and Molecular Physics,
Wuhan Institute of Physics and Mathematics,
The Chinese Academy of Sciences, Wuhan,
P.R. China

1. Introduction

Since hyperpolarized ^{129}Xe MRI was first demonstrated in the lung, air space imaging using hyperpolarized noble gases (^{129}Xe and ^{3}He) has progressed at a rapid rate (Goodson, 2002; Zhou, 2011c). Owing to high lipid solubility, absence of background signal in biological tissue, non-invasiveness, lack of radioactivity, different relaxation to oxygenated and deoxygenated blood, and larger chemical shift to the neighbor environment, hyperpolarized ^{129}Xe magnetic resonance imaging (MRI) has a great potential as a tool for studying the brain, especially for the assessment of cerebral blood flow (CBF) related to the brain function and activities.

In this chapter, we will review the progress of recent research on hyperpolarized xenon brain MRI, and compare this novel technique with the conventional proton MRI in order to comment the possible innovation and development in the future. This chapter contains six main parts as follows:

2. Properties of xenon

Xenon, with the chemical element symbol Xe and atomic number 54, is a member of the zero-valence elements that are called noble gases or inert gases. Xenon was discovered in the residue left over from evaporating components of liquid air by William Ramsay and Morris Travers in England in 1898, then was named by Ramsay from Greek word *ξένον*, with the meaning 'foreign' and 'strange'. Natural abundant xenon is made of nine stable isotopes, and more than 35 unstable isotopes have been characterized. Nuclei of two isotopes, ^{129}Xe and ^{131}Xe, have non-zero spin quantum number: 26.4% of ^{129}Xe with a nuclear spin $I=1/2$; and 21.2% of ^{131}Xe with a nuclear spin $I=3/2$ (^{133}Xe is used as a radioisotope in nuclear medicine). These two isotopes are both detectable by NMR with sensitivities of 0.021 (^{129}Xe, per nucleus relative to proton assuming thermal polarization) and 2.7×10^{-3} (^{131}Xe). The highly enhanced signal of hyperpolarized xenon and extremely long relaxation time greatly simplified and enhanced NMR experiments, and it is the fundamental for possible biological application in MRI.

Xenon, chemically inert with the external electronic orbits fully occupied, is well known as a noble gas at room temperature and an atmospheric pressure. However, the liquid and solid phases of Xenon can be easily obtained within an experimentally accessible range of temperatures and pressures (Cook, 1961) (Fig. 1).

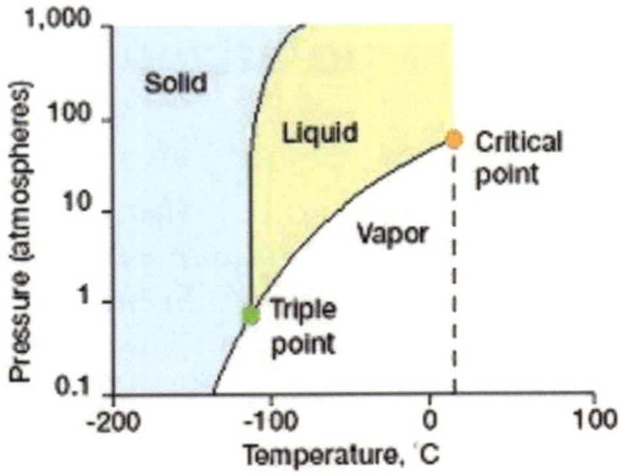

Fig. 1. Phase diagram of xenon.
(Figure from: http://science.nasa.gov/science-news/science-at-nasa/2008/25apr_cvx2/)

Furthermore, the large and highly polarizable electron cloud makes xenon highly lipid soluble in solution, without chemically or structurally damage during interactions with other molecules. Ostwald solubility is defined as the ratio of the volume of the gas absorbed to the volume of the absorbing liquid, measured at same temperature and a pressure of 1 atm (101,325 Pa) (Cherubini, 2003; Oros, 2004) (Table 1).

Compound		Ostwald solubility
	T=25 °C	
Water		0.11
Hexane		4.8
Benzene		3.1
Fluorobenzene		3.3
Carbon disulphide		4.2
	T=37 °C	
Water		0.08
Saline		0.09
Plasma		0.10
Erythrocytes (98%)		0.20
Human albumin (100%,extrapolated)		0.15
Blood		0.14
Oil		1.9
Fat tissue		1.3
DMSO (dimethyl sulfoxide)		0.66
Intralipid (20%)		0.4
PFOB (perflubron)		1.2
PFOB (90% w/v, estimated)		0.62

Table 1. Solubilities of xenon gas in various compounds. (Data taken from Cherubini, 2003)

Owing to the inter-atomic collisions distortion of xenon electron cloud during the interactions with different chemical environment, the chemical shift of ^{129}Xe is extremely sensitive. Total solvent effect on the Xe resonance frequency is over 7500 ppm, very large compared with most other NMR sensitive nuclei (^{1}H : 20 ppm 、^{13}C : 300 ppm). A few examples are shown in Figure 2, the natural reference point for xenon chemical shift in the gas phase; with respect to the gas resonance (0 ppm), peaks at 70 ppm corresponding to cryptophane-bound xenon; around 197 ppm, five dissolved peaks can be observed, a dominant peak at 194.7 ppm and another discriminable peak at 189 ppm are identified as dissolved hyperpolarized ^{129}Xe in the brain tissue and non-brain tissue, respectively, two small peaks at 191.6 ppm and 197.8 ppm are still unknown, and a smaller broad peak at 209.5 ppm comes from the dissolved hyperpolarized ^{129}Xe in the blood (Zhou et al., 2008).

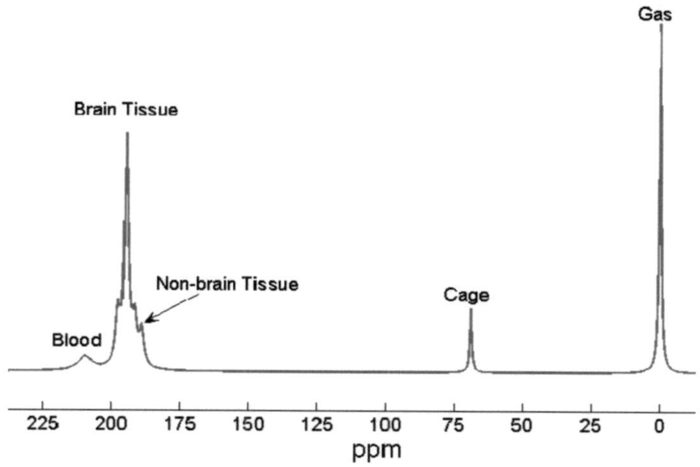

Fig. 2. Chemical shift of ^{129}Xe in biosensor and biological system (Data taken from Zhou et al., 2011c)

As a closed shelled noble gas, xenon has a peculiar large polarizable electron cloud, it can be easily interacted with biological materials, including water 'lipids' and proteins and so on; meanwhile, ^{129}Xe NMR parameters like relaxation time and chemical shift are very sensitive to local chemical environment, these biochemical physiological characters make xenon a very interesting NMR probe for biological applications. Arising from large increase in sensitivity associated with hyperpolarized ^{129}Xe, the biological NMR applications have been dramatically extended. Being Chemically Inert, xenon can be safely delivered into living organisms, associated with another advantage of no background signal, thus *in vivo* MR imaging and spectroscopy is possible using hyperpolarized ^{129}Xe technique.

3. Signal enhanced MRI with hyperpolarized ^{129}Xe

Nuclear magnetic resonance (NMR) has been widely used in most fields of natural sciences, such as physics, chemistry, biology, and medicine. Because of the intrinsic low nuclear spin polarization at the thermal equilibrium, NMR is relatively insensitive. The normal ^{129}Xe MRI, i.e., at the thermal equilibrium, is not able to get enough signal to visualize tissues or organs. The polarization can be moderately increased by using lower temperature or higher magnetic fields (Navon et al., 1996), whereas the nuclear spin polarizations of noble gases can be increased by four or five orders of magnitude via the spin-exchange optical pumping (SEOP) techniques (Walker, 1997). Therefore, it enables a very high sensitive detection of hyperpolarized ^{129}Xe MRI. This subsection will describe how to produce hyperpolarized ^{129}Xe, which is the basis for the brain imaging.

^{3}He and ^{129}Xe are generally selected for hyperpolarized lung gas imaging, because ^{3}He and ^{129}Xe are the only noble gas nuclei with nuclear spin 1/2, which results in the longitudinal relaxation time of many hours or even days at the standard temperature and pressure. However, hyperpolarized ^{3}He could not be used for the brain study due to the extremely low solubility in blood and tissue, while hyperpolarized ^{129}Xe is a novel contrast agent for the cerebral research. Hyperpolarized ^{129}Xe is generally generated by employing the technique of SEOP.

For SEOP, the first step is to transfer the anglar momentum of the cicularly polarized laser light to the electronic spin, i.e., optical pumping. In principal, any alkali metal vapor can be optically pumped. Rb is normally used as the corresponding pumping laser diode arrays (LDA), which are routinely manufactured in high power configurations. When the Rb vapor experiences an external magnetic field of 20-30 Gauss, the ground state $5^2S_{1/2}$ is split into two Zeeman sublevels, M_J=-1/2 and M_J=1/2, i.e., electronic spin "down" or "up". These two Zeeman states have a nearly equal population at room temperature. After the Rb vapor absorbs the circularly polarized laser light (σ+) centered at 795nm, the Rb D1 transition occurs, i.e., $5^2S_{1/2} \rightarrow 5^2P_{1/2}$. Accordingly, the ground state with a sublevel M_J=-1/2 is pumped into the excited state, M_J=1/2. The nitrogen gas quenches the excited state back to the ground state. Because the M_J=-1/2 sublevel continues to absorb the circularly polarized light (σ+) an excess of Rb atoms are optically pumped into the Zeeman sublevel M_J=1/2 while the other sublevel M_J=-1/2 is depleted. Therefore, an Rb electronic spin polarization of roughly 100% is able to be achieved.

The second step of SEOP is spin exchange, which occurs between the polarized electronic spins of Rb and the xenon nucleus. The collision between polarized Rb atoms and xenon atoms induces the transfer of angular momentum from the electronic spin to the nuclear spin. During this collision, the electron wave function of the Rb overlaps the nuclear wave function of xenon, which results in the spin exchange between the electronic spin and nuclear spin. Binary collisions dominate the spin exchange at high pressure, while three-body collision (by forming a Rb/Xe van der Waals molecule) dominate at low pressure (a few tens of torr).

Generally, Rb atoms and nitrogen gas are employed for optical pumping, however, Cs may be proposed as a better candidate for spin exchange with ^{129}Xe due to several advantages: the natural abundance of ^{133}Cs is 100% while Rb has two isotopes (^{85}Rb and ^{87}Rb), so that Cs is more convenient than Rb for wide applications of hyperpolarized ^{129}Xe, particularly in the clinic application; optical pumping cells for Cs are operated at lower temperatures with correspondingly fewer chemical corrosion problems; according to the previous experimental results, the spin-exchange rate of Cs-Xe is about 10% higher than the Rb-Xe rate (Zhou et al., 2004a). When the polarization of hyperpolarized ^{129}Xe is high enough, the observed radiation damping has been reported (Zhou, 2004b). The xenon polarizer with a flow feature can be readily extended to produce larger quantities of hyperpolarized ^{129}Xe for not only medical imaging but also materials science and biology (Zhou, 2004c; Zhou, 2009a).

4. Longitudinal relaxation time (T_1) of hyperpolarized ^{129}Xe in the brain

Hyperpolarized ^{129}Xe magnetization enhanced by SEOP is non-recoverable, and the T_1 of an hyperpolarized gas is the time elapsed for the signal to decay, because its thermal equilibrium polarization is almost zero relative to the hyperpolarized polarization. Usually, small flip angles has to be used to ration the hyperpolarized magnetization, and it is very important to have a T_1 as long as possible to ensure that the signal lasts long enough for the acquisition. Therefore, the T_1 of hyperpolarized ^{129}Xe in the brain is a critical parameter. This subsection will discuss the aspects that affect T_1 of hyperpolarized xenon, and describe the methods to accurately measure the T_1 in the brain (Zhou et. al, 2008).

4.1 T_1 of hyperpolarized ^{129}Xe

For conventional MRI, the magnetization at thermal equilibrium is induced by the magnetic field, and the longitudinal relaxation time (T_1) is the time for the magnetization, i.e. the magnetic resonance signal, to recover back to the thermal equilibrium. However, hyperpolarized noble gas magnetization produced by SEOP is unable to recover back to the hyperpolarized magnetization by itself, and the T_1 of an hyperpolarized noble gas is the decay time of magnetization, because the thermal polarized magnetization is almost zero related to the hyperpolarized magnetization. The longitudinal relaxation time of hyperpolarized ^{129}Xe in the brain is a critical parameter for developing hyperpolarized ^{129}Xe brain imaging and spectroscopy and optimizing the pulse sequences, especially in the case of cerebral blood flow measurements. Various studies have produced widely varying estimates of hyperpolarized ^{129}Xe T_1 in the rat brain (Choquet, 2003; Wakai, 2005).

The hyperpolarized magnetization is generally tipped by a pulse with a small flip angle, and it is very challenging to make the T_1 as long as possible in order to ensure the signal lasts long enough for the acquisition. Therefore, when considering hyperpolarized ^{129}Xe as a marker for brain perfusion by MRI, evaluation of tissue characterization and pulse sequence optimization, the T_1 of hyperpolarized ^{129}Xe in the brain is a critical parameter. Previous attempts to measure T_1 in the rat brain have yielded strikingly disparate results. Wilson et al. found that T_1 measured in rat brain homogenates in vitro ranged from 18±1 to 22±2 s (mean ± SD) (Wilson et. al , 2009) depending on the oxygenation level of the tissue, and T_1 values from measurements in rat brain *in vivo* have ranged from 3.6±2.1 (Choquet et al, 2003) to 26±4 s (Wakai et. al, 2005). Part of the discrepancy is believed to be due to the protocols used in T_1 determination. The attempt of Choquet et al. used a multi-pulse protocol during the uptake and washout process by injecting hyperpolarized ^{129}Xe in a lipid emulsion, whereas the estimation of Wakai et al. used a two-pulse protocol during the washout process after the rat had breathed hyperpolarized ^{129}Xe gas. Under the condition of typically achieved polarizations (5 - 21%) (Zook et. al, 2001), low signal-to-noise ratio (SNR) due to the low concentration of the dissolved hyperpolarized ^{129}Xe in tissue is an important factor in making T_1 measurements in the rat brain (Cherubinia et. al, 2003; Ruppert et. al, 2000). The maximum SNR in the above two measurements in vivo was only 30 (Choquet et. al, 2003) and 46 (Wakai et. al, 2005), and the noise effect was not considered in these studies. When the SNR is low, noise will dominate the measured signal and result in large differences between the true T_1 and the measured T_1. Thus, low SNR might be a large contributor of error in the published T_1 values.

4.2 Multi-pulse and two-pulse washout protocols for measurements of T_1

Hyperpolarized ^{129}Xe transport in the brain has been modeled using appropriate adaptations of the Kety–Schmidt theory (Martin et al., 1997; Peled et al., 1996). Martin and co-workers derived the equation of the cerebral xenon concentration during hyperpolarized ^{129}Xe delivery to the lungs as follow:

$$\frac{dC_{brain}}{dt} = FC_{cereb} - (\frac{F}{p} + \frac{1}{T_{1brain}})C_{brain} \qquad (1)$$

where C_{cereb} is the xenon concentration in the cerebral artery, C_{brain} is the xenon concentration in brain parenchyma, F is the tissue perfusion in units of (volume blood)/(volume tissue)/time, p is the brain/blood partition coefficient for xenon, and T_{1brain} is the longitudinal relaxation time of xenon in the brain. In this equation, the first term on the right describes xenon transport to the brain, and the second term describes the loss of xenon signal due to both perfusion and T_1 decay. Xenon signal observed from the brain is proportional to C_{brain}. During the washout phase of the xenon signal, there is no transport of hyperpolarized ^{129}Xe by the cerebral artery, and hence C_{cereb} is zero. Accordingly, the xenon concentration in the brain during washout ($C_{brainwashout}$) is given by the following equation:

$$\frac{dC_{brainwashout}}{dt} = -(\frac{F}{p} + \frac{1}{T_{1brain}})C_{brainwashout} \qquad (2)$$

This equation can be solved to yield an analytical solution for the concentration of xenon in the brain during the washout of signal. The decay time constant (τ) of hyperpolarized ^{129}Xe during the washout from the rat brain is given by:

$$\tau = \frac{1}{(\frac{F}{p} + \frac{1}{T_{1brain}})} \qquad (3)$$

Thus, τ can be calculated from a series of pulse excitations (multi-pulse protocol) after compensating for the hyperpolarized xenon signal losses resulted from radio frequency (RF) excitation, as described below. To compare the results obtained using the multi-pulse protocol, a two-pulse protocol has also been adopted to measure τ (Wakai et al., 2005). Both protocols were performed on each rat during the washout phase of the ^{129}Xe signal.

Table 2 shows individual T_1 values of hyperpolarized ^{129}Xe and their mean from the six rat brains using the two protocols, with and without the SNR threshold. The mean T_1 value calculated using the improved two-pulse method is larger than that using its conventional counterpart, whereas the mean T_1 value calculated using the improved multi-pulse method is less than that using its conventional counterpart. These T_1 values were named 'group 1' to 'group 4' for easy reference during discussion.

In this subsection, we investigated the error in T_1 measurement as a result of low SNR of the ^{129}Xe signal *in vivo*. Correcting for these errors allowed us to more accurately measure the T_1 of hyperpolarized ^{129}Xe in the rat brain *in vivo*. Our calculations produced highly consistent

T_1 results independent of the measurement protocol and offer a resolution to the discrepancy between previously reported values.

Rat	Multi-pulse protocol		2-pulse protocol	
	Conventional	Improved	Conventional	Improved
	T_1(s) (group 1)	T_1(s) (group 2)	T_1(s) (group 3)	T_1(s) (group 4)
1	14.2	12.9	19.5	17.6
2	12.2	15.1	18.2	16.4
3	11.5	16.1	16.3	14.9
4	11.7	15.5	18.0	16.5
5	12.7	16.4	18.8	16.6
6	12.1	15.7	17.2	15.4
Mean	12.4	15.3	18.0	16.2
Std. Deviation	1.0	1.2	1.1	0.9

Table 2. T_1 values of hyperpolarized ^{129}Xe from six rat brains. The mean T_1 value and standard deviation obtained from the multi-pulse and two-pulse protocols before (conventional method) and after (improved method) setting a threshold of SNR=5.5 are also given. (Zhou et al., 2008)

5. Stroke MRI with hyperpolarized ^{129}Xe

Because there is no background signal from xenon in biological tissue, and because the inhaled xenon is delivered to the brain by the blood flow, we would expect a perfusion deficit, such as could be seen in stroke, to reduce xenon concentration in the region of the deficit. Thermal polarization yields negligible xenon signal relative to hyperpolarized xenon; therefore, hyperpolarized xenon can be used as a tracer of cerebral blood flow (CBF). This subsection will describe that hyperpolarized ^{129}Xe MRI is able to detect, *in vivo* hypoperfused area of focal cerebral ischemia—i.e., the ischemic core area of stroke, by using a rat permanent right middle cerebral artery occlusion (MCAO) model (Zhou et al., 2011a).

Stroke is the single most common reason for permanent disability and is the third leading cause of death in developed countries. During acute ischemic stroke, a core of brain cells at the center of the affected region dies quickly, and the damage subsequently spreads to surrounding tissue over the next few hours. Because they allow for the delineation of areas of ischemic neuronal injury and hypoperfusion within minutes after the induction of cerebral ischemia, conventional proton MRI, especially diffusion-weighted imaging (DWI) and perfusion weighted imaging (PWI), have been particularly useful in the diagnosis of acute ischemic stroke. The target of acute stroke therapy is the portion of the ischemic region which is still potentially salvageable, that is the ischemic penumbra. MRI operationally defines the ischemic penumbra by the mismatch area of PWI–DWI. DWI detects changes in the apparent diffusion coefficient (ADC) of water molecules associated with early cytotoxic edema in ischemic stroke. Arterial spin labeling (ASL)-based PWI methods provide excellent anatomical information for the measurement of tissue perfusion. The ASL technique shows numerous advantages, such as noninvasive measurements of cerebral blood flow (CBF) quantifiable in standard units of mL/g/min, and is able to image multi-slices and multi-regions of the brain. However, in some situations, PWI methods require the injection of gadolinium containing contrast agents to map relative CBF in order to identify the hypoperfused tissue. In addition to the conventional DWI and PWI techniques, van Zijl and coworkers have developed pH-weighted MRI to study stroke and ischemic penumbra. However, proton imaging has a large background signal in biological tissue, and contrast injection is an invasive approach. Moreover, contrast-associated nephrogenic systemic fibrosis has been reported after the use of gadolinium-based agents, and many patients with impaired renal function are not eligible to receive contrast media. In contrast, hyperpolarized ^{129}Xe MRI shows great potential and advantages for the identification of hypoperfused brain tissue. Xenon is highly lipid soluble and lacks an intrinsic background signal in biological tissue (Albert et al., 1994). Duhamel and co-workers have studied CBF using intra-arterial injection of hyperpolarized ^{129}Xe dissolved in a lipid emulsion (Duhamel et al., 2000). Alternatively, hyperpolarized ^{129}Xe can be administered noninvasively by inhalation; following inhalation, ^{129}Xe is absorbed into the bloodstream and delivered to the brain through the circulation. Because the spin-exchange optical pumping technique can enhance the ^{129}Xe MR signal 10,000–100,000 times over thermal polarization, the dissolved-phase hyperpolarized ^{129}Xe signal in the brain can be detected even at low concentrations. Because the xenon signal is proportional to CBF (Zhou et al., 2008), a decrease in the signal is expected to occur in areas of decreased CBF after the inhalation of hyperpolarized xenon gas. Hyperpolarized xenon imaging currently can not achieve a slice as thin as that obtained by ASL. In addition, ASL can be performed with substantially higher spatial resolution than hyperpolarized xenon imaging in brain tissue. However, the ASL technique requires two experiments (arterial spin labeled and controlled) to obtain CBF information. In this subsection, we report, for the first time, that hyperpolarized ^{129}Xe MRI is able to detect areas of decreased CBF following middle cerebral artery occlusion (MCAO) in a single scan. These findings show the great potential and utility of hyperpolarized ^{129}Xe MRI for stroke imaging, and further demonstrate that hyperpolarized ^{129}Xe is a safe and noninvasive signal source for imaging diseases and function of the brain.

Figure 3a shows a representative proton ADC map obtained 90 min following MCAO. There is a large ischemic core within the ipsilesional (right) MCA territory, as indicated by ADC values below the critical threshold of 5.3×10^{-4} mm^2/s for infarction (Meng et al., 2004). [The normal ADC value of rat brain tissue in the contralesional (left) hemisphere is $(7.5\pm1.8)\times10^{-4}$ mm^2/s.] Figure 3b depicts the corresponding hyperpolarized ^{129}Xe CSI, indicating signal reduction in large parts of the right hemisphere, consistent with the area typically experiencing decreased CBF following right MCAO in the model used (Duhamel et al., 2002). Figure 3c shows the TTC-stained brain section of the same animal as illustrated in Fig. 3a, b; the black line in this figure delineates the infracted brain tissue. Xenon CSI, shown in Fig. 3b, demonstrates reduced perfusion in brain tissue, ultimately leading to infarction, as shown by TTC staining in Fig. 3c. In Fig. 3d, the blue area represents the difference between the ADC lesion and TTC lesion areas, and the green area shows the nonischemic region. ROI analyses were performed to further characterize the Xe CSI tissue signals within the different observed tissue compartments defined by their respective ADC and TTC signatures.

Xenon signals from each ROI in the contralesional (left) hemisphere were set as a reference (100%), and xenon signals from each ROI in the ipsilesional (right) hemisphere were normalized to these signals. The xenon signal in the ischemic core (ROI_1) dropped to 8.4±0.4% of the contralesional side signal, and the xenon signal in normal tissue (ROI_2) remained the same. Moreover, the xenon signal in ROI_1 was reduced significantly relative to the corresponding con-tralesional ROIs in the MCAO group, as well as the corresponding ipsilateral ROIs in control animals. Within the control group, no significant differences in the xenon signal were observed between the corresponding ROIs of both hemispheres.

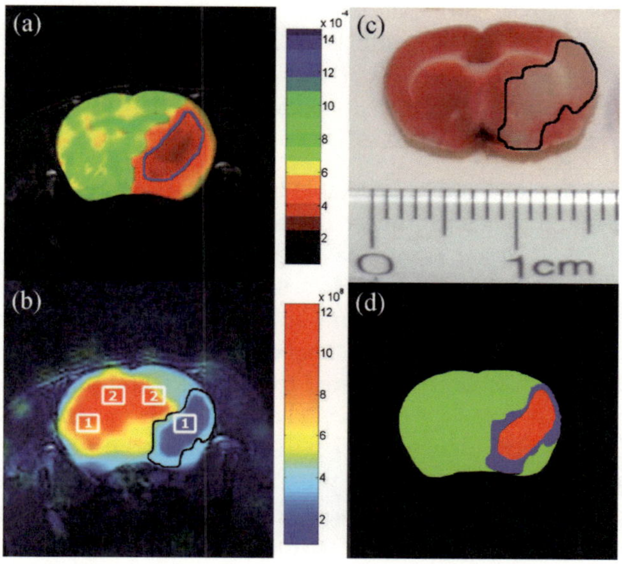

Fig. 3. (a) Representative proton apparent diffusion coefficient (ADC) map image obtained 90 min after right middle cerebral artery occlusion (MCAO). The ischemic core is indicated by ADC values below 5.3 × 10^{-4} mm^2/s (circled by a blue line). (b) Corresponding hyperpolarized ^{129}Xe chemical shift image (CSI). There is a large signal void in the ipsilesional (right) hemisphere. The defined regions of interest (ROIs) are labeled as follows: ROI1, core; ROI2, normal tissue. The xenon signal intensity is given in arbitrary units. (c) Corresponding 2,3,5-triphenyltetrazolium chloride (TTC)-stained brain section of the same animal as in (a) and (b). (d) Tricolor map based on the ADC and TTC images shown in (a) and (c). Green, red and blue represent nonischemic tissue, core and penumbra, respectively.

Using a rat permanent right middle cerebral artery occlusion model, it has demonstrated that hyperpolarized ^{129}Xe MRI is able to detect, *in vivo*, the hypoperfused area of focal cerebral ischemia, that is the ischemic core area of stroke. To the best of our knowledge, this is the first time that hyperpolarized ^{129}Xe MRI has been used to explore normal and abnormal cerebral perfusion. The study shows a novel application of hyperpolarized ^{129}Xe

MRI for imaging stroke, and further demonstrates its capacity to serve as a complementary tool to proton MRI for the study of the pathophysiology during brain hypoperfusion. More importantly, these results indicate the possibility of the use of *in vivo* MRI to diagnose brain disease employing inhaled hyperpolarized gas, eliminating the potential adverse effects to the patient resulting from the injection of gadolinium-based contrast agents.

6. Functional MRI with hyperpolarized ^{129}Xe

As hyperpolarized xenon is a MRI signal source with properties very different from those generated from water-protons, hyperpolarized ^{129}Xe MRI may yield structural and functional information not detectable by conventional proton-based MRI methods. This subsection shows that the differential distribution of hyperpolarized ^{129}Xe in the cerebral cortex of the rat following a pain stimulus evoked in the animal's forepaw. Areas of higher hyperpolarized ^{129}Xe signal corresponded to those areas previously demonstrated by conventional functional MRI (fMRI) methods as being activated by a forepaw pain stimulus. It demonstrated that the percent increase in hyperpolarized ^{129}Xe signal over baseline was 13 - 28%, which is more sensitive than the conventional fMRI based on the blood oxygen level dependence (BOLD) (2-4%) (Zhou et al., 2011b).

Ex-vivo hyperpolarization of ^{129}Xe is detectable by magnetic resonance spectroscopy (MRS) and MRI in animals and humans, although the resulting *in vivo* signal to noise ratio (SNR) of the hyperpolarized ^{129}Xe signal is not as great as the signal produced by protons in conventional MRI, hyperpolarized ^{129}Xe has several unique characteristics which may endow it with advantages in some imaging applications, including brain imaging (Zhou et.al, 2011a). The nuclear magnetic resonance frequency range (chemical shift) of hyperpolarized ^{129}Xe *in vivo* is large compared to protons (200 ppm vs. 5 ppm respectively) and is also substantially affected by the local chemical environment, providing a means to detect localized physiological changes and biochemical binding events. In particular, the chemical shift experienced by ^{129}Xe in the presence of oxygen (O_2) is substantial and may offer a means to image changes in tissue O_2 concentration that result from changes in neuronal activity. Xenon is also an ideal perfusion tracer (Betz, 1972) and inhaled non-radioactive xenon gas has been used to detect disease induced alterations in cerebral blood flow with high anatomical specificity (Gur, 1982). Because xenon is not intrinsic to biological tissue, hyperpolarized ^{129}Xe produces virtually no background signal, which, in turn, results in high contrast hyperpolarized ^{129}Xe MR images (Swanson, 1997).

6.1 Rat brain functional hyperpolarized ^{129}Xe imaging experiment

In the rat brain function study, hyperpolarized ^{129}Xe MRI was performed in rats to investigate the distribution of the hyperpolarized ^{129}Xe signal following a well-established paradigm for producing anatomically localized neuronal activity. Six rats were intubated and connected to a ventilator that controlled the delivery of oxygen and hyperpolarized ^{129}Xe gas. Male Spragur-Dawley rats weighing between 200-250g were placed on animal respirator, with tidal volume of 3ml O_2 (3% isoflurane included) supplied for each breath. Immediately prior to the acquisition of CSI images, the animal was ventilated with alternate breaths of 100% hyperpolarized ^{129}Xe and 98% O_2: 2% isoflurane. The breath-hold period during the delivery of each hyperpolarized ^{129}Xe breath was 2 seconds.

High resolution proton images were taken of the rat head to provide an anatomical reference for hyperpolarized ^{129}Xe images. In order to evaluate the distribution of hyperpolarized ^{129}Xe in brain following an external sensory stimulus, we acquired MRS images before and after a pain producing stimulus that has a well-defined functional response that can be measured using traditional fMRI techniques. A baseline hyperpolarized ^{129}Xe spectroscopic image was acquired from a coronal slice centered at the level of the anatomical reference slice.

The maximal, steady-state ^{129}Xe brain signal occurred within 15 seconds after starting the ventilation with hyperpolarized ^{129}Xe. Once verification of the xenon signal in the brain, a baseline ^{129}Xe chemical shift image (CSI) was acquired that was centred in the plane corresponding to the proton reference image. Low flip angle used for CSI acquisition insured minimal loss of hyperpolarized ^{129}Xe signal due to RF destruction, and the relatively long TR allowed continuous delivery of hyperpolarized ^{129}Xe to the tissue, a steady-state concentration of hyperpolarized ^{129}Xe was maintained in the brain thereby insuring constant signal intensity across the k-space. In a subset of animals (n=3) the animal's left forepaw was injected with a vehicle solution during baseline. Following acquisition of the baseline CSI image, the animal was ventilated for 10 minutes with O_2 (isoflurane to allow for complete clearance of ^{129}Xe magnetization from the brain). After that, the chemical irritant capsaicin (20 ul of 3 mg/ml) was injected into the animal's right forepaw (n= 6), and a second CSI was acquired.

6.2 Experiment results and discussion

A robust hyperpolarized ^{129}Xe spectroscopic signal with one primary peak at 194.7 ppm developed within 15 seconds after starting the ventilation with hyperpolarized ^{129}Xe. In order to determine the extent of hyperpolarized ^{129}Xe distribution throughout the rat brain, a magnetic resonance spectroscopic image was acquired of the primary peak during the administration of hyperpolarized ^{129}Xe (Figure 4). The four smaller resonances did not have sufficient SNR to produce spectroscopic images. Figure 4a shows an hyperpolarized ^{129}Xe image taken in the axial plane. Addition of a color look-up table (Figure 4b) aided in visually delineating areas of low and high SNR. Figure 4c show a 1 mm proton slice in which the olfactory bulbs and cerebellum are visible. Overlay of the hyperpolarized ^{129}Xe spectroscopic image onto the proton reference image (Figure 4d) revealed that the steady-state hyperpolarized ^{129}Xe signal originated from within the brain tissue and further demonstrated a pattern of hyperpolarized ^{129}Xe distribution throughout the brain with varying signal intensity in different brain regions.

Three of the six animals studied received a vehicle injection (saline) to the left forepaw immediately prior to the acquisition of the baseline image. 10 minutes after acquisition of the baseline hyperpolarized ^{129}Xe MRS, the animal's right forepaw was injected with the chemical irritant capsaicin (20 ml of 3 mg/ml), and a second hyperpolarized ^{129}Xe spectroscopic image was acquired. Responses from three individual animals are shown in Figure 5. Whereas baseline images showed some hyperpolarized ^{129}Xe signal intensity in cortical and sub-cortical brain regions (Figure 5, left panel), images acquired following administration of capsaicin showed both higher hyperpolarized ^{129}Xe signal intensity and an increased area of distribution within the brain (Figure 5, right panel). Superimposition of a rat brain atlas (Figure 5a) revealed that areas of hyperpolarized ^{129}Xe signal increase occurred both bilaterally and contralaterally in areas of the brain known to be involved in the processing of forepaw pain information, including the anterior cingulate and somatosensory cortices.

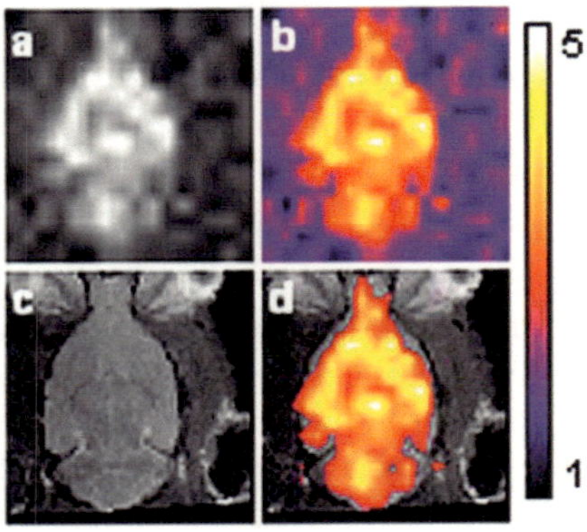

Fig. 4. Hyperpolarized ^{129}Xe signal distribution in the rat brain. (3a) hyperpolarized ^{129}Xe CSI image acquired with a 2D CSI pulse sequence from rat head under normal breathing conditions (slice thickness 10 mm). (3b) same image with false color applied. Warmer colors indicate increased hyperpolarized ^{129}Xe signal intensity. (3c) Proton MRI of a rat head showing a 1 mm coronal slice through the brain acquired with a RARE pulse sequence. (3d) Proton image shown with overlay of hyperpolarized ^{129}Xe MRI, in which only hyperpolarized ^{129}Xe signal with an SNR above 2 are shown. FOV was 25 mm.

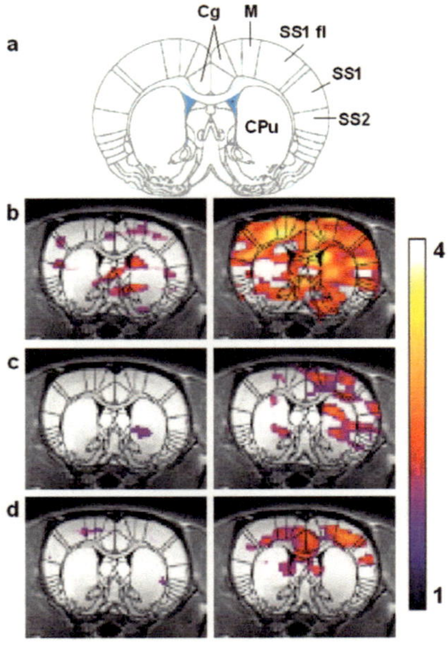

Fig. 5. Hyperpolarized ^{129}Xe fMRI data from three animals. The hyperpolarized ^{129}Xe signal is shown as a false color overlay on the corresponding 1 mm thick coronal proton reference image taken from the same animal. The left panel shows hyperpolarized ^{129}Xe signal intensity during baseline and the right panel shows hyperpolarized ^{129}Xe signal intensity after injection of capsaicin 20 ul (3 mg/ml) into the right forepaw. Color scale represents SNR and only signal with SNR above 2 are shown.

In spite of the as yet unrefined nature of this imaging modality, our results indicate that hyperpolarized ^{129}Xe MRI may have use as a probe for brain physiology and function. Because xenon is not inherent in the body, the substantial challenges resulting from high background signal in ^{1}H fMRI may be somewhat reduced. Extracting meaningful data from ^{1}H fMRI experiments is labour intensive, and requires a large number of subjects and image acquisitions. Extensive image post-processing is required and the influence that different post-processing steps play on the final data set achieved is actively debated. Conversely, hyperpolarized ^{129}Xe MRI showed patterns of brain activation consistent with those obtained using ^{1}H fMRI, using only a single set of images (one baseline and one post stimulus image) obtained from six animals. The magnitude of the signal difference between baseline and stimulus conditions for hyperpolarized ^{129}Xe (13–28%) was comparable to differences typically obtained with conventional BOLD fMRI (2 to 29%) (Bock et al., 1998; Silva et al., 1999; Mandeville et al., 1999; Tuor et al., 2000) using a rat forepaw activation paradigm.

7. Outlook of hyperpolarized ^{129}Xe brain MRI

This subsection will summarize the current progress as previously described, and comment the future research directions and applications in the brain imaging. Conventional MRI focuses mainly on the nuclear spin of the proton because it is ubiquitous in most parts of the human body. However, certain organs have a low proton spin density attributable to the large volume of air dispersed throughout the tissue. The low sensitivity of traditional magnetic resonance has motivated the development of techniques using hyperpolarized noble gases for NMR and MRI. Xenon has the unique characteristic of being soluble in many fluids and biological tissues, such as water, blood, lung tissue, and white and gray matter. Being a trace element in the atmosphere, xenon has no natural background signal in the human body. Therefore, dissolved-phase xenon MRI and molecular imaging could provide rich information related to biological and physiological changes beyond void space lung imaging. Efforts have demonstrated the value of dissolved xenon MRI in the study of lung gas exchange (Swanson et.al, 1999), and brain perfusion (Swanson et al., 1997; Kilian et al., 2004; Zhou et al., 2008, 2011a, 2011b) and function (Mazzanti et al., 2011). Recently, xenon-based molecular imaging has been demonstrated by using cryptophane-containing biosensors (Hilty et al., 2006). Sensitivity enhancement using a chemical amplification technique, hyperpolarized xenon chemical exchange saturation transfer (Hyper-CEST) (Schröder et al., 2006), allows imaging at low concentrations; however, for *in vivo* applications the small filling factor of a region of interest in the body relative to the NMR coil is a significant factor limiting sensitivity. In such cases remote detection methods (Hilty et.al, 2005) can provide dramatic improvements in sensitivity. In remote detection, the normal NMR coil that contains the full region of interest is used to encode spectroscopic and spatial information, then stores it as longitudinal magnetization. These encoded spins then flow into a second coil with an optimized filling factor for detection.

Remote detection can overcome the filling factor issue of dissolved xenon MRI, although a low concentration of xenon in solution can be another significant impediment to highly sensitive detection. It has been shown that the solvated xenon signal can be amplified by xenon polarization transfer contrast, in which the dissolved-phase xenon from either lungs or brains is selectively saturated, and through exchange, the gas-phase signal is attenuated.

This method is able to indirectly image dissolved-phase xenon, but is limited to tissue in direct exchange with the air in the lungs. The gas exchange process could be similarly exploited for direct signal amplification of dissolved xenon with the remote detection technique, which extends the study area from lung to brain. Xenon gas can be extracted from the dissolved solutions and concentrated in the gas phase for detection. Furthermore, with the long longitudinal relaxation time of gas-phase xenon, extracted xenon gas from solution can be compressed or liquefied while preserving the encoded information. The xenon density in the liquid state is approximately four orders of magnitude higher than in aqueous solutions, which in principle could result in up to 10,000 times enhancement of spin density, thus allowing substantial signal amplification

We have demonstrated the hyperpolarized xenon signal amplification by gas extraction (Hyper-SAGE) method (Zhou et al., 2009b) with enhanced NMR spectra and time-of-flight (TOF) images by using recently commercialized membrane technology for high-efficiency xenon dissolution (Baumer et.al, 2006). The Hyper-SAGE technique relies on physical amplification by exploiting a phase change and is completely distinct from chemical amplification. In combination with additional amplification techniques such as Hyper-CEST, this method promises to dramatically decrease the detection threshold of MRI and has the potential to benefit molecular imaging applications and brain imaging.

Recent innovations in the production of highly polarized ^{129}Xe and novel method of signal enhancement should make feasible the emergence of hyperpolarized ^{129}Xe MRI as a viable adjunct method to conventional MRI for the study of brain function and disease. The high sensitivity of hyperpolarized noble gas signal and non-background noise in biological tissue offer xenon as an important and promising contrast agent to study the brain. Because the polarization of hyperpolarized xenon does not depend on the magnetic field strength, the technique for brain imaging could also be applied for use with low field portable MRI devices (Appelt, 2007; Blümich, 2008; Paulsen, 2008).

8. Acknowledgments

This work was supported by the Chinese Academy of Sciences (the 100 talents program and KJCX2-EW-N06-04), Natural Science Foundation of China (11004228), and Innovation Method Fund of China (2010IM030600).

9. References

Albert MS, et al. (1994). Biological magnetic resonance imaging using laser-polarized ^{129}Xe. *Nature*, Vol. 370, pp.(199–201).

Andrea & Angelo (2003), Hyperpolarised xenon in biology. *Nucl. Magn. Reson. Spectr.*, Vol. 4, pp.(1–30).

Appelt S, et al. (2005). Mobile high-resolution xenon nuclear magnetic resonance spectroscopy in the Earth's magnetic field. *Phys Rev Lett,* Vol.94, pp.(197602).

Baumer D, et al. (2006). NMR spectroscopy of laser-polarized ^{129}Xe under continuous flow: A method to study aqueous solutions of biomolecules. *Angew Chem Int Ed*, Vol. 45, pp.(7282–7284).

Betz E .(1972). Cerebral blood flow: Its measurement and regulation. *Physiol. Rev.*, Vol. 52: 595–630

Bock C, et al. (1998). Functional MRI of somatosensory activation in rat: effect of hypercapnic upregulation on perfusion- and BOLD-imaging. *Magn. Reson. Med.*, Vol. 39, pp.(457–461).

Blümich B, et al. (2008). Mobile single-sided NMR. *Prog. Nucl. Magn. Reson. Spectr.*, Vol.52, pp.(197–269).

Cherubini A & Bifone A. (2003). Hyperpolarized xenon in biology. *Prog. Nucl. Magn. Reson. Spectr.*, Vol. 42, pp.(1–30).

Choquet P, et al. (2003) Method to determine *in vivo* the relaxation time T1 of hyperpolarized xenon in rat brain. *Magn. Reson. Med.*, Vol. 49, pp.(1014–1018).

Cook GE. (1961). Argon, Helium and the Rare Gases, Interscience Publishers, New York

Duhamel G, et al. (2000). *In vivo* ^{129}Xe NMR in rat brain during intra-arterial injections of hyperpolarized ^{129}Xe dissolved in a lipid emulsion. *C.R. Acad. Sci. III*, Vol. 323, pp. (529-536).

Duhamel G, et al. (2002). Global and regional cerebral blood flow measurements using NMR of injected hyperpolarized xenon-129. *Acad. Radiol.*, Vol. suppl 2, pp.(S498-S500).

Goodson BM. (2002). Nuclear magnetic resonance of laser-polarized noble gases in molecules, materials, and organisms. *J. Magn. Reson.*, Vol.155, pp.(157–216).

Gur D & Good WF.(1982). *In vivo* mapping of local cerebral blood flow by xenon-enhanced computed tomography. *Science,* Vol.215, pp.(1267–1268).

Hilty C, et al. (2006). Spectrally resolved magnetic resonance imaging of a xenon biosensor. *Angew. Chem. Int. Ed.* Vol.45, pp.(70–73).

Hilty C, et al. (2005). Microfluidic gas-flow profiling using remote-detection NMR. *Proc. Natl. Acad. Sci. USA,* Vol.102, pp.(14960–14963).

Kilian W, et al. (2004). Dynamic NMR spectroscopy of hyperpolarized ^{129}Xe in human brain analyzed by an uptake model. *Magn. Reson. Med.*, Vol. 51, pp.(843–847).

Mandeville JB, et al. (1999). MRI measurement of the temporal evolution of relative CMRO2 during rat forepaw stimulation. *Magn. Reson. Med.*, Vol. 42, pp.(944–951).

Martin CC, et al. (1997). The pharmacokinetics of hyperpolarized xenon: implications for cerebral MRI. *J. Magn. Reson. Imag.*, Vol. 7, pp.(848–854).

Mazzanti M, et al. (2011). Distribution of hyperpolarized xenon in the brain following sensory stimulation: preliminary MRI findings. *PLoS ONE*, Vol. 6, pp.(e21607).

Meng X, et al. (2004). Characterizing the diffusion/perfusion mismatch in experimental focal cerebral ischemia. *Ann. Neurol.*, Vol. 55, pp.(207-212).

Navon et al. (1996). Enhancement of solution NMR and MRI with laser-polarized xenon. *Science*, Vol. 271, pp.(1848-1851).

Oros A-M & Shah NJ. (2004). Hyperpolarized xenon in NMR and MRI. *Phys. Med. Biol.*, Vol. 49, pp.(R105–R153).

Paulsen JL, et al. (2008). Volume-selective magnetic resonance imaging using an adjustable, single-sided, portable sensor. *Proc. Natl. Acad. Sci. USA*, Vol.105, pp.(20601–20604).

Peled S, et al. (1996). Determinants of tissue delivery for ^{129}Xe magnetic resonance in humans. *Magn. Reson. Med.*, Vol. 36, pp.(340–344).

Ruppert K, et al. (2000). Probing lung physiology with xenon polarization transfer contrast (XTC). *Magn. Reson. Med.*, Vol. 44, pp.(349–357).

Swanson SD & Rosen MS. (1997). Brain MRI with laser-polarized ^{129}Xe. *Magn. Reson. Med.*, Vol.38, pp.695–698,

Swanson SD & Rosen MS. (1999). Distribution and dynamics of laser-polarized ^{129}Xe agnetization *in vivo*. *Magn. Reson. Med.,* 42:1137–1145.

Saam BT, et al. (2000). MR imaging of diffusion of ^{3}He gas in healthy and diseased lungs. *Magn. Reson. Med.,* Vol.44, pp.(174–179).

Schöder L, et al. (2006). Molecular imaging using a targeted magnetic resonance hyperpolarized biosensor. *Science,* Vol. 314, pp.(446–449).

Silva AC, et al. (1999). Simultaneous blood oxygenation level-dependent and cerebral blood flow functional magnetic resonance imaging during forepaw stimulation in the rat. *J. Cereb. Blood. F. Met.,* Vol. 19, pp.(871–879).

Tuor UI, et al. (2000). Functional magnetic resonance imaging in rats subjected to intense electrical and noxious chemical stimulation of the forepaw. *Pain,* Vol. 87, pp.(315–324).

Walker TG & Happer W. (1997). Spin-exchange optical pumping of noble-gas nuclei. *Rev. Mod. Phys.,* Vol. 69, pp.(629–642).

Wakai A, et al. (2005). A method for measuring the decay time of hyperpolarized ^{129}Xe magnetization in rat brain without estimation of RF flip angles. *Magn. Reson. Med. Sci.,* Vol. 4, pp.(19–25).

Wilson GJ, et al. (1999). Longitudinal relaxation times of ^{129}Xe in rat tissue homogenates at 9.4 T. *Magn. Reson. Med.,* Vol. 41, pp.(933–938).

Zhou X , et al. (2004a). Production of Hyerpolarized ^{129}Xe Gas without Nitrogen by Optical Pumping at ^{133}Cs D_2 Line in Flow System. *Chin. Phys. Lett.,* Vol.21, pp.(1501-1503).

Zhou X, et al. (2004b). Experimental and Dynamic Simulations of Radiation Damping of Laserpolarized Liquid ^{129}Xe at Low Magnetic Field in a Flow System. *Appl. Magn. Reson.,* Vol. 26, pp.(327-337).

Zhou X, et al. (2004c). Enhancement of Solid-state Proton NMR via SPINOE with Laser-polarized Xenon. *Phys. Rev. B,* Vol. 70, pp.(052405-1-052405-4).

Zhou X, et al. (2008). Reinvestigating Hyperpolarized ^{129}Xe Longitudinal Relaxation Time in the Rat Brain with Noise Considerations. *NMR in Biomedicine,* Vol.21, pp.(217-225).

Zhou X. et al. (2009a). Quantitative Estimation of SPINOE Enhancement in Solid State. *J. Magn. Reson.,* Vol. 196, pp.(200-203).

Zhou X , et al. (2009b). Hyperpolarized Xenon NMR and MRI Signal Amplification by Gas Extraction. *Proc. Natl. Acad. Sci. USA,* Vol.106, pp.(16903-16906).

Zhou X , et al. (2011a). MRI of Stroke using Hyperpolarized ^{129}Xe. *NMR in Biomedicine,* Vol. 24, pp.(170-175).

Zhou X , et al. (2011b). Distribution of Hyperpolarized Xenon in the Brain Following Sensory Stimulation: Preliminary MRI Findings. *PLoS ONE,* Vol. 6, pp.(e21607).

Zhou X, et al. (2011c). Hyperpolarized ^{129}Xe magnetic resonance imaging and its applications in biomedicine. *Physics* (review article in Chinese), Vol. 40, pp.(379-388).

http://science.nasa.gov/science-news/science-at-nasa/2008/25apr_cvx2/

8

Segmentation of Brain MRI

Rong Xu[1], Limin Luo[2] and Jun Ohya[1]
[1]Waseda University,
[2]Southeast University,
[1]Japan,
[2]China

1. Introduction

Effective, precise and consistent brain cortical tissue segmentation from magnetic resonance (MR) images is one of the most prominent issues in many applications of medical image processing. These applications include surgical planning (Kikinis et al., 1996), surgery navigation (Grimson et al., 1997), multimodality image registration (Saeed, 1998), abnormality detection (Rusinek et al., 1991), multiple sclerosis lesion quantification (Udupa et al., 1997), brain tumour detection (Vaidyanathan et al., 1997), functional mapping (Roland et al., 1993), etc. Traditionally, the purpose of segmentation is to partition the image into non-overlapping, constituent regions (or called classes, clusters, subsets or sub-regions) that are homogeneous with respect to intensity and texture (Gonzalez & Woods, 1992). If the domain of the image is given by Ω, then the segmentation problem is to determine the sets $S_k \subset \Omega$, whose union is the entire domain Ω. Thus, the sets that make up a segmentation must satisfy

$$\Omega = \bigcup_{k=1}^{K} S_k \tag{1}$$

where $S_k \cap S_j = \emptyset$ for $k \neq j$, and each S_k is connected. Ideally, a segmentation method is to find those sets that correspond to distinct anatomical structures or regions of interest in the image (Pham et al., 2000).

For brain MR image segmentation, some studies aim to identify the entire image into sub-regions such as white matter (WM), grey matter (GM), and cerebrospinal fluid spaces (CSF) of the brain (Lim & Pfefferbaum, 1989), whereas others aim to extract one specific structure, for instance, brain tumour (M.C. Clark et al., 1998), multiple sclerosis lesions (Mortazavi et al., 2011), or subcortical structures (Babalola et al., 2008). Due to varying complications in segmenting human cerebral cortex, the manual methods for brain tissues segmentation might easily lead to errors both in accuracy and reproducibility (operator bias), and are exceedingly time-consuming, we thus need fast, accurate and robust semi-automatic (i.e., supervised classification explicitly needs user interaction) or completely automatic (i.e., non-supervised classification) techniques (Suri, Singh, et al., 2002b).

1.1 MR imaging (MRI)

MR imaging (MRI), invented by Raymond V. Damadian in 1969, and was firstly done on a human body in 1977 (Damadian et al., 1977). MR imaging is a popular medical imaging technique used in radiology to visualize detailed internal structures. It provides good contrast between different soft tissues of the body, which makes it especially useful in imaging the brain, muscles, the heart and cancers when compared with other medical imaging techniques, such as computed tomography (CT) or X-rays (Novelline & Squire, 2004). According to different magnetic signal weighting with particular values of the echo time (T_E) and the repetition time (T_R), three different images can be achieved from the same body: T_1-weighted, T_2-weighted, and PD-weighted (proton density).

In the clinical diagnosis, one patient's head is examined from 3 planes showed in Fig.1 (a), and they are axial plane, sagittal plane and coronal plane. The T_1-weighted brain MR images from different planes are respectively showed in Fig.1 (b), (c), and (d).

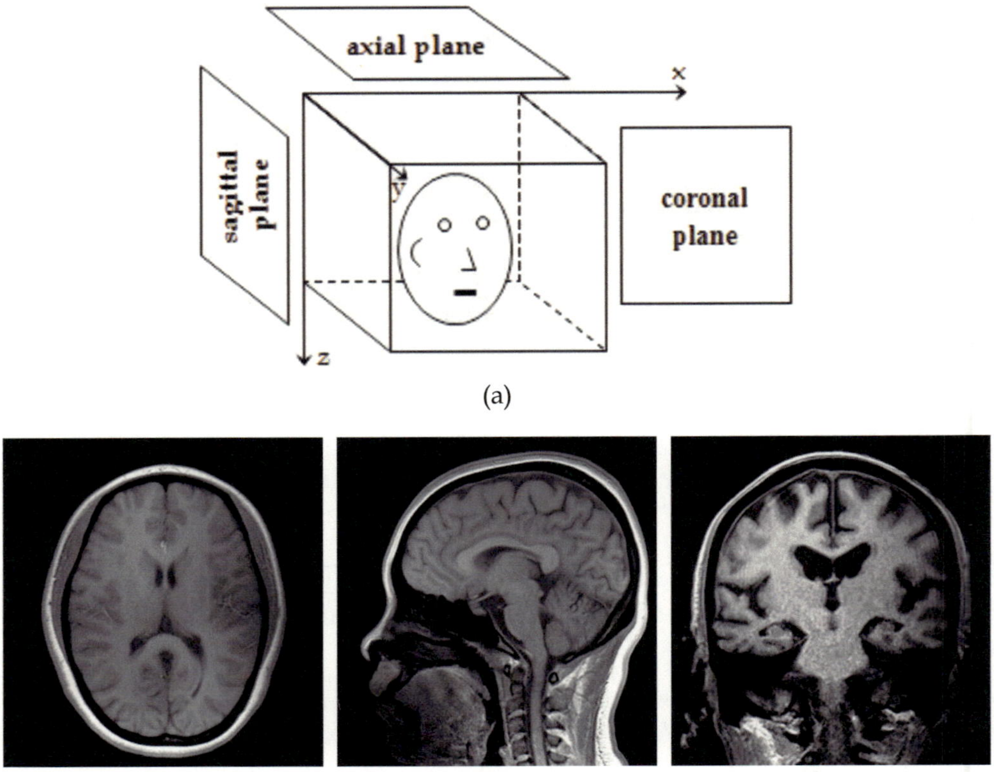

(a)

(b) (c) (d)

Fig.1. Brain MR images from (b) axial plane, (c) sagittal plane and (d) coronal plane.

1.2 Difficulties in segmentation of brain MRI

Even though cortical segmentation has developed for many years in medical research, it is not regarded as an automated, reliable, and high speed technique because of magnetic field inhomogeneities:

1. Noise: random noise associated with the MR imaging system, which is known to have a Rician distribution (Prima et al., 2001);
2. Intensity inhomogeneity (also called bias field, or shading artefact): the non-uniformity in the radio frequency (RF) field during data acquisition, resulting in the shading of effect (X. Li et al., 2003);
3. Partial volume effect: more than one type of class or tissue occupies one pixel or voxel of an image, which are called partial volume effect. These pixels or voxels are usually called mixels (Ruan et al., 2000).

1.3 Evaluation of segmentation techniques

The evaluation of brain tissue classification also is a complex issue in medical image processing. Visual inspection and comparison with manual segmentation are very strenuous and are not reliable since the amount of data to be processed is usually large. Tissue classification methods can also be validated by using synthetic data and real brain MR images. The simulated brain MR data with different noise levels and different levels of intensity inhomogeneity, have been provided by Brainweb simulated brain phantom (Collins et al., 1998; Kwan et al., 1999) (http://www.bic.mni.mcgill.ca/brainweb/), and the ground truth for both the classification and partial volumes within the images is also available to estimate different methods quantitatively. The real brain MRI datasets with expert segmentations can be obtained from Internet Brain Segmentation Repository (IBSR) (http://www.cma.mgh.harvard.edu/ibsr/). A few surveys on this topic have been provided in (H. Zhang et al., 2008; Y.J. Zhang, 1996, 2001). Here, we depict three different measures for quantitatively evaluating segmentation results.

(1) The misclassification rate (MCR) is the percentage of misclassified pixels and is computed as (background pixels were ignored in the MCR computation) (Bankman, 2000)

$$MCR = \frac{number\ of\ misclassified\ pixels}{total\ number\ of\ all\ pixels} \times 100\% \tag{2}$$

(2) The root mean squared error (RMSE) is to quantify the difference between the true partial volumes and the algorithm estimations. The RMSE of an estimator $\hat{\theta}$ with respect to the estimated parameter θ is defined as (Bankman, 2000):

$$RMSE(\hat{\theta}) = \sqrt{MSE(\hat{\theta})} = \sqrt{E[(\hat{\theta} - \theta)^2]} \tag{3}$$

(3) Let N_{fp} be the number of pixels that do not belong to a cluster and are segmented into the cluster, N_{fn} be the number of pixels that belong to a cluster and are not segmented into the cluster, N_p be the number of all pixels that belong to a cluster, and N_n be the total number of pixels that do not belong to a cluster. Three parameters in this evaluation system may now be defined as follows (Shen et al., 2005).

- Under segmentation (UnS): $UnS = N_{fp}/N_n$, representing the percentage of negative false segmentation;
- Over segmentation (OvS): $OvS = N_{fn}/N_p$, representing the percentage of positive false segmentation;

- Incorrect segmentation (InC): $InC = (N_{fp} + N_{fn})/N$, representing the total percentage of false segmentation.

The purpose of this chapter is to render a review about existing segmentation techniques and the work we have done in the segmentation of brain MR images. The rest of this chapter is organized as follows: In Section 2, existing techniques for human cerebral cortical segmentation and their applications are reviewed. In Section 3, a new non-homogeneous Markov random field model based on fuzzy membership is proposed for brain MR image segmentation. In Section 4, image pre-processing, such as de-noising, the correction of intensity inhomogeneity and the estimation of partial volume effect are summarized. In Section 5, the conclusion of this chapter is given.

2. Image segmentation methods

A wide variety of segmentation techniques have been reviewed in (Balafar et al., 2010; Bankman, 2000; Bezdek et al., 1993; Clarke et al., 1995; Dubey et al., 2010; Pal & Pal, 1993; Pham et al., 2000; Saeed, 1998; Suri, Singh, et al., 2002b, 2002a; Zijdenbos & Dawant, 1994). We separate these techniques into 9 categories based on the classification scheme in (Pham et al., 2000): (1) thresholding, (2) region growing, (3) edge detection, (4) classifiers, (5) clustering, (6) statistical models, (7) artificial neural networks, (8) deformable models, and (9) atlas-guided approaches. Other notable methods that do not belong to any of these categories are described at the end of this section. Though each technique is presented separately, multiple techniques are often used in conjunction to solve various applications.

2.1 Thresholding

The simplest operation in this category is image thresholding (Pal & Pal, 1993). In this technique a threshold is selected, and an image is divided into groups of pixels having value less than the threshold and groups of pixels with values greater or equal to the threshold. There are several thresholding methods: global thresholding, adaptive thresholding, optimal global and adaptive thresholding, local thresholding, and thresholds based on several variables (Bankman, 2000). Thresholding is a very simple, fast and easily implemented procedure that works reasonably well for images with very good contrast between distinctive sub-regions. A typical example is to separate CSF from highly T2-weighted brain images (Saeed, 1998). However, the distribution of intensities in brain MR images is usually very complex, and determining a threshold is difficult. In most cases, thresholding is combined with other methods (Brummer et al., 1993; Suzuki & Toriwaki, 1991).

2.2 Region growing

Region growing (or region merging) is a procedure that looks for groups of pixels with similar intensities. It starts with a pixel or a group of pixels (called seeds) that belong to the structure of interest. Subsequently the neighbouring pixels with the same properties as seeds (or based on a homogeneity criteria) are appended gradually to the growing region until no more pixels can be added (Dubey et al., 2010). The object is then represented by all pixels that have been accepted during the growing procedure. The advantage of region growing is that it is capable of correctly segmenting regions that have the same properties and are spatially separated, and also it generates connected regions (Bankman, 2000). Instead of region merging, it is possible to start with some initial segmentation and subdivide the regions that do not satisfy a given uniformity test. This technique is called splitting (Haralick & Shapiro, 1985). A combination of splitting and merging adds together the advantages of both approaches (Zucker, 1976). However, the results of region growing depend strongly on the selection of homogeneity criterion. Another problem is that different starting points may not grow into identical regions (Bankman, 2000). Region growing has been exploited in many clinical applications (Cline et al., 1987; Tang et al., 2000).

2.3 Edge detection techniques

In edge detection techniques, the resulting segmented image is described in terms of the edges (boundaries) between different regions. Edges are formed at intersection of two regions where there are abrupt changes in grey level intensity values. Edge detection works well on images with good contrast between regions. A large number of different edge operators can be used for edge detection. These operations are generally named after their inventors. The most popular ones are the Marr-Hildreth or LoG (Laplacian-of-Gaussian), Sobel, Roberts, Prewitt, and Canny operators. Binary mathematical morphology and Watershed algorithm are often used for edge detection purposed in the segmentation of brain MR images (Dogdas et al., 2002; Grau et al., 2004). However, the major drawbacks of these methods are over-segmentation, sensitivity to noise, poor detection of significant areas with low contrast boundaries, and poor detection of thin structures, etc. (Grau et al., 2004).

2.4 Classifiers

Classifier methods are known as supervised methods in pattern recognition, which seek to partition the image by using training data with known labels as references. The simplest classifier is nearest-neighbour classifier (NNC), in which each pixel is classified in the same class as the training datum with closest intensity (Boudraa & Zaidi, 2006). Other examples of classifiers are *k*-nearest neighbour (*k*-NN) (Duda & Hart, 1973; Fukunaga, 1990), Parzen window (Hamamoto et al., 1996), Bayes classifier or maximum likelihood (ML) estimation (Duda & Hart, 1973), Fisher's linear discriminant (FLD) (Fisher, 1936), the nearest mean classifier (NMC) (Skurichina & Duin, 1996), support vector machine (SVM) (Vapnik, 1998). The weakness of classifiers is that they generally do not perform any spatial modelling. This weakness has been addressed in recent work extending classifier methods to segment images corrupted by intensity in-homogeneities (Wells III et al., 1996). Neighbourhood and geometric information was also incorporated into a classifier approach in (Kapur et al., 1998). In addition, it requires manual interaction to obtain training data. Training sets for each image can be time consuming and laborious (Pham et al., 2000).

2.5 Clustering

Clustering is the process of organizing objects into groups whose members are similar in certain ways, whose goal is to recognize structures or clusters presented in a collection of unlabelled data. It is a method of unsupervised learning, and a common technique for statistical data analysis used in many fields.

2.5.1 K-means clustering

K-means clustering (or Hard C-means clustering, HCM) (MacQueen, 1967) is one of the simplest unsupervised clustering method, aiming to partition N samples into K clusters by minimizing an objective function so that the within-cluster sum of squares is minimized. It starts with defined initial K cluster centers and keeps reassigning the samples to clusters based on the similarity between the sample and the cluster centers until a convergence criterion is met. Given a set of samples $(x_1, x_2, \dots, x_N)$, where each sample is a M-dimensional real vector, N_k is the num of samples in cluster k denoted by Γ_k, v_k is the mean value of these samples, and then the objective function is defined as:

$$J_m = \sum_{k=1}^{K}\sum_{i=1}^{N} ||x_i - v_k||^2 \tag{4}$$

$$v_k = \frac{1}{N_k}\sum_{x_i \in \Gamma_k} x_i \tag{5}$$

where $||x_i - v_k||$ is a distance measure between point x_i and the cluter center v_k. The common distance measures are Euclidean distance, chessboard distance, city block distance, Mahalanobis distance, or Hamming distance. The K-means algorithm has been used widely in brain MR image segmentation (Abras & Ballarin, 2005; Vemuri et al., 1995), because of its easy implementation and simple time complexity. A major problem of this algorithm is that it is sensitive to the selection of K cluster centers, and may converge to a local minimum of the criterion function value (Jain et al., 1999). Dozens of optimal solutions have been proposed for selecting better initial K cluster centers to find the global minimum value (Bradley & Fayyad, 1998; Khan & Ahmad, 2004).

2.5.2 Fuzzy c-means clustering (FCM)

Fuzzy c-means clustering (FCM) (Bezdek, 1981; Dunn, 1973) is based on the same idea of finding cluster centers by iteratively adjusting their positions and minimizing an objective function as K-means algorithm. Meanwhile it allows more flexibility by introducing multiple fuzzy membership grades to multiple clusters. The objective function is defined as:

$$J_m = \sum_{k=1}^{K}\sum_{i=1}^{N} u_{ik}^m ||x_i - v_k||^2, 1 \le m < \infty \tag{6}$$

where m is constant to control clustering fuzziness, generally $m = 2$. u_{ik} is the fuzzy membership of x_i in the cluster k and satisfying ① $0 \le u_{ik} \le 1$, ② $\sum_{k=1}^{K} u_{ik} = 1$. x_i is the i-th sample in measured data. v_k is the cluster center, and $\|*\|$ is a distance measure. Fuzzy partitioning is carried out through an iterative optimization of the objective function shown above, with the update of membership u_{ik} and cluster centers v_k by:

$$u_{ik} = \frac{1}{\sum_{l=1}^{K}\left(\frac{||x_i - v_k||}{||x_i - v_l||}\right)^{2/(m-1)}} \tag{7}$$

$$v_k = \frac{\sum_{i=1}^{N} u_{ik}^m x_i}{\sum_{i=1}^{N} u_{ik}^m} \tag{8}$$

This iteration will stop when $max\left\{\left|u_{ik}^{(p)} - u_{ik}^{(p-1)}\right|\right\} \leq \varepsilon$, ε is a termination criterion between 0 and 1, and p is the iteration step (Kannan et al., 2010). Although clustering algorithms do not require training data, they do require an initial segmentation (or equivalently, initial parameters). Clustering algorithms do not directly incorporate spatial modeling and can therefore be sensitive to noise and intensity inhomogeneities. This lack of spatial modeling, however, can provide significant advantages for fast computation (Hebert, 1997). Some work on improving the robustness of clustering algorithms to intensity inhomogeneities in MR images have been carried out (Pham & Prince, 1999). Robustness to noise can be incorporated with spatial correlations in an image based on k-nearest neighbor model (R. Xu & Ohya, 2010) or Markov random field (MRF) modeling (Liu et al., 2005).

2.6 Statistical models

Statistical classification methods usually solve the segmentation problem by either assigning a class label to a pixel or by estimating the relative amounts of the various tissue types within a pixel (Noe et al., 2001). Statistical inference enables us to make statements about which element(s) of this set are likely to be the true ones.

2.6.1 Expectation maximization (EM)

Expectation maximization (EM) algorithm (Dempster et al., 1977) is a method for finding the maximum likelihood or maximum a posteriori (MAP) estimator of a hidden parameter θ with a probability distribution. EM is an iterative method which alternates between performing an expectation (E) step, in which each pixel is classified into one cluster according to the current estimates of the posterior distributions over hidden variables, and a maximization (M) step, in which the hidden parameters are re-estimated by maximizing the likelihood function, according to the current classification. These parameter-estimates are then used to determine the distribution over hidden variables in the next E step. Convergence is assured since the increase of likelihood after each iteration (Zaidi et al., 2006). The underlying model in EM algorithm can be specified according the specific requirements of the given task (Wells III et al., 1996; Y. Zhang et al., 2001). In spite of these achievements, they have a few deficiencies: a good prior distribution and the known number of classes are required, and it has extensive computations.

2.6.2 Markov random field model (MRF)

Markov random field (S.Z. Li, 1995) model is a statistical model that can be used within segmentation methods. MRFs model spatial interactions among neighboring or nearby pixels. In medical imaging, they are typically used because most pixels belong to the same class as their neighboring pixels (Pham et al., 2000). Let a finite lattice I as a 2D image, $i \in I$ is the pixel i in this image, which is denoted by $Y = \{Y_i, i \in I\}$, where Y_i is the gray value of pixel i. For each pixel, the region-type (or pixel class) that the pixel belongs to is specified by a class label $X = \{X_i, i \in I\}$ (i.e., image segmentation results). $X_i \in \Lambda$, $\Lambda = \{1,2,\dots,K\}$ is a set of labels and K is the number of classes. So X (label filed) and Y (gray field) will be random fields in lattice I and the purpose of MRF model is to establish the relationship between X and Y, then the image model is defined as:

$$Y_i = v_{X_i} + e_i, i \in I \tag{9}$$

where v_{X_i} is the gray mean value of class X_i, and e_i is a random variable meeting Gaussian distribution. If $X_i = k, k \in \Lambda$, $e_i - N(0, \sigma_k^2)$, in which σ_k^2 is the variance of e_i for k, then the conditional probability density is defined as:

$$P(Y_i = y_i \mid X_i = k) = \frac{1}{\sqrt{2\pi\sigma_k^2}} \exp[-\frac{(y_i - v_k)^2}{2\sigma_k^2}] \tag{10}$$

Subsequently, $X = \{X_i, i \in I\}$, the priori model of image segmentation results is a 2D MRF. According to Hammersley-Clifford theorem in (Hammersley & Clifford, 1971), the priori probability of MRF meets Gibbs distribution, and so the priori model is defined as:

$$P(X = x) = \frac{1}{Z} \exp[-\sum_{c \in C} V_c(x)] \tag{11}$$

where $Z = \sum_{x \in \Lambda} \exp[-\sum_{c \in C} V_c(x)]$ is a normalizing constant called *partition function* and $V_c(x)$ denotes the potential function of clique $c \in C$, which only depends on $\delta(i), i \in c$. C is the set of second order cliques (i.e. doubletons), and $\delta(i)$ indicates the neighborhood of pixel i. If multi-level logistic (MLL) model is adopted and the second order neighborhood system and the dual potential function are only considered, energy function is defined as:

$$U(x) = \sum_{i \in I} \sum_{j \in \delta(i)} V(x_i, x_j) \tag{12}$$

$$V(x_i, x_j) = \begin{cases} -\beta, & if \quad x_i = x_j \\ \beta, & if \quad x_i \neq x_j \end{cases} \tag{13}$$

Note that the energies of singletons (i.e. pixel $i \in I$) directly reflect the probabilistic modeling of labels without context, while doubleton clique potentials express relationship between neighboring pixel label. On the basis of maximum a posteriori (MAP) estimation (Geman & Geman, 1993) and Bayes' theorem, the optimal solution $X = X^*$ is defined as:

$$\begin{aligned} X^* &= \arg\max_X P(X \mid Y) \\ &= \arg\max_X P(Y \mid X) P(X) \end{aligned} \tag{14}$$

In order to facilitate the solution, the objective function takes natural logarithm to be

$$X^* = \arg\min_{x \in \Lambda} \{U(y \mid x; \theta) + U(x)\} \tag{15}$$

$$U(y \mid x;\theta) = \sum_{i \in I} U(y_i \mid x_i) = \sum_{i \in I} [\frac{(y_i - v_k)}{2\sigma_k^2} + \frac{1}{2}\log(\sigma_k^2)] \tag{16}$$

$$\theta = \{v_k, \sigma_k \mid k \in \Lambda\} \tag{17}$$

In this way, the segmentation problem in MRF model is reduced to the minimization of the above energy function, which is usually computed by iterated conditional modes (ICM) algorithm (Besag, 1986). The ICM method uses the 'greedy' strategy in the iterative local minimization and convergence is guaranteed after only a few iterations (Boudraa & Zaidi, 2006). By importing spatial relations among pixels, non-supervised and nonparametric MRF model can effectively decrease the influence of image noise, and undertake fine stable and satisfied segmentation results for low SNR images. This model has been widely applied in human cerebral cortical segmentation (Held et al., 1997; Y. Zhang et al., 2001). Contrarily a difficulty associated with MRF models is proper selection of the parameters controlling the strength of spatial interaction (S.Z. Li, 1995). A setting that is too high can result in an excessively smooth segmentation and a loss of important structural details. Some researchers have proposed several schemes for the estimation of MRF parameters (Descombes et al., 1999; Salzenstein & Pieczynski, 1997; R. Xu & Luo, 2009). In addition, MRF methods usually require computationally intensive algorithms (Pham et al., 2000).

2.7 Artificial neural networks (ANNs)

Artificial neural networks (ANNs) are parallel networks of processing elements or nodes to simulate biological neural networks. Each node in an ANN is capable of performing elementary computations. Learning is achieved through the adaptation of weights assigned to the connections between nodes. The massive connectionist architecture usually makes the system robust while the parallel processing enables the system to produce output in real time. To simulate biological neural network, the neurons and connections in ANNs model comprise the following components and variables in Fig. 2 (Kriesel, 2007). A thorough treatment of ANNs can be found in (J.W. Clark, 1991).

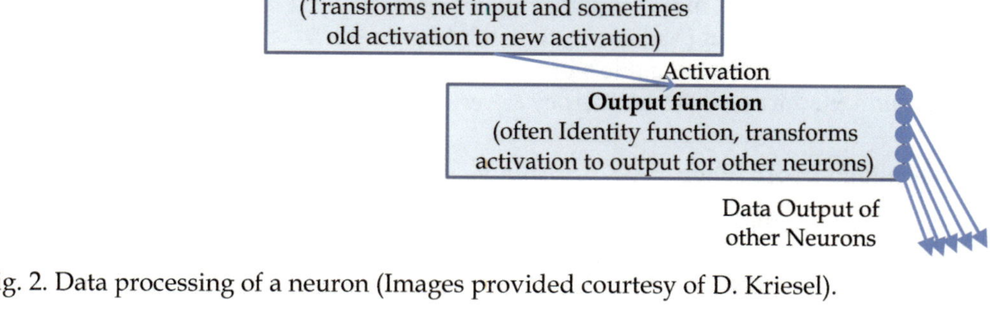

Fig. 2. Data processing of a neuron (Images provided courtesy of D. Kriesel).

The most widely application in medical imaging is as a classifier (Gelenbe et al., 1996; Hall et al., 1992), in which the weights are determined by training data and the ANN is then used to segment new data. ANNs can also be used in an unsupervised fashion as a clustering method (Bezdek et al., 1993; Reddick et al., 1997), as well as for deformable models (Vilarino et al., 1998). Because of the many interconnections used in a neural network, spatial information can be easily incorporated into its classification procedures (Pham et al., 2000). However, the major disadvantage of the artificial neural networks (ANNs) is that it requires training data. For large neural networks, it also requires high processing time because its processing is usually simulated on a standard serial computer.

2.8 Deformable models

Deformable models are physically motivated, model-based techniques for detecting region boundaries by using closed parametric curves or surfaces that deform under the influence of internal and external forces. To delineate an object boundary in an image, a closed curve or surface must first be placed near the desired boundary and then be allowed to undergo an iterative relaxation process. Internal forces are computed from within the curve or surface to keep it smooth throughout the deformation. External forces are usually derived from the image to drive the curve or surface toward the desired feature of interest (Pham et al., 2000). The original deformable, called *snake* model, was introduced in (Kass et al., 1988), in which the contour deforms to minimize the contour energy that includes the internal energy from the contour and the external energy from the image. A number of improvements have also been proposed, such as snake variations (Cohen, 1991; McInerney & Terzopoulos, 2000; C. Xu & Prince, 1998). *Level set* is another important deformable contour method and it was firstly proposed for image segmentation in (Malladi et al., 1995). Some researchers applied level set formulation with a contour energy minimization for obtaining a better convergence (Siddiqi et al., 1998; Wang et al., 2004).

Deformable models are quite helpful for cerebral cortical segmentation in MR images (Davatzikos & Bryan, 1996; C. Xu et al., 1998). The advantages are that they are capable of generating closed parametric curves or surfaces from images and incorporating a smoothness constraint that provides robustness to noise and spurious edges. The disadvantage is that they require manual interaction to place an initial model and choose appropriate parameters. The successes in reducing sensitivity to initialization have been made in (Cohen, 1991; Malladi et al., 1995; C. Xu & Prince, 1998). Standard deformable models can also exhibit poor convergence to concave boundaries. This difficulty can be alleviated somewhat through the use of pressure forces (Cohen, 1991) and other modified external-force models (C. Xu & Prince, 1998). Another important extension of deformable models is the adaptivity of model topology by using an implicit representation rather than an explicit parameterization (Malladi et al., 1995; McInerney & Terzopoulos, 1995). Several general reviews on deformable models in medical image analysis can be found in (He et al., 2008; Heimann & Meinzer, 2009; McInerney & Terzopoulos, 1996; Suri, Liu, et al., 2002).

2.9 Atlas-guided approaches

Atlas-guided approaches are a powerful tool for medical image segmentation when a standard atlas or template is available. The whole idea of using the brain atlas was to provide a priori knowledge, which can help in grouping the segments into anatomical structures. This helps to obtain fully automatic cortical segmentation procedures. The standard atlas-guided approach treats segmentation as a registration problem. It first finds a one-to-one transformation that maps a pre-segmented atlas image to the target image. This process is often referred to as 'atlas warping'. The warping can be performed with linear transformations (Talairach & Tournoux, 1988), or nonlinear transformations (Collins et al., 1995; Davatzikos, 1996). Atlas-guided approaches have been applied mainly in brain MRI segmentation (Collins et al., 1995), as well as in extracting the brain volume from head scans (Aboutanos & Dawant, 1997). One advantage is that labels as well as the segmentation are transferred. They also provide a standard system for studying morphometric properties (Thompson & Toga, 1997). Atlas-guided approaches are generally better suited for segmentation of structures that are stable over the population of study. One method that helps model anatomical variability is to use probabilistic atlases (Thompson & Toga, 1997), but these require additional time and interaction to accumulate data. Another method is to use manually selected landmarks (Davatzikos, 1996) to constrain transformation.

2.10 Other techniques

Texture segmentation is to segment an image into regions according to the textures of the regions. It was in the late 1970s when Haralick et al (Haralick et al., 1973) published an extensive paper on texture. Later, Peleg et al (Peleg et al., 1984) and Cross et al (Cross & Jain, 1983) also published work in texture analysis applied to computer vision images. Application of texture in brain segmentation started in the early 1990s, when Lachmann et al (Lachmann & Barillot, 1992) developed a method for the classification of WM, GM and CSF. This method, however, did not discuss the validation schemes, and it was hard to judge the performance of such a segmentation algorithm. Besides, it seemed sensitive to initial textural properties, and no such discussion was carried out in the paper (Suri, Singh, et al., 2002b).

Self-organizing maps (SOM), introduced by Kohonen in early 1981 (Kohonen, 1990), is a type of artificial neural network, whose precursor is *learning vector quantization* (LVQ) invented by T. Kohonen (Kohonen, 1997). It is able to convert complex, nonlinear statistical relationships between high-dimensional data items into simple geometric relationships on a low-dimensional display via using unsupervised learning. The applications of SOM method can be found in (Y. Li & Chi, 2005; Tian & Fan, 2007). However, SOM algorithms are, firstly, highly dependent on the training data representatives and the initialization of the connection weights. Secondly, they are very computationally expensive if the dimensions of the data increases (Y. Li & Chi, 2005).

Wavelet transform, adventured in medical imaging research in 1991 (Weaver et al., 1991), is a tool that cuts up data or functions or operators into different frequency components, and then studies each component with a resolution matched to its scale (Daubechies, 2004). Modern wavelet analysis was considered to be proposed by Grossmann and Morlet in their milestone paper (Morlet & Grossman, 1984). In medical image segmentation, wavelet transforms have been employed to combine texture analysis, edge detection, classifiers, statistical models, and deformable models, etc. Many works benefit through using image features within a spatial-frequency domain after wavelet transform to assist the segmentation (Barra & Boire, 2000; Bello, 1994).

Multispectral segmentation is a method for differentiating tissue classes having similar characteristics in a single imaging modality by using several independent images of the same anatomical slice in different modalities (e.g., T1, T2, proton density, etc.). As a consequence of different responses of the tissues to particular pulse sequences, this increases the capability of discrimination between different tissues (Fletcher et al., 1993; Vannier et al., 1985). The most common approach for multispectral MR image segmentation is pattern recognition (Bezdek et al., 1993; Suri, Singh, et al., 2002b). These techniques generally appear to be successful particularly for brain MR images (Reddick et al., 1997; Taxt & Lundervold, 1994), but much work remains in the area of validation.

3. A new non-homogeneous Markov random field model

As we introduced in Section 2.6.2, Markov random field (MRF) theory (S.Z. Li, 1995) has been widely used in the field of medical image processing with the advantages, including non-supervision, fine stability and satisfied segmentation effect for the image with low SNR. MRF theory provides a convenient and consistent way for modeling context among image pixels. This is achieved through characterizing mutual influences among such entities using conditional MRF distributions. The practical use of MRF models is largely ascribed to the equivalence between MRF and Gibbs distributions established by Hamersley and Clifford (Hammersley & Clifford, 1971) and is further developed by Besag (Besag, 1974) for the joint distribution of MRF. This enables us to model vision problems by a mathematically sound yet tractable means for image segmentation in Bayesian framework (Geman & Geman, 1993; Grenander, 1983).

In traditional MRF model, Gibbs random field (GRF) uses the parameter β to determine spatial correlation among dependent image pixels. The greater the parameter β is, the stronger the spatial correlation would be; the smaller the parameter β is, the weaker the spatial correlation would be. Generally, MRF model is assumed to be homogeneous, which means the parameter β is constant. Plenty of previous researches have offered a series of methods to accurately estimate this parameter, which advance the effect of image segmentation (Deng & Clausi, 2004; Descombes et al., 1999). Due to its own features of medical image, homogeneous MRF model often leads to over-segmentation and induces higher misclassification rate. In this section, we propose a new non-homogeneous MRF model (called Modified-MRF or M-MRF model) using fuzzy membership to accurately estimate the parameter β and the experimental results show our model effectively reduces over-segmentation and enhances segmentation precision (R. Xu & Luo, 2009).

3.1 Fuzzy sets

Fuzzy sets are sets whose elements have degrees of membership, which firstly were proposed by L.A. Zedeh in 1965 (Zadeh, 1965) as an extension of the classical notion of set. Classical set theory only describes precise phenomenon, because an element belonging to a classic set contains only two cases: yes or no. By contrast, fuzzy set theory permits the gradual assessment of the membership of elements in a set; this is described with the aid of a membership function valued in the real unit interval *[0, 1]*. Fuzzy sets generalize classical sets, since the indicator functions of classical sets are special cases of the membership functions of fuzzy sets, if the latter only take values 0 or 1 (DuBois & Prade, 1980).

The fuzzy set is defined as: Given a domain X, x denotes its element, the mapping u_F is defined as $u_F : X \rightarrow [0,1]$, $x \rightarrow u_F(x)$, which means u_F confirms a fuzzy set F in domain X, u_F is called F's membership function and $u_F(x)$ is x's membership for F. The greater the membership, the greater the degree of one element pertaining to one fuzzy set. As a consequence, F is a subset in domain X, which does not have undefined border.

3.2 Modified non-homogeneous MRF model

In terms of the features in brain MR images, the spatial correlation of adjacent pixels varies with the positions of image space, which indicates the parameter β should be a variable changing with space site. Consequently, the corresponding MRF model should be considered as non-homogeneous.

3.2.1 The β Function based on fuzzy membership

Let y be the gray value of pixels, and x be the classification of pixels in image I. If pixel i is marked by class k (v_k is the clustering center of class k, $k = 1, \dots, K$), the parameter β will be a decreasing function of u_{ik}, which denotes the membership of pixel i belonging to class k. The smaller the u_{ik} is, the less the degree of pixel i in class k would be, which implies the attribute of pixel i should be decided by the state of neighborhood. The larger the u_{ik} is, the larger the degree of pixel i in class k would be, which implies the attribute of pixel i should be decided by the gray value of itself. Thus, the β function is defined as:

$$\beta_i = 1 - 0.8 \cdot u_{ik} \tag{18}$$

3.2.2 The modified MRF model (M-MRF model)

In traditional MRF model (see Section 2.6.2), the parameter β is used to calculate the *energy function* $U(x)$ and *clique potentials* $V_c(x)$ over all possible cliques $c \in C$, which only depends on the neighborhood of pixel i: $\delta(i), i \in c$. According to the β function, the energy function and clique potentials through considering multi-level logistic (MLL) model, second-order neighborhood system and dual potential function, can be modified as

$$U(x) = \sum_{i \in I} \sum_{j \in \delta(i)} V_c(x_i, x_j) \tag{19}$$

$$V(x_i, x_j) = \begin{cases} -\beta_i, & if \ \ x_i = x_j \\ \beta_i, & if \ \ x_i \neq x_j \end{cases} \tag{20}$$

And the new non-homogeneous MRF (M-MRF) model has been improved into

$$U(y \mid x) = \sum_{i \in I} U(y_i \mid x_i) = \sum_{i \in I} [\frac{(y_i - v_k)^2}{2\sigma_k^2} + \frac{1}{2}\log(\sigma_k^2)] \tag{21}$$

Therefore, the segmentation problem is reduced to minimize the above energy function, which is generally solved by iterated conditional modes (ICM) algorithm (Besag, 1986). The algorithm of M-MRF model for image segmentation is designed as follows:

1. Initialize the number of class K, the clustering center v_k, the smallest error ε, and $p = 0$;
2. Get the initial segmentation results via KFCM algorithm (L. Zhang et al., 2002), and estimate the parameter β by Eq.(18);
3. Segment the initial image based on maximum-likelihood criterion and M-MRF model, and calculate the global energy E of whole image;
4. Calculate local conditional energy of every pixel for all possible classification by Eq.(19) and Eq.(21), and update the classification of every pixel following the principle of minimizing local conditional energy.
5. Calculate the global energy E of whole image again by the new classification of every pixel, $p = p + 1$;
6. if $\max[|E^{(p)} - E^{(p-1)}|] \leq \varepsilon$, then go to (7), else return (4);
7. Output image segmentation results and stop.

3.2.3 Smoothing of image

Owing to complexity of brain MR images and their own reasons of segmentation algorithms, segmentation results are often accompanied by burrings, stains, rugged edges, etc. By smoothing, isolated burrings and stains of image can be removed, edges of regions can be smoothed and holes of areal objects can be filled. Sequentially, the quality of segmentation results can be further improved. In the processing of image smoothing, matrix template of $n \times n$(n is customarily assigned by 3~5) is currently employed to march image via lines and columns. If the image matches successfully, the segmentation result of the pixel in the center of matrix template will be replaced by the same segmentation results around this pixel.

3.2.3.1 Deburring

The 3×3 deburring matrix in (a) is frequently betaken, where $a, b, x \in L, a \neq b$(L is the set of labels) and 'x' is arbitrary which figures the segmentation results of x's sites can be left out of account. When the image segmentation results in 3×3 matrix march the deburring matrix in Fig. 3 (a), 'b' in the center of matrix will become 'a'.

a	a	a
a	b	a
x	x	x

a	a	x
a	b	x
a	a	x

x	x	x
a	b	a
a	a	a

x	a	a
x	b	a
x	a	a

(a)

x	a	x
a	b	a
x	a	x

(b)

Fig. 3. The matrix for deburring and smoothing. (a) the deburring matrices; (b) the matrix of smoothing of lines.

3.2.3.2 Smoothing of lines and filling of holes

The methods of smoothing of lines and filling of holes are the same as that of deburring, just the matrices are different. The 3×3 matrix of smoothing of lines in Fig. 3 (b) is utilized as a rule. In the same way, When the image segmentation results in 3×3 matrix march the 3×3 matrix in Fig. 3 (b), 'b' in the center of matrix will become 'a'.

3.3 Experimental results

In order to verify the effect of M-MRF model in image segmentation, KFCM algorithm (L. Zhang et al., 2002), traditional MRF model (S.Z. Li, 1995) and M-MRF model are applied in the segmentation of simulated brain MR images. During the experiments, brain MR images are divided into four regions: gray matter (GM), white matter (WM), cerebrospinal fluid (CSF) and background (BG). All experiments are operated by VS.Net 2003 in PC of Intel® Core™2 CPU 6600 @ 2.40GHZ with 2GB memory.

The simulated brain MR images from Brainweb (http://www.bic.mni.mcgill.ca/brainweb/) are applied in the experiments, and we call them gold standard of image segmentation. Each data set is composed of 258 × 258 pixels, thickness of layer is *1mm*, T_1 weighted. Herein, the lay images used in experiments are the $Z = 16.5mm$'s ones of image sequences. Fig. 4 is a comparison of the segmentation results of several algorithms for a simulated brain MRI superposed 9% noise. The experimental results demonstrate that, even for images of lower signal-to-noise ratio (SNR), M-MRF model also achieves more satisfied segmentation results.

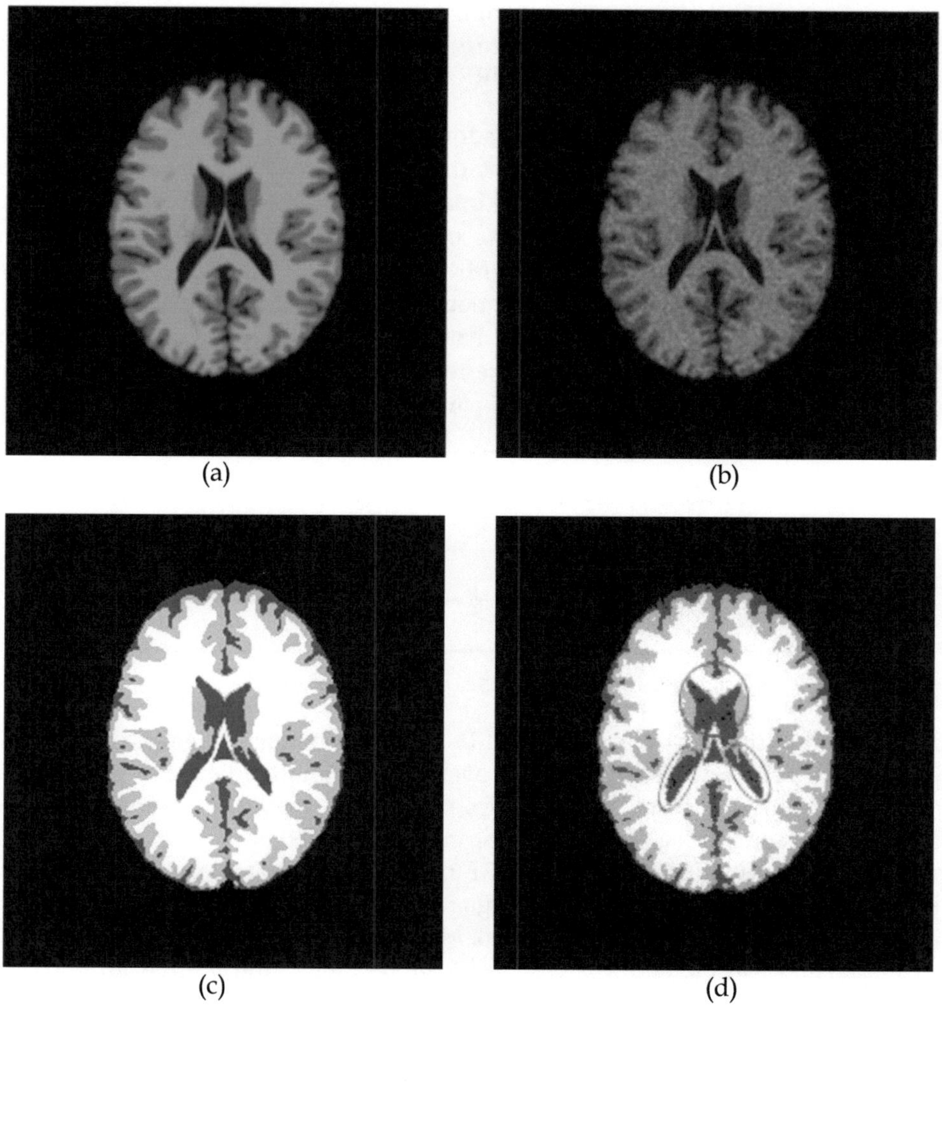

(a) (b)

(c) (d)

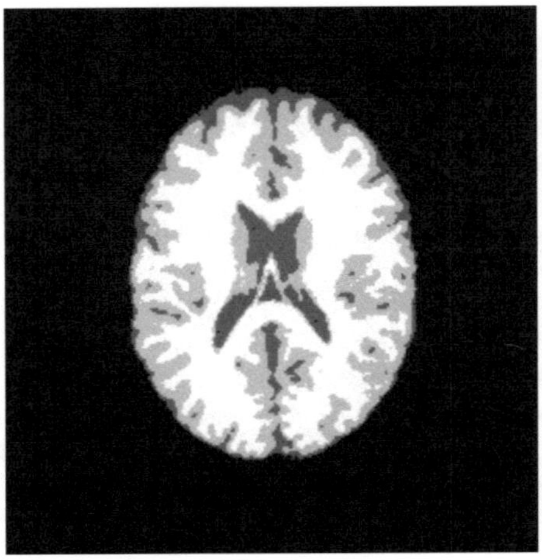

(e)

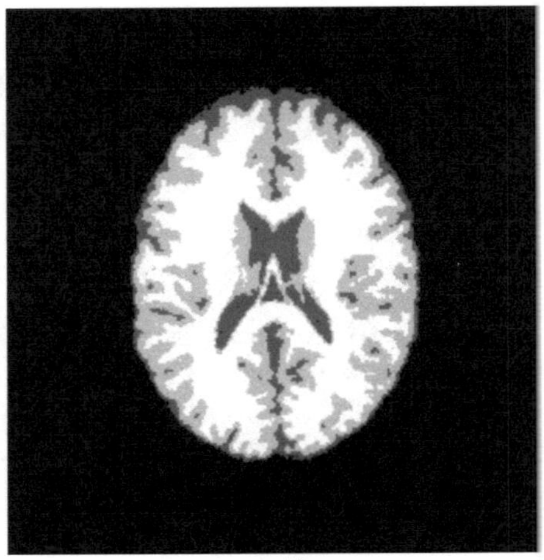

(f)

Fig. 4. A comparison of the segmentation results for several algorithms. (a) a simulated brain MR image; (b) a simulated brain MR image superposed 9% noise; (c) ground truth; (d) the results of KFCM method; (e) the results of MRF model; (f) the results of M-MRF model.

Table 1 presents MCRs of several algorithms for simulated brain MRIs superposed noise of distinct intensity in image segmentation (see the definition of MCR in Section 1.3), whose data are average segmentation results of 20 images. From table 1, MCRs of M-MRF model for all simulated brain MRIs are lower than other algorithms. In addition, segmentation effect of M-MRF model for simulated brain MRI superposed 7% and 9% noise is obviously better than other algorithms, while segmentation effect of M-MRF model for simulated brain MRI superposed 3% and 5% noise only has slight ascendancy compared with other algorithms. For this reason, the stronger the intensity of noise in image is, the better the segmentation performance of M-MRF model would be.

The intensity of noise(%)	3%	5%	7%	9%
MCRs of KFCM(%)	4.88	5.65	6.64	8.19
MCRs of MRF(%)	4.21	5.24	6.30	7.64
MCRs of M-MRF(%)	4.06	5.00	5.80	6.67

Table 1. MCRs (%) of images superposed noise of distinct intensity

In consideration of its own traits of brain MRIs, a new non-homogeneous MRF model (M-MRF model) is put forward for reducing over-segmentation, where the parameter β is estimated to an inch by fuzzy membership, so that the spatial relativities among each pixel will be reasonably set up. The experimental results prove our model not only inherits the superiorities of traditional MRF model, e.g., non-supervision, fine stability and satisfied robustness for image of low signal-to-noise ratio (SNR), but also significantly enhance the accuracy of image segmentation. Meanwhile, the algorithm of this new model is also simple and feasible and it is easy to be applied into clinical application by fusing de-bias field model.

4. Image pre-processing

Due to the inherent technical limitations of the MR image process, uncertainties are inserted into MR images, including random noise, intensity inhomogeneity, and partial volume effect, etc. A more complete and comprehensive coverage of the contributing sources of error inherent in MR images can be found in (Plante & Turkstra, 1991). The image pre-processing techniques reviewed here mainly focus on reducing the detrimental effects of the artifacts mentioned for the purpose of applying segmentation methods.

It is difficult to remove noise from MR images, which is known to have a *Rician distribution* (Prima et al., 2001), and state-of-art methods in removing noise are substantial. Methods vary from standard filters to more advanced filters, from general methods to specific MR image de-noising methods, such as linear filtering, nonlinear filtering, adaptive filtering, anisotropic diffusion filtering, wavelet analysis, total variation regularization, bilateral filter, trilateral filtering, and non-local means models (NL-means), etc. A worthy survey of image de-noising algorithms can be seen in (Buades et al., 2006).

Intensity inhomogeneity (also called bias field, or shading artefact) in MRI, which arises from the imperfections of the image acquisition process, manifests itself as a smooth intensity variation across the image (Fig. 5). Because of this phenomenon, the intensity of the same tissue varies with the location of the tissue within the image. Although intensity inhomogeneity is usually hardly noticeable to a human observer, many medical image analysis methods, such as segmentation and registration, are highly sensitive to the spurious variations of image intensities. This is why a large number of methods for the correction of intensity inhomogeneity in MR images have been proposed in the past (Vovk et al., 2007). Early publications on MRI intensity inhomogeneity correction date back to 1986 (Haselgrove & Prammer, 1986; McVeigh et al., 1986). Since then, sources of intensity inhomogeneity in MRI have been studied extensively (Alecci et al., 2001; Keiper et al., 1998; Liang & Lauterbur, 2000; Simmons et al., 1994) and can be generally divided into two groups: prospective methods and retrospective methods. According to the classification proposed by U. Vovk (Vovk et al., 2007), we may further classify the prospective methods into those that are based on phantoms, multi-coils, and special sequences. The retrospective methods are further classified into filtering, surface fitting, segmentation-based, and histogram-based, etc. Additionally, several valuable reviews about this topic can be found in (Arnold et al., 2001; Belaroussi et al., 2006; Hou, 2006; Sled et al., 1997; Velthuizen et al., 1998; Vovk et al., 2007).

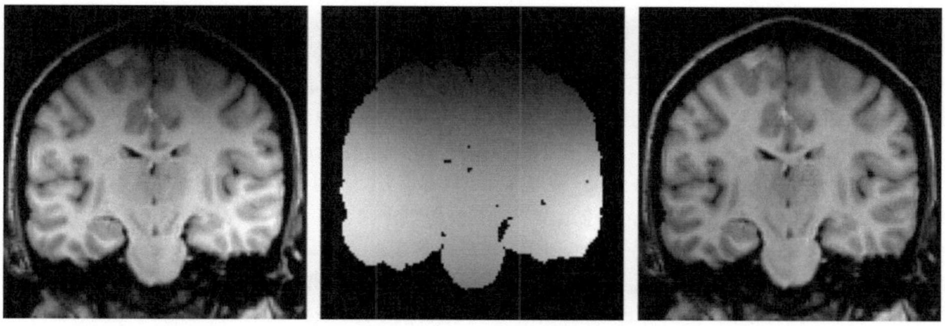

Fig. 5. Intensity inhomogeneity in MR brain image (Images provided courtesy of U. Vovk).

Partial volume effect (PVE) means artefacts that occur where multiple tissue types contribute to a single pixel, resulting in a blurring of intensity across boundaries, which is common in medical images, particularly for 3D MRI data. Fig. 6 illustrates how the sampling process can result in PVE, leading to ambiguities in structural definitions. In Fig. 6 (Right), it is difficult to precisely determine the boundaries of the two objects. The most common approach to addressing partial volume effect is to produce segmentations that allow regions or classes to overlap, called soft segmentations. Standard approaches use 'hard segmentations' that enforce a binary decision on whether a pixel is inside or outside the object. Soft segmentations, on the other hand, retain more information from the original image by allowing for uncertainty (such as membership for every pixel) in the location of object boundaries. Generally, membership functions can be derived by fuzzy clustering and classifier algorithms (Herndon et al., 1996; Pham & Prince, 1999) or statistical algorithms, in which case the membership functions are probability functions (Wells III et al., 1996), or can be computed as estimates of partial volume fractions (Choi et al., 1991). Soft segmentations based on membership functions can be easily converted to hard segmentations by assigning a pixel to its class with the highest membership value (Pham et al., 2000). The growing attention have been given to estimate partial volume effect in the last decade (Choi et al., 1991; Gage et al., 1992; Gonzalez Ballester et al., 2002; Roll et al., 1994; Soltanian-Zadeh et al., 1993; Thacker et al., 1998; Tohka et al., 2004).

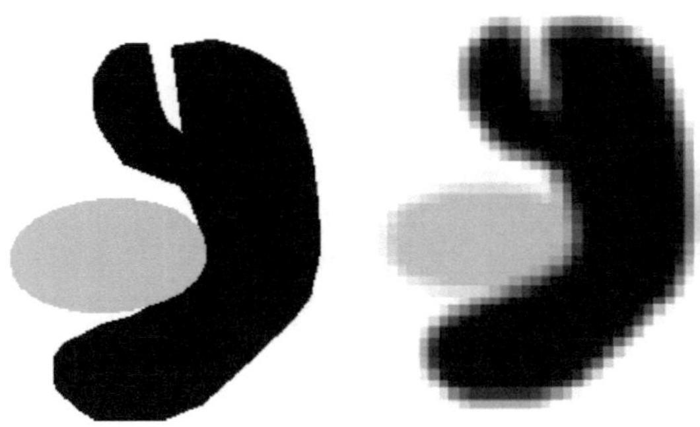

Fig. 6. Illustration of partial volume effect. (Left) Ideal image; (Right) Acquired image (Images provided courtesy of D.L. Pham).

5. Conclusion

A great number of medical image segmentation techniques have been used for analysis of MRI data of human brain, whose performance is affected by the characteristics of MRI data, which include a number of artifacts, such as random noise, intensity inhomogeneity and partial volume effect, etc. On the other hand, the inherent multispectral character of MRI gives it a distinct advantage over other imaging techniques. Many of the approaches described here explore ways to correct the artifacts in MRI and to fully exploit the multi-spectral character of this imaging modality. In this chapter, we have given a brief introduction to the fundamental concepts of these techniques, and presented our work on brain MR image segmentation, as well as a descripted the pre-processings such as de-noising, the correction of intensity inhomogeneity and the estimation of partial volume effect.

The future researches in the segmentation of human brain MRI will focus upon improving the accuracy, precision, and execution speed of segmentation methods, as well as reducing the amount of manual interaction. Accuracy and precision can be improved by incorporating prior information from atlases and by the fusion of different methods. For the sake of advancing execution efficiency, multi-scale processing, graphic processing unit (GPU) technique and parallelizable methods such as neural networks can be used promisingly. In order to raise the current acceptance of routine clinical applications for segmentation methods, extensive efficient validation is required. Furthermore, one must be able to demonstrate some significant performance advantage (e.g. more accurate diagnosis or earlier detection of pathology) over traditional methods to guarantee the less cost of training and equipment. It is impossible that automated methods will replace the physicians, but they are likely to become crucial elements in medical image analysis.

6. Acknowledgment

Special thanks to go the group of Ohya Laboratory, Global Information and Telecommunication Studies (GITS), Waseda University, Japan, and the group of the Laboratory of Image Science and Technology (LIST), School of Computer Science and Engineering, Southeast University, China, for their contribution and discussion on various aspects and projects associated with image segmentation. The authors would like to thank the reviewers for their valuable suggestions for improving this manuscript.

7. References

Aboutanos, G.B. & Dawant, B.M. (1997). Automatic Brain Segmentation and Validation: Image-Based Versus Atlas-Based Deformable Models, *Processings of SPIE*, Vol.3034, pp.299, DOI: 10.1117/12.274098.

Abras, G.N. & Ballarin, V.L. (2005). A Weighted K-Means Algorithm Applied to Brain Tissue Classification. *Journal of Computer Science & Technology*, Vol.5, No.3, pp.121-126.

Alecci, M., Collins, C.M., Smith, M.B. & Jezzard, P. (2001). Radio Frequency Magnetic Field Mapping of a 3 Tesla Birdcage Coil: Experimental and Theoretical Dependence on Sample Properties. *Magnetic Resonance in Medicine*, Vol.46, No.2, pp.379-385, ISSN: 1522-2594.

Arnold, J.B., Liow, J.S., Schaper, K.A., Stern, J.J., Sled, J.G., Shattuck, D.W., Worth, A.J., Cohen, M.S., Leahy, R.M. & Mazziotta, J.C. (2001). Qualitative and Quantitative Evaluation of Six Algorithms for Correcting Intensity Nonuniformity Effects. *NeuroImage*, Vol.13, No.5, pp.931-943, ISSN: 1053-8119.

Babalola, K., Patenaude, B., Aljabar, P., Schnabel, J., Kennedy, D., Crum, W., Smith, S., Cootes, T., Jenkinson, M. & Rueckert, D. (2008). Comparison and Evaluation of Segmentation Techniques for Subcortical Structures in Brain MRI, *Processings of Medical Image Computing and Computer-Assisted Intervention (MICCAI' 2008)*, Vol.5241, pp.409-416, DOI: 10.1007/978-3-540-85988-8_49.

Balafar, M.A., Ramli, A.R., Saripan, M.I. & Mashohor, S. (2010). Review of Brain MRI Image Segmentation Methods. *Artificial Intelligence Review*, Vol.33, No.3, pp.261-274, ISSN: 0269-2821.

Bankman, I.N. (2000). *Handbook of Medical Imaging: Processing and Analysis*, Academic Press, ISBN 0120777908.

Barra, V. & Boire, J.Y. (2000). Tissue Segmentation on MR Images of the Brain by Possibilistic Clustering on a 3D Wavelet Representation. *Journal of Magnetic Resonance Imaging*, Vol.11, No.3, pp.267-278, ISSN: 1522-2586.

Belaroussi, B., Milles, J., Carme, S., Zhu, Y.M. & Benoit-Cattin, H. (2006). Intensity Non-Uniformity Correction in MRI: Existing Methods and Their Validation. *Medical Image Analysis*, Vol.10, No.2, pp.234-246, ISSN: 1361-8415.

Bello, M.G. (1994). A Combined Markov Random Field and Wave-Packet Transform-Based Approach for Image Segmentation. *IEEE Transactions on Image Processing*, Vol.3, No.6, pp.834-846, ISSN: 1057-7149.

Besag, J. (1974). Spatial Interaction and the Statistical Analysis of Lattice Systems. *Journal of the Royal Statistical Society. Series B (Methodological)*, Vol.36, No.2, pp.192-236, ISSN: 0035-9246.

Besag, J. (1986). On the Statistical Analysis of Dirty Pictures. *Journal of the Royal Statistical Society. Series B (Methodological)*, Vol.48, No.3, pp.259-302, ISSN: 0035-9246.

Bezdek, J.C. (1981). *Pattern Recognition with Fuzzy Objective Function Algorithms*, Kluwer Academic Publishers, ISBN 0306406713.

Bezdek, J.C., Hall, L.O. & Clarke, L.P. (1993). Review of MR Image Segmentation Techniques Using Pattern Recognition. *Medical Physics*, Vol.20, No.4, pp.1033-1048, ISSN: 0094-2405.

Boudraa, A.O. & Zaidi, H. (2006). Image Segmentation Techniques in Nuclear Medicine Imaging. *Quantitative Analysis in Nuclear Medicine Imaging*, pp.308-357.

Bradley, P.S. & Fayyad, U.M. (1998). Refining Initial Points for K-Means Clustering, *Processings of the 15th International Conference on Machine Learing (ICML' 98)*, pp.91-99, Morgan Kaufmann, San Francisco, 1998.

Brummer, M.E., Mersereau, R.M., Eisner, R.L. & Lewine, R.R.J. (1993). Automatic Detection of Brain Contours in MRI Data Sets. *IEEE Transactions on Medical Imaging*, Vol.12, No.2, pp.153-166, ISSN: 0278-0062.

Buades, A., Coll, B. & Morel, J.M. (2006). A Review of Image Denoising Algorithms, with a New One. *Multiscale Modeling and Simulation*, Vol.4, No.2, pp.490-530, ISSN: 1540-3459.

Choi, H.S., Haynor, D.R. & Kim, Y. (1991). Partial Volume Tissue Classification of Multichannel Magnetic Resonance Images-A Mixel Model. *IEEE Transactions on Medical Imaging*, Vol.10, No.3, pp.395-407, ISSN: 0278-0062.

Clark, J.W. (1991). Neural Network Modelling. *Physics in Medicine and Biology*, Vol.36, pp.1259.

Clark, M.C., Hall, L.O., Goldgof, D.B., Velthuizen, R., Murtagh, F.R. & Silbiger, M.S. (1998). Automatic Tumor Segmentation Using Knowledge-Based Techniques. *IEEE Transactions on Medical Imaging*, Vol.17, No.2, pp.187-201, ISSN: 0278-0062.

Clarke, L.P., Velthuizen, R.P., Camacho, M.A., Heine, J.J., Vaidyanathan, M., Hall, L.O., Thatcher, R.W. & Silbiger, M.L. (1995). MRI Segmentation: Methods and Applications. *Magnetic Resonance Imaging*, Vol.13, No.3, pp.343-368, ISSN: 0730-725X.

Cline, H.E., Dumoulin, C.L., Hart Jr, H.R., Lorensen, W.E. & Ludke, S. (1987). 3D Reconstruction of the Brain from Magnetic Resonance Images Using a Connectivity Algorithm. *Magnetic Resonance Imaging*, Vol.5, No.5, pp.345-352, ISSN: 0730-725X.

Cohen, L.D. (1991). On Active Contour Models and Balloons. *CVGIP: Image understanding*, Vol.53, No.2, pp.211-218, ISSN: 1049-9660.

Collins, D.L., Holmes, C.J., Peters, T.M. & Evans, A.C. (1995). Automatic 3-D Model-Based Neuroanatomical Segmentation. *Human Brain Mapping*, Vol.3, No.3, pp.190-208, ISSN: 1097-0193.

Collins, D.L., Zijdenbos, A.P., Kollokian, V., Sled, J.G., Kabani, N.J., Holmes, C.J. & Evans, A.C. (1998). Design and Construction of a Realistic Digital Brain Phantom. *IEEE Transactions on Medical Imaging*, Vol.17, No.3, pp.463-468, ISSN: 0278-0062.

Cross, G.R. & Jain, A.K. (1983). Markov Random Field Texture Models. *IEEE Transactions on Pattern Analysis and Machine Intelligence*, Vol.PAMI-5, No.1, pp.25-39, ISSN: 0162-8828.

Damadian, R., Goldsmith, M. & Minkoff, L. (1977). NMR in Cancer: XVI. FONAR Image of the Live Human Body. *Physiological Chemistry and Physics*, Vol.9, No.1, pp.97-100, ISSN: 0031-9325.

Daubechies, I. (2004). *Ten Lectures on Wavelets*, Society for Industrial and Applied Mathematics, ISBN 0898712742.

Davatzikos, C. (1996). Spatial Normalization of 3D Brain Images Using Deformable Models. *Journal of Computer Assisted Tomography*, Vol.20, No.4, pp.656-665, ISSN: 0363-8715.

Davatzikos, C. & Bryan, N. (1996). Using a Deformable Surface Model to Obtain a Shape Representation of the Cortex. *IEEE Transactions on Medical Imaging*, Vol.15, No.6, pp.785-795, ISSN: 0278-0062.

Dempster, A.P., Laird, N.M. & Rubin, D.B. (1977). Maximum Likelihood from Incomplete Data Via the EM Algorithm. *Journal of the Royal Statistical Society. Series B (Methodological)*, Vol.39, No.1, pp.1-38, ISSN: 0035-9246.

Deng, H. & Clausi, D.A. (2004). Unsupervised Image Segmentation Using a Simple MRF Model with a New Implementation Scheme. *Pattern Recognition*, Vol.37, No.12, pp.2323-2335, ISSN: 0031-3203.

Descombes, X., Morris, R.D., Zerubia, J. & Berthod, M. (1999). Estimation of Markov Random Field Prior Parameters Using Markov Chain Monte Carlo Maximum Likelihood. *IEEE Transactions on Medical Imaging*, Vol.8, No.7, pp.954-963, ISSN: 1057-7149.

Dogdas, B., Shattuck, D.W. & Leahy, R.M. (2002). Segmentation of the Skull in 3D Human MR Images Using Mathematical Morphology, *Processings of SPIE*, Vol.4684, pp.1553-1562.

Dubey, R.B., Hanmandlu, M. & Gupta, S.K. (2010). The Brain MR Image Segmentation Techniques and Use of Diagnostic Packages. *Academic Radiology*, Vol.17, No.5, pp.658-671, ISSN: 1076-6332.

DuBois, D. & Prade, H.M. (1980). *Fuzzy Sets and Systems: Theory and Applications*, Academic Press, ISBN 0122227506, New York.

Duda, R.O. & Hart, P.E. (1973). *Pattern Classification and Scene Analysis*, New York: Wiley.

Dunn, J.C. (1973). A Fuzzy Relative of the Isodata Process and Its Use in Detecting Compact Well-Separated Clusters. *Cybernetics and Systems*, Vol.3, No.3, pp.32-57, ISSN: 0196-9722.

Fisher, R.A. (1936). The Use of Multiple Measurements in Taxonomic Problems. *Annals of Human Genetics*, Vol.7, No.2, pp.179-188, ISSN: 1469-1809.

Fletcher, L.M., Barsotti, J.B. & Hornak, J.P. (1993). A Multispectral Analysis of Brain Tissues. *Magnetic Resonance in Medicine*, Vol.29, No.5, pp.623-630, ISSN: 1522-2594.

Fukunaga, K. (1990). *Introduction to Statistical Pattern Recognition*, Academic Press Professional, ISBN 0122698517.

Gage, H.D., Santago II, P. & Snyder, W.E. (1992). Quantification of Brain Tissue through Incorporation of Partial Volume Effects, *Processings of SPIE*, Vol.1652, pp.84, DOI: 10.1117/12.59414.

Gelenbe, E., Feng, Y. & Krishnan, K.R.R. (1996). Neural Network Methods for Volumetric Magnetic Resonance Imaging of the Human Brain. *Proceedings of the IEEE 1996*, Vol.84, No.10, pp.1488-1496, ISSN: 0018-9219.

Geman, S. & Geman, D. (1993). Stochastic Relaxation, Gibbs Distributions and the Bayesian Restoration of Images*. *Journal of Applied Statistics*, Vol.20, No.5, pp.25-62, ISSN: 0266-4763.

Gonzalez Ballester, M.A., Zisserman, A.P. & Brady, M. (2002). Estimation of the Partial Volume Effect in MRI. *Medical Image Analysis*, Vol.6, No.4, pp.389-405, ISSN: 1361-8415.

Gonzalez, R.C. & Woods, R.E. (1992). *Digital Image Processing*, Addison Wisley.

Grau, V., Mewes, A.U.J., Alcaniz, M., Kikinis, R. & Warfield, S.K. (2004). Improved Watershed Transform for Medical Image Segmentation Using Prior Information. *IEEE Transactions on Medical Imaging*, Vol.23, No.4, pp.447-458, ISSN: 0278-0062.

Grenander, U. (1983). Tutorials in Pattern Synthesis. *Brown University, Division of Applied Mathematics*.

Grimson, W.E.L., Ettinger, G.J., Kapur, T., Leventon, M.E., Wells, W.M. & Kikinis, R. (1997). Utilizing Segmented MRI Data in Image-Guided Surgery. *International Journal of Pattern Recognition and Artificial Intelligence*, Vol.11, No.8, pp.1367-1397.

Hall, L.O., Bensaid, A.M., Clarke, L.P., Velthuizen, R.P., Silbiger, M.S. & Bezdek, J.C. (1992). A Comparison of Neural Network and Fuzzy Clustering Techniques in Segmenting Magnetic Resonance Images of the Brain. *IEEE Transactions on Neural Networks*, Vol.3, No.5, pp.672-682, ISSN: 1045-9227.

Hamamoto, Y., Fujimoto, Y. & Tomita, S. (1996). On the Estimation of a Covariance Matrix in Designing Parzen Classifiers. *Pattern Recognition*, Vol.29, No.10, pp.1751-1759, ISSN: 0031-3203.

Hammersley, J.M. & Clifford, P. (1971). Markov Field on Finite Graphs and Lattices. Unpublished.

Haralick, R.M., Shanmugam, K. & Dinstein, I. (1973). Textural Features for Image Classification. *IEEE Transactions on Systems, Man and Cybernetics*, Vol.3, No.6, pp.610-621, ISSN: 0018-9472.

Haralick, R.M. & Shapiro, L.G. (1985). Image Segmentation Techniques. *Computer Vision, Graphics, and Image Processing*, Vol.29, No.1, pp.100-132, ISSN: 0734-189X.

Haselgrove, J. & Prammer, M. (1986). An Algorithm for Compensation of Surface-Coil Images for Sensitivity of the Surface Coil. *Magnetic Resonance Imaging*, Vol.4, No.6, pp.469-472, ISSN: 0730-725X.

He, L., Peng, Z., Everding, B., Wang, X., Han, C.Y., Weiss, K.L. & Wee, W.G. (2008). A Comparative Study of Deformable Contour Methods on Medical Image

Segmentation. *Image and Vision Computing*, Vol.26, No.2, pp.141-163, ISSN: 0262-8856.

Hebert, T.J. (1997). Fast Iterative Segmentation of High Resolution Medical Images. *IEEE Transactions on Nuclear Science*, Vol.44, No.3, pp.1362-1367, ISSN: 0018-9499.

Heimann, T. & Meinzer, H.P. (2009). Statistical Shape Models for 3D Medical Image Segmentation: A Review. *Medical Image Analysis*, Vol.13, No.4, pp.543-563, ISSN: 1361-8415.

Held, K., Kops, E.R., Krause, B.J., Wells III, W.M., Kikinis, R. & Muller-Gartner, H.W. (1997). Markov Random Field Segmentation of Brain MR Images. *IEEE Transactions on Medical Imaging*, Vol.16, No.6, pp.878-886, ISSN: 0278-0062.

Herndon, R.C., Lancaster, J.L., Toga, A.W. & Fox, P.T. (1996). Quantification of White Matter and Gray Matter Volumes from T1 Parametric Images Using Fuzzy Classifiers. *Journal of Magnetic Resonance Imaging*, Vol.6, No.3, pp.425-435, ISSN: 1522-2586.

Hou, Z. (2006). A Review on Mr Image Intensity Inhomogeneity Correction. *International Journal of Biomedical Imaging*, Vol.2006, pp.1-11.

Jain, A.K., Murty, M.N. & Flynn, P.J. (1999). Data Clustering: A Review. *ACM Computing Surveys (CSUR)*, Vol.31, No.3, pp.264-323, ISSN: 0360-0300.

Kannan, S.R., Ramathilagam, S., Sathya, A. & Pandiyarajan, R. (2010). Effective Fuzzy C-Means Based Kernel Function in Segmenting Medical Images. *Computers in Biology and Medicine*, Vol.40, No.6, pp.572-579, ISSN: 0010-4825.

Kapur, T., Grimson, W.E.L., Kikinis, R. & Wells, W.M. (1998). Enhanced Spatial Priors for Segmentation of Magnetic Resonance Imagery. *Medical Image Computing and Computer-Assisted Interventation (MICCAI' 98)*, pp.457.

Kass, M., Witkin, A. & Terzopoulos, D. (1988). Snakes: Active Contour Models. *International Journal of Computer Vision*, Vol.1, No.4, pp.321-331, ISSN: 0920-5691.

Keiper, M.D., Grossman, R.I., Hirsch, J.A., Bolinger, L., Ott, I.L., Mannon, L.J., Langlotz, C.P. & Kolson, D.L. (1998). MR Identification of White Matter Abnormalities in Multiple Sclerosis: A Comparison between 1.5 T and 4 T. *American Journal of Neuroradiology*, Vol.19, No.8, pp.1489-1493.

Khan, S.S. & Ahmad, A. (2004). Cluster Center Initialization Algorithm for K-Means Clustering. *Pattern Recognition Letters*, Vol.25, No.11, pp.1293-1302, ISSN: 0167-8655.

Kikinis, R., Shenton, M.E., Iosifescu, D.V., McCarley, R.W., Saiviroonporn, P., Hokama, H.H., Robatino, A., Metcalf, D., Wible, C.G. & Portas, C.M. (1996). A Digital Brain Atlas for Surgical Planning, Model-Driven Segmentation, and Teaching. *IEEE Transactions on Visualization and Computer Graphics*, Vol.2, No.3, pp.232-241, ISSN: 1077-2626.

Kohonen, T. (1990). The Self-Organizing Map. *Proceedings of the IEEE*, Vol.78, No.9, pp.1464-1480, ISSN: 0018-9219.

Kohonen, T. (1997). Self-Organizing Maps. *Springer, Berlin.*

Kriesel, D.: A Brief Introduction to Neural Networks, 2007, Available from: <http://www.dkriesel.com/en/science/neural_networks>.

Kwan, R.K.S., Evans, A.C. & Pike, G.B. (1999). MRI Simulation-Based Evaluation of Image-Processing and Classification Methods. *IEEE Transactions on Medical Imaging*, Vol.18, No.11, pp.1085-1097, ISSN: 0278-0062.

Lachmann, F. & Barillot, C. (1992). Brain Tissue Classification from MRI Data by Means of Texture Analysis, *Processings of SPIE*, Vol.1652, pp.72, DOI: 10.1117/12.59413.

Li, S.Z. (1995). *Markov Random Field Modeling in Image Analysis*, Springer-Verlag, ISBN 1848002785, New York.

Li, X., Li, L., Lu, H., Chen, D. & Liang, Z. (2003). Inhomogeneity Correction for Magnetic Resonance Images with Fuzzy C-Mean Algorithm, *Processings of SPIE*, Vol.5032, 2003.

Li, Y. & Chi, Z. (2005). MR Brain Image Segmentation Based on Self-Organizing Map Network. *International Journal of Information Technology*, Vol.11, No.8, pp.45-53.

Liang, Z.P. & Lauterbur, P.C. (2000). *Principles of Magnetic Resonance Imaging: A Signal Processing Perspective*, Wiley: IEEE press, ISBN 0780347234.

Lim, K.O. & Pfefferbaum, A. (1989). Segmentation of MR Brain Images into Cerebrospinal Fluid Spaces, White and Gray Matter. *Journal of Computer Assisted Tomography*, Vol.13, No.4, pp.588-593, ISSN: 0363-8715.

Liu, S., Li, X. & Li, Z. (2005). A New Image Segmentation Algorithm Based the Fusion of Markov Random Field and Fuzzy C-Means Clustering, *Processings of IEEE International Symposium on Communications and Information Technology 2005 (ISCIT' 2005)*, pp.144-147.

MacQueen, J.B. (1967). Some Methods for Classification and Analysis of Multivariate Observations, *Processings of Proceedings of the 5th Berkeley Symposium on Mathematical Statistics and Probability*, Vol.1, pp.281-297, Berkeley.

Malladi, R., Sethian, J.A. & Vemuri, B.C. (1995). Shape Modeling with Front Propagation: A Level Set Approach. *IEEE Transactions on Pattern Analysis and Machine Intelligence*, Vol.17, No.2, pp.158-175, ISSN: 0162-8828.

McInerney, T. & Terzopoulos, D. (1995). Topologically Adaptable Snakes, *Processings of the 5th International Conference on Computer Vision 1995*, pp.840-845, Cambridge, MA , USA

McInerney, T. & Terzopoulos, D. (1996). Deformable Models in Medical Image Analysis: A Survey. *Medical Image Analysis*, Vol.1, No.2, pp.91-108, ISSN: 1361-8415.

McInerney, T. & Terzopoulos, D. (2000). T-Snakes: Topology Adaptive Snakes. *Medical Image Analysis*, Vol.4, No.2, pp.73-91, ISSN: 1361-8415.

McVeigh, E.R., Bronskill, M.J. & Henkelman, R.M. (1986). Phase and Sensitivity of Receiver Coils in Magnetic Resonance Imaging. *Medical Physics*, Vol.13, No.6, pp.806-814.

Morlet, J. & Grossman, A. (1984). Decomposition of Hardy Functions into Square Integrable Wavelets of Constant Shape. *SIAM Journal on Mathematical Analysis*, Vol.15, No.4, pp.723-736.

Mortazavi, D., Kouzani, A.Z. & Soltanian-Zadeh, H. (2011). Segmentation of Multiple Sclerosis Lesions in MR Images: A Review. *Neuroradiology*, pp.1-22, ISSN: 0028-3940.

Noe, A., Kovacic, S. & Gee, J.C. (2001). Segmentation of Cerebral Mri Scans Using a Partial Volume Model, Shading Correction and an Anatomical Prior, *Processings of SPIE*, pp.1466-1477.

Novelline, R.A. & Squire, L.F. (2004). *Squire's Fundamentals of Radiology*, Harvard Univ Press, ISBN 0674012798.

Pal, N.R. & Pal, S.K. (1993). A Review on Image Segmentation Techniques. *Pattern Recognition*, Vol.26, No.9, pp.1277-1294, ISSN: 0031-3203.

Peleg, S., Naor, J., Hartley, R. & Avnir, D. (1984). Multiple Resolution Texture Analysis and Classification. *IEEE Transactions on Pattern Analysis and Machine Intelligence*, Vol.PAMI-6, No.4, pp.518-523, ISSN: 0162-8828.

Pham, D.L. & Prince, J.L. (1999). An Adaptive Fuzzy C-Means Algorithm for Image Segmentation in the Presence of Intensity Inhomogeneities. *Pattern Recognition Letters*, Vol.20, No.1, pp.57-68, ISSN: 0167-8655.

Pham, D.L., Xu, C. & Prince, J.L. (2000). Current Methods in Medical Image Segmentation. *Annual Review of Biomedical Engineering*, Vol.2, No.1, pp.315-337, ISSN: 1523-9829.

Plante, E. & Turkstra, L. (1991). Sources of Error in the Quantitative Analysis of MRI Scans. *Magnetic Resonance Imaging*, Vol.9, No.4, pp.589-595, ISSN: 0730-725X.

Prima, S., Ayache, N., Barrick, T. & Roberts, N. (2001). Maximum Likelihood Estimation of the Bias Field in MR Brain Images: Investigating Different Modelings of the Imaging Process, *Processings of Medical Image Computing and Computer-Assisted Intervention (MICCAI' 2001)*, Vol.2208, pp.811-819, DOI: 10.1007/3-540-45468-3_97.

Reddick, W.E., Glass, J.O., Cook, E.N., Elkin, T.D. & Deaton, R.J. (1997). Automated Segmentation and Classification of Multispectral Magnetic Resonance Images of Brain Using Artificial Neural Networks. *IEEE Transactions on Medical Imaging*, Vol.16, No.6, pp.911-918, ISSN: 0278-0062.

Roland, P.E., Graufelds, C.J., Wahlin, J., Ingelman, L., Andersson, M., Ledberg, A., Pedersen, J., Akerman, S., Dabringhaus, A. & Zilles, K. (1993). Human Brain Atlas: For High-Resolution Functional and Anatomical Mapping. *Human Brain Mapping*, Vol.1, No.3, pp.173-184, ISSN: 1097-0193.

Roll, S.A., Colchester, A.C.F., Summers, P.E. & Griffin, L.D. (1994). Intensity-Based Object Extraction from 3D Medical Images Including a Correction for Partial Volume Errors, *Processings of the 5th British Machine Vision Conference (BMVC' 94)*, Vol.94, pp.205-214, Guildford, UK.

Ruan, S., Jaggi, C., Xue, J., Fadili, J. & Bloyet, D. (2000). Brain Tissue Classification of Magnetic Resonance Images Using Partial Volume Modeling. *IEEE Transactions on Medical Imaging*, Vol.19, No.12, pp.1179-1187, ISSN: 0278-0062.

Rusinek, H., De Leon, M.J., George, A.E., Stylopoulos, L.A., Chandra, R., Smith, G., Rand, T., Mourino, M. & Kowalski, H. (1991). Alzheimer Disease: Measuring Loss of Cerebral Gray Matter with MR Imaging. *Radiology*, Vol.178, No.1, pp.109-114, ISSN: 0033-8419.

Saeed, N. (1998). Magnetic Resonance Image Segmentation Using Pattern Recognition, and Applied to Image Registration and Quantitation. *NMR in Biomedicine*, Vol.11, No.4-5, pp.157-167, ISSN: 1099-1492.

Salzenstein, F. & Pieczynski, W. (1997). Parameter Estimation in Hidden Fuzzy Markov Random Fields and Image Segmentation. *Graphical Models and Image Processing*, Vol.59, No.4, pp.205-220, ISSN: 1077-3169.

Shen, S., Sandham, W., Granat, M. & Sterr, A. (2005). MRI Fuzzy Segmentation of Brain Tissue Using Neighborhood Attraction with Neural-Network Optimization. *IEEE Transactions on Information Technology in Biomedicine*, Vol.9, No.3, pp.459-467, ISSN: 1089-7771.

Siddiqi, K., Lauziere, Y.B., Tannenbaum, A. & Zucker, S.W. (1998). Area and Length Minimizing Flows for Shape Segmentation. *IEEE Transactions on Image Processing*, Vol.7, No.3, pp.433-443, ISSN: 1057-7149.

Simmons, A., Tofts, P.S., Barker, G.J. & Arridge, S.R. (1994). Sources of Intensity Nonuniformity in Spin Echo Images at 1.5 T. *Magnetic Resonance in Medicine*, Vol.32, No.1, pp.121-128, ISSN: 1522-2594.

Skurichina, M. & Duin, R.P.W. (1996). Stabilizing Classifiers for Very Small Sample Sizes, *Processings of the 13th International Conference on Pattern Recognition*, Vol.2, pp.891-896, 1996.

Sled, J., Zijdenbos, A. & Evans, A. (1997). A Comparison of Retrospective Intensity Non-Uniformity Correction Methods for MRI, *Processings of Information Processing in Medical Imaging*, Vol.1230, pp.459-464, Springer, DOI: 10.1007/3-540-63046-5_43.

Soltanian-Zadeh, H., Windham, J.P. & Yagle, A.E. (1993). Optimal Transformation for Correcting Partial Volume Averaging Effects in Magnetic Resonance Imaging. *IEEE Transactions on Nuclear Science*, Vol.40, No.4, pp.1204-1212, ISSN: 0018-9499.

Suri, J.S., Liu, K., Singh, S., Laxminarayan, S.N., Zeng, X. & Reden, L. (2002). Shape Recovery Algorithms Using Level Sets in 2-D/3-D Medical Imagery: A State-of-the-Art Review. *IEEE Transactions on Information Technology in Biomedicine*, Vol.6, No.1, pp.8-28, ISSN: 1089-7771.

Suri, J.S., Singh, S. & Reden, L. (2002a). Fusion of Region and Boundary/Surface-Based Computer Vision and Pattern Recognition Techniques for 2-D and 3-D MR Cerebral Cortical Segmentation (Part-II): A State-of-the-Art Review. *Pattern Analysis & Applications*, Vol.5, No.1, pp.77-98, ISSN: 1433-7541.

Suri, J.S., Singh, S. & Reden, L. (2002b). Computer Vision and Pattern Recognition Techniques for 2-D and 3-D Mr Cerebral Cortical Segmentation (Part I): A State-of-the-Art Review. *Pattern Analysis & Applications*, Vol.5, No.1, pp.46-76, ISSN: 1433-7541.

Suzuki, H. & Toriwaki, J. (1991). Automatic Segmentation of Head MRI Images by Knowledge Guided Thresholding. *Computerized Medical Imaging and Graphics*, Vol.15, No.4, pp.233-240, ISSN: 0895-6111.

Talairach, J. & Tournoux, P. (1988). *Co-Planar Stereotaxic Atlas of the Human Brain: 3-Dimensional Proportional System: An Approach to Cerebral Imaging*, Thieme, ISBN 0865772932.

Tang, H., Wu, E.X., Ma, Q.Y., Gallagher, D., Perera, G.M. & Zhuang, T. (2000). MRI Brain Image Segmentation by Multi-Resolution Edge Detection and Region Selection. *Computerized Medical Imaging and Graphics*, Vol.24, No.6, pp.349-357, ISSN: 0895-6111.

Taxt, T. & Lundervold, A. (1994). Multispectral Analysis of the Brain Using Magnetic Resonance Imaging. *IEEE Transactions on Medical Imaging*, Vol.13, No.3, pp.470-481, ISSN: 0278-0062.

Thacker, N., Jackson, A., Zhu, X.P. & Li, K.L. (1998). Accuracy of Tissue Volume Estimation in NMR Images, *Processings of MIUA' 98*, Leeds, UK.

Thompson, P.M. & Toga, A.W. (1997). Detection, Visualization and Animation of Abnormal Anatomic Structure with a Deformable Probabilistic Brain Atlas Based on Random Vector Field Transformations. *Medical Image Analysis*, Vol.1, No.4, pp.271-294, ISSN: 1361-8415.

Tian, D. & Fan, L. (2007). A Brain MR Images Segmentation Method Based on SOM Neural Network, *Processings of The 1st International Conference on ICBBE' 2007*, pp.686-689, Wuhan.

Tohka, J., Zijdenbos, A. & Evans, A. (2004). Fast and Robust Parameter Estimation for Statistical Partial Volume Models in Brain MRI. *NeuroImage*, Vol.23, No.1, pp.84-97, ISSN: 1053-8119.

Udupa, J.K., Wei, L., Samarasekera, S., Miki, Y., Van Buchem, M.A. & Grossman, R.I. (1997). Multiple Sclerosis Lesion Quantification Using Fuzzy-Connectedness Principles. *IEEE Transactions on Medical Imaging*, Vol.16, No.5, pp.598-609, ISSN: 0278-0062.

Vaidyanathan, M., Clarke, L.P., Hall, L.O., Heidtman, C., Velthuizen, R., Gosche, K., Phuphanich, S., Wagner, H., Greenberg, H. & Silbiger, M.L. (1997). Monitoring Brain Tumor Response to Therapy Using MRI Segmentation. *Magnetic Resonance Imaging*, Vol.15, No.3, pp.323-334, ISSN: 0730-725X.

Vannier, M.W., Butterfield, R.L., Jordan, D., Murphy, W.A., Levitt, R.G. & Gado, M. (1985). Multispectral Analysis of Magnetic Resonance Images. *Radiology*, Vol.154, No.1, pp.221-224, ISSN: 0033-8419.

Vapnik, V.N. (1998). *Statistical Learning Theory*, Wiley-Interscience, ISBN 0471030031, New York.

Velthuizen, R.P., Heine, J.J., Cantor, A.B., Lin, H., Fletcher, L.M. & Clarke, L.P. (1998). Review and Evaluation of MRI Nonuniformity Corrections for Brain Tumor Response Measurements. *Medical physics*, Vol.25, pp.1655.

Vemuri, B., Rahman, S. & Li, J. (1995). Multiresolution Adaptive K-Means Algorithm for Segmentation of Brain MRI. *Image Analysis Applications and Computer Graphics*, Vol.1024, pp.347-354.

Vilarino, D.L., Brea, V.M., Cabello, D. & Pardo, J.M. (1998). Discrete-Time CNN for Image Segmentation by Active Contours. *Pattern Recognition Letters*, Vol.19, No.8, pp.721-734, ISSN: 0167-8655.

Vovk, U., Pernus, F. & Likar, B. (2007). A Review of Methods for Correction of Intensity Inhomogeneity in MRI. *IEEE Transactions on Medical Imaging*, Vol.26, No.3, pp.405-421, ISSN: 0278-0062.

Wang, X., He, L. & Wee, W. (2004). Deformable Contour Method: A Constrained Optimization Approach. *International Journal of Computer Vision*, Vol.59, No.1, pp.87-108, ISSN: 0920-5691.

Weaver, J.B., Xu, Y., Healy Jr, D.M. & Cromwell, L.D. (1991). Filtering Noise from Images with Wavelet Transforms. *Magnetic Resonance in Medicine*, Vol.21, No.2, pp.288-295, ISSN: 1522-2594.

Wells III, W.M., Grimson, W.E.L., Kikinis, R. & Jolesz, F.A. (1996). Adaptive Segmentation of Mri Data. *IEEE Transactions on Medical Imaging*, Vol.15, No.4, pp.429-442, ISSN: 0278-0062.

Xu, C., Pham, D.L., Prince, J.L., Etemad, M.E. & Yu, D.N. (1998). Reconstruction of the Central Layer of the Human Cerebral Cortex from MR Images, *Processings of Medical Image Computing and Computer-Assisted Interventation (MICCAI' 98)*, Vol.1496/1998, pp.481-488, DOI: 10.1007/BFb0056233.

Xu, C. & Prince, J.L. (1998). Snakes, Shapes, and Gradient Vector Flow. *IEEE Transactions on Image Processing*, Vol.7, No.3, pp.359-369, ISSN: 1057-7149.

Xu, R. & Luo, L.M. (2009). A New Nonhomogeneous Markov Random Field Model Based on Fuzzy Membership for Brain MRI Segmentation, *Processings of SPIE*, Vol.7497, pp.74972F, Yichang, China, DOI: 10.1117/12.832160.

Xu, R. & Ohya, J. (2010). An Improved Kernel-Based Fuzzy C-Means Algorithm with Spatial Information for Brain MR Image Segmentation, *Processings of 25th International Conference of Image and Vision Computing New Zealand* (IVCNZ' 2010), Queenstown, New Zealand.

Zadeh, L.A. (1965). Fuzzy Sets. *Information and Control*, Vol.8, No.3, pp.338-353, ISSN: 0019-9958.

Zaidi, H., Ruest, T., Schoenahl, F. & Montandon, M.L. (2006). Comparative Assessment of Statistical Brain MR Image Segmentation Algorithms and Their Impact on Partial Volume Correction in PET. *NeuroImage*, Vol.32, No.4, pp.1591-1607, ISSN: 1053-8119.

Zhang, H., Fritts, J.E. & Goldman, S.A. (2008). Image Segmentation Evaluation: A Survey of Unsupervised Methods. *Computer Vision and Image Understanding*, Vol.110, No.2, pp.260-280, ISSN: 1077-3142.

Zhang, L., Zhou, W.D. & Jiao, L.C. (2002). Kernel Clustering Algorithm. *Chinese Journal of Computers*, Vol.25, No.6, pp.587-590, ISSN: 0254-4164.

Zhang, Y., Brady, M. & Smith, S. (2001). Segmentation of Brain MR Images through a Hidden Markov Random Field Model and the Expectation-Maximization Algorithm. *IEEE Transactions on Medical Imaging*, Vol.20, No.1, pp.45-57, ISSN: 0278-0062.

Zhang, Y.J. (1996). A Survey on Evaluation Methods for Image Segmentation. *Pattern Recognition*, Vol.29, No.8, pp.1335-1346, ISSN: 0031-3203.

Zhang, Y.J. (2001). A Review of Recent Evaluation Methods for Image Segmentation, *Processings of the Sixth International Symposium on Signal Processing and its Applications 2001*, Vol.1, pp.148-151, Kuala Lumpur.

Zijdenbos, A.P. & Dawant, B.M. (1994). Brain Segmentation and White Matter Lesion Detection in MR Images. *Critical Review in Biomedical Engineering*, Vol.22, No.5-6, pp.401-465.

Zucker, S.W. (1976). Region Growing: Childhood and Adolescence. *Computer Graphics and Image Processing*, Vol.5, No.3, pp.382-399, ISSN: 0146-664X.

9

Comparison of Granulometric Studies of Brain Slices from Normal and Dissociated Strabismus Subjects Through Morphological Transformations

Jorge D. Mendiola-Santibañez[1], Martín Gallegos-Duarte[2], Domingo J. Gómez-Meléndez[1], Angélica R. Jiménez-Sánchez[3] and Israel M. Santillán-Méndez[1]

[1]*División de Investigación y Posgrado de la Facultad de Ingeniería, Universidad Autónoma de Querétaro, Centro Universitario S/N, CP. 76010, Querétaro*

[2]*Posgrado de la Facultad de Medicina, Departamento de Investigación, Universidad Autónoma de Querétaro, Clavel # 200, Fraccionamiento Prados de la Capilla, Santiago de Querétaro*

[3]*Universidad Politécnica de Querétaro, Carretera Estatal 420 S/N, El Rosario, El Marqués, CP. 76240 Querétaro*

México

1. Introduction

Notation

μ, λ scalars (i.e. positive numbers)

B structuring element

$\check{B}$ transposed of the structuring element B, i.e., $\check{B}=\{-x : x \in B\}$

$\wedge$ inf operator

$\vee$ sup operator

Z^+ integer and positive numbers space

$f(x), g(x)$ numerical function of x

$\varepsilon_\mu(f)(x)$ morphological erosion size μ

$\delta_\mu(f)(x)$ morphological dilation size μ

$\gamma_\mu(f)(x)$ morphological opening size μ

$\varphi_\mu(f)(x)$ morphological closing size μ

$\tilde{\gamma}_\mu(f)(x)$ opening by reconstruction size μ

$\tilde{\varphi}_\mu(f)(x)$ closing by reconstruction size μ

$(\psi_\lambda)_{\lambda \in Z^+}$ a family of transformations depending on an unique positive parameter λ

χ_{WM} normalized volumetric measure of granulometric residues of clear structures conforming the image

ζ_{GM} normalized volumetric measure of granulometric residues of dark structures conforming the image

CS Control subject

SS subjects with dissociated strabismus

$SSAV$ Strabismus syndrome of angular variability

WM, GM white and grey matter, respectively.

DHD Dissociated horizontal deviation

$SSAV1$, $SSAV2$ subject 1 and subject 2 with strabismus syndrome of angular variability

$DHD1$, $DHD2$ subject 1 and subject 2 with dissociated horizontal deviation

DBM Digitized brain mapping

CT Computed tomography

Occipital lobe is located in the posterior portion of brain, contiguous to parietal and temporal lobes. Brain lobes present at their most superficial portions, pyramidal as well as starred neurons forming nuclei conforming GM. These neurons are ordered in six laminae on the brain surface to form the brain cortex. The cellular groups in this cortical regions are disposed in an orderly fashion forming columns; their axons extend deeper into the WM (1).

WM is composed by neuronal axons interconnecting cortical zones with other nuclei, for example, magnocellular (great size) and parvocellular (small size) cells, whose projections go to the geniculate lateral bodies toward the cerebral cortex of the occipital lobes (1).

GM, as well as WM, are part of the visual pathway, but only the most superficial layer of the brain that contains cellular nuclei conforming the GM is known as brain cortex; whereas the WM is basically constituted by the axons of these cells (2)(3).

The cerebral cortex is traversed by circumvolutions (gyrus and sulcus) of varied aspects, making it difficult to identify with precision where a brain specific cortical area begins and ends, when it is first observed by means of conventional neuroimaging studies, as is the case of MRI or computed tomography (CT) (1)(2)(3). In spite of this difficulty, it has been possible to obtain important advances in cerebral cortex morphometric studies by means of voxel-based morphometry (VBM). In (4), the authors find a GM diminution in the calcarine sulcus containing the primary visual cortex; they also demonstrate reductions in parieto-occipital areas and in the ventral temporal cortex in children and adult patients with amblyopia. This condition is characterized by dimness of vision with no-improvement in spite of using the best optical correction. In the same way, but using a MR-based morphometric technique, a study on adult patients with exotropia (5), reports a GM increase in motor cortical regions, in conjunction with a diminution in visual cortex, suggesting morphometric changes related to cerebral plasticity. In spite of these morphometric advances, no studies are available in which alterations in the WM and GM in child cerebral cortex with congenital strabismus are compared with that of healthy children of the same age.

On the other hand, congenital strabismus affects 3% of the world-wide population. Nevertheless, it is not known with precision, the anatomical site or microstructural damage underlying the origin of the disease and the zones or nuclei involved. This situation arises from the difficulty of applying morphometric studies in vivo, which would provide an accurate identification of the involved zones and nuclei and would give a better description of diseases such as dissociated strabismus, which is a form of congenital strabismus (6)(7)(8). Therefore, evidence related to the etiology of this disease has been collected from neurofunctional studies (6)(7)(8)(9).

Some forms of dissociated strabismus, besides presenting alterations in the digitized brain mapping (DBM), show ocular movements with angles of variable presentation. When movement is directed in ward, the condition is called SSAV, when it is directed outward it is known as DHD. This last visual alteration is generally symmetrical and concomitant with posterior electroencephalographic alterations, while SSAV tends to present more anterior and asymmetric alterations (6)(7)(8)(9).

Cortical areas in dissociated strabismus can be observed and differentiated with high accuracy by means of techniques of optical dissector as those employed in (10). These authors show, in rodents, changes in cortical cellular density related to visual activity using optical dissector techniques or in vitro methods such as cytochrome oxidase (11)(12)(13). As a result of these studies, the authors demonstrate the presence of structural changes in monkey's cerebral cortex with strabismus and amblyopia; however, given the nature of these methods, it is not possible to apply them to strabismic children.

Up to the present moment, no morphological alterations have been described in any of the varieties of strabismus. But based on the experience drawn from neurofunctional studies of patients with dissociated strabismus, using DBM (6)(7)(8), single photon emission computerized tomography (SPECT) (14)(15) and nuclear proton magnetic resonance spectroscopy (H-NMRS) (9) it is expected that forthcoming evidence on this subject will soon allow the identification of microstructural changes.

Moreover, for the first time, by means of DBM (7)(8), the participation of the cerebral cortex in dissociated strabismus was demostrated. This finding was lately verified by means of SPECT studies. This technique enabled the localization of cortical areas involved in dissociated strabismus and in an epilepsy case. SPECT results (14)(15) showed neuroadaptive changes consistent with the improvement of glucose consumption in the cerebral cortex of patients with strabismus treated with the botulinic toxin or surgery.

The combined application of DBM and H-NMRS methods has demonstrated that cortical regions in dissociated strabismus patients present neuroelectric and biochemical alterations compatible with epileptogenous disease (9). The difficulty lies in identifying, by means of neuroimage studies applied to live subjects, the microstructural alterations related to the origin of dissociated strabismus in children; these micro-alterations cannot be determined with conventional methods of imagenology such as CT or MRI. So far, one alternative for identifying structural changes in cortical regions would be by means of a granulometric analysis of the diverse regions under study.

Granulometric analysis is a methodology developed within mathematical morphology. Mathematical morphology is a technique widely used in image processing. This technique was initially used to solve a real problem applied to the study of porous means in materials science (16). Currently, one of its multiple applications is the processing of medical images.

In this paper we present a methodology to segment brain MRI [1] by using the morphological opening by reconstruction (17; 18). In particular, the segmentation of regions included in the occipital lobe and areas nearest to this brain structure is performed. Subsequently, two granulometric studies are carried out in a similar way to that followed in granulometric density studies (19). The first study, consists in analyzing clear and dark structures in the segmented deskulling brain for SS and CS groups. Subsequently, a similar procedure is done but on the WM and GM for the subject under study. In each of the granulometric studies, mean patterns are obtained and compared against the granulometric patterns belonging to the CS group. This comparison enables the establishment of volumetric differences, and the introduction of an index, which is useful to understand the behavior of the structures detected in the WM and GM for CS and SS.

It is important to mention not only that the age of the six participants in this study is seven years old; but also that, the GM and WM are segmented by using the methodology followed in (20). From the latter procedure, only some output images are presented to illustrate such segmentations.

This paper is organized as follows. In section 2, a background of the different transformations and concepts related to mathematical morphology are presented. The morphological opening and closing are defined in subsection 2.1. While the opening and closing by reconstruction are presented in subsection 2.2. In subsection 2.3, the granulometry notion, as well as the equations that work in a way similar to those in granulometric density are given. On the other hand, a methodology to segment regions of interest from MRI by using morphological transformations is provided in section 3. In subsection 3.1 several patterns describing the granulometric density of clear structures, dark regions, WM and GM are introduced. The intervals considered for the different structure sizes and a volumetric analysis based on a given index are reported in section 4. Finally, conclusions are presented in section 5.

2. Background on morphological transformations

As follows a background on morphological transformations employed for the treatment of MRIs is presented.

2.1 Definitions of some morphological transformations

In mathematical morphology increasing and idempotent transformations are frequently used. Morphological transformations fulfilling these properties are known as morphological filters (16; 21; 22). The basic morphological filters are the morphological opening $\gamma_{\mu B}(f)(x)$ and closing $\varphi_{\mu B}(f)(x)$ using a given structural element. In this paper, a square structuring element is employed, where B represents the structuring element of size 3×3 pixels, which contains its origin. While $\check{B}$ is the transposed set ($\check{B}= \{-x : x \in B\}$) and μ is a homothetic parameter.

[1] The MRIs used in this paper were obtained from an equipment Philips Intera of 1.5 T (Philips Medical Systems Best Netherlands), using a sequence fast feel echo (FFE), with echo time TE = 6.9 ms, repetition time TR = 25 ms, deviation angle FA = 30 degrees, excitation number NSA = 1, vision field FOV = 230 mm and slice number = 120.

Formally, the morphological opening $\gamma_{\mu B}(f)(x)$ and closing $\varphi_{\mu B}(f)(x)$ are expressed as follows:

$$\gamma_{\mu B}(f)(x) = \delta_{\mu \check{B}}(\varepsilon_{\mu B}(f))(x) \quad and \quad \varphi_{\mu B}(f)(x) = \varepsilon_{\mu \check{B}}(\delta_{\mu B}(f))(x) \tag{1}$$

where the morphological erosion $\varepsilon_{\mu B}(f)(x)$ and the morphological dilation $\delta_{\mu B}(f)(x)$ are $\varepsilon_{\mu B}(f)(x) = \wedge\{f(y) : y \in \mu \check{B}_x\}$ and $\delta_{\mu B}(f)(x) = \vee\{f(y) : y \in \mu \check{B}_x\}$. Here, $\wedge$ is the inf operator and $\vee$ is the sup operator.

The morphological opening and closing can be interpreted in the following way, both morphological transformations allow the elimination of components that can not be contained by the structuring element. Morphological opening works in the interior of the function, while the morphological closing in the complement of the function.

On the other hand, throughout the paper, we will use size 1, or size μ of the structuring element. Size 1 means a square of 3×3 pixels, while size μ means a square of $(2\mu + 1)(2\mu + 1)$ pixels. For example, if the structuring element is size 3, then the square will be 7×7 pixels, i.e, 49 neighbors are analyzed. In any size of the structuring element the origin is located at its center.

In Fig.1 the erosion, dilation, opening and closing are illustrated by using a size 5 structuring element.

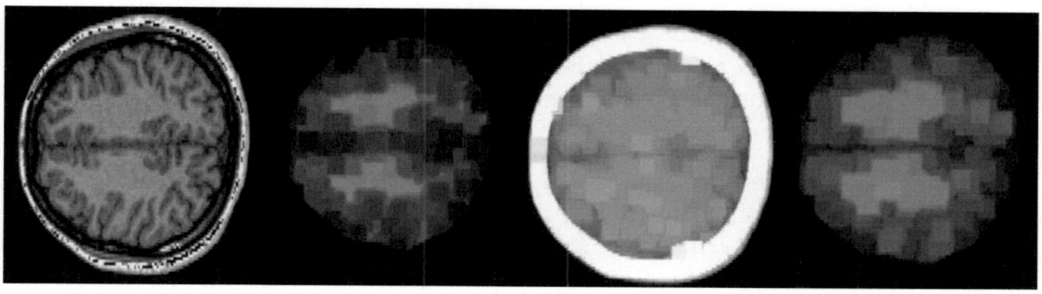

(a) (b) (c) (d)

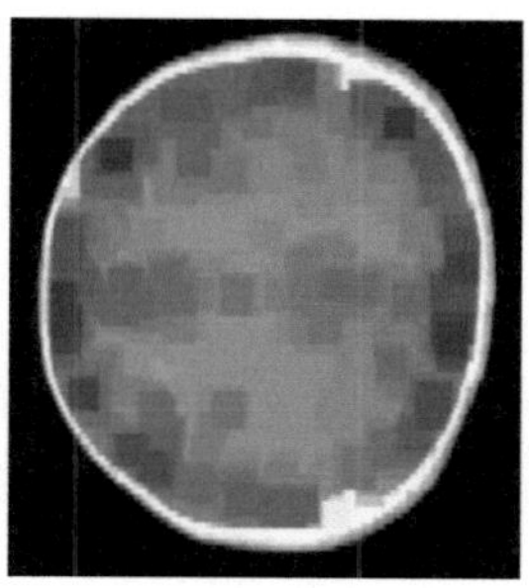

(e)

Fig. 1. Images illustrating several morphological operators using a structuring element size 5. a) Input image, b) erosion, c) dilation, d) opening, and e) closing.

2.2 Opening and closing by reconstruction

The reconstruction transformation notion is a useful concept introduced by mathematical morphology. These transformations allow the elimination of undesirable regions without considerably affecting the remaining structures of the image. This characteristic is due to the fact that these transformations are built by means of geodesic transformations (19). The geodesic dilation $\delta_f^1(g)(x)$ and the geodesic erosion $\varepsilon_f^1(g)(x)$ of size one are given by $\delta_f^1(g)(x)=f(x) \wedge \delta(g)(x)$ with $g(x) \leq f(x)$ and $\varepsilon_f^1(g)(x)=f(x) \vee \varepsilon(g)(x)$ with $g(x) \geq f(x)$, respectively. When the function $g(x)$ is equal to the erosion or the dilation of the original function, we obtain the opening $\tilde{\gamma}_{\mu B}(f)(x)$ and the closing $\tilde{\varphi}_{\mu B}(f)(x)$ by reconstruction (17; 18; 23):

$$\tilde{\gamma}_{\mu B}(f)(x) = \lim_{n\to\infty} \delta_f^n(\varepsilon_{\mu B}(f))(x) \quad and \quad \tilde{\varphi}_{\mu B}(f)(x) = \lim_{n\to\infty} \varepsilon_f^n(\delta_{\mu B}(f))(x) \tag{2}$$

In Fig. 2 the performance of the opening and closing by reconstruction is illustrated. Note in Figs. 2(c) and 2(d) that some components have been eliminated, while the remaining are maintained equal to those in the original image.

2.3 Granulometry

Granulometry is the distribution by sizes of particles that constitute an aggregate; it is employed in diverse areas to describe the qualities of size and shape of individual grains within a product. The concept of granulometry was introduced by G. Matheron at the end of the sixties and is presented as follows (24).

Definition 1 (Granulometry). *Let $(\psi_{\lambda\geq 0})_{\lambda\in Z^+}$ be a family of transformations depending on an unique positive parameter λ. This family constitutes a granulometry if and only if the next three properties are verified: (i) $\forall$ positive λ, ψ_λ is increasing; (ii) $\forall$ positive λ, ψ_λ is antiextensive, and (iii) $\forall$ positive λ and μ, $\psi_\lambda\psi_\mu = \psi_\mu\psi_\lambda = \psi_{max(\lambda,\mu)}$*

The family of morphological openings and closings for the numerical case $\{\gamma_{\mu B}\}$, $\{\varphi_{\mu B}\}$ with $\mu = \{1,..,n\}$ fulfils this last definition.

In this paper, we try to detect some characteristics of the different structures conforming the image by means of plots; which are obtained in a way similar to a granulometric density (19). Equations 3 and 4 are used in this article to deduce the granulometric plots. Such equations enable us to obtain a normalized volumetric measure of the granulometric residues of clear (χ_{Clear}) and dark (ζ_{Dark}) structures conforming the image (25; 26). Note that the structures of different dimensions are detected from the diverse μ sizes of the structuring element.

$$\chi_{Clear} = \frac{vol(\gamma_{(\mu-1)B}(f)(x)) - vol(\gamma_{\mu B}(f)(x))}{vol(f(x)) + 1} \tag{3}$$

$$\zeta_{Dark} = \frac{vol(\varphi_{\mu B}(f)(x)) - vol(\varphi_{(\mu-1)B}(f)(x))}{vol(f(x)) + 1} \tag{4}$$

Where vol represents the volume; the unit has been added in the denominator of equations 3 and 4 to avoid any indetermination.

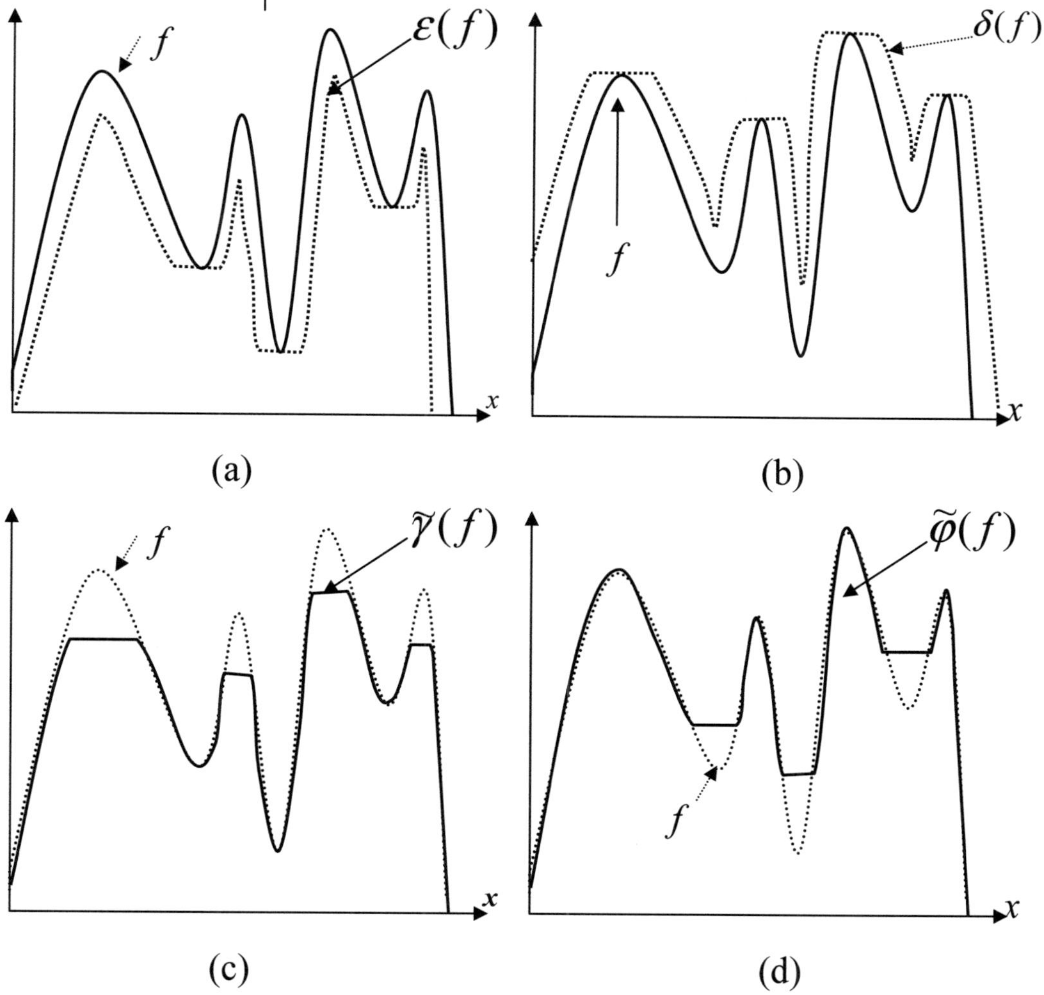

Fig. 2. a) Original image f and the marker $g = \varepsilon(f)$, b) Original image f and the marker $g = \delta(f)$, c) Opening by reconstruction, which uses erosion as marker, d) Closing by reconstruction, which uses dilation as marker.

In Fig. 3 the procedure to find χ_{Clear} on one slice is illustrated; this procedure is the same in the case of equation 4. On the other hand, in the last image of Fig. 3, the arithmetic difference is calculated between openings of sizes 5 and 6. This last image illustrates well some components that are not visible at first sight; however, they are detected by a granulometric process.

3. MRI processing through morphological transformations

In Fig. 4 we present a set of brain MRI slices belonging to a patient with dissociated strabismus classified as SSAV (in the following, in order to simplify the notation we will use for example,

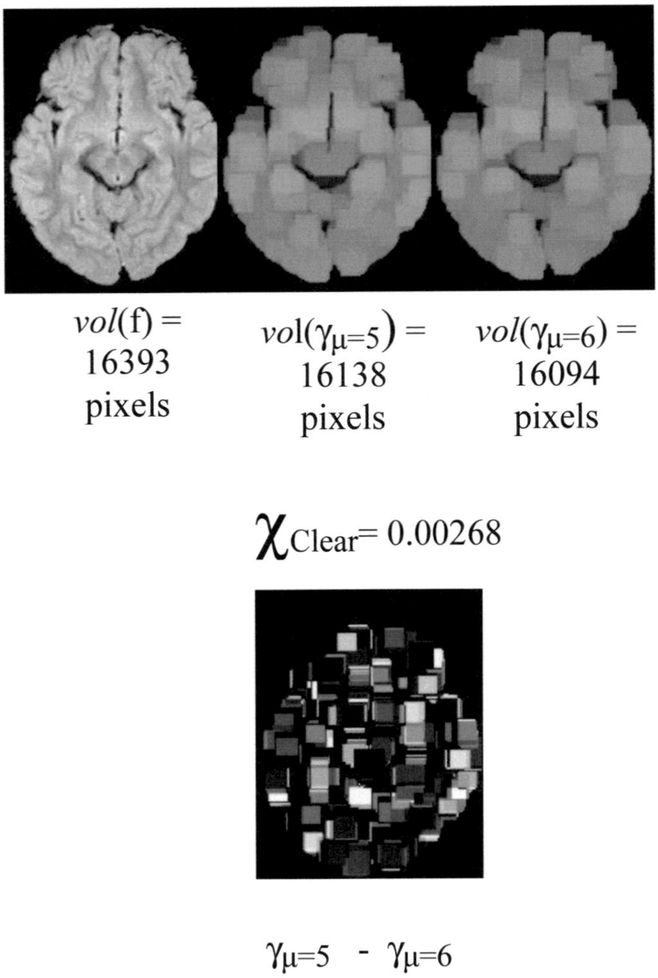

Fig. 3. Exemplification of the procedure followed to obtain the χ_{Clear} value of one slice. Bottom image illustrates the arithmetic difference between openings.

the acronym SSAV1 to denote subject 1 with dissociated strabismus classified as SSAV; and the same is extended for DHD subjects.)

The interest in analyzing the regions nearest and within the occipital lobe comes from the finding that in patients with dissociated strabismus, using DBM, an important increment in the electrical activity in the alpha rhythm has been observed (7; 8; 14; 15). This rhythm has been associated with an occipital distribution. An example of these maps is provided in Fig. 5, in which we can note, in black color, an increment in the electrical activity in the alpha rhythm, in accordance with the scale situated at the right and top of the images. In this way, ten axial slices are considered for analysis. The slices are parallel and within the visual via.

On the other hand, images in Fig. 4 are useful to present examples of output images, after the algorithm to carry out the deskulling step is applied.

As follows, we introduce the algorithm to achieve the deskulling step for the regions under study. This algorithm was applied to images acquired from the subjects in this study (CS and SS).

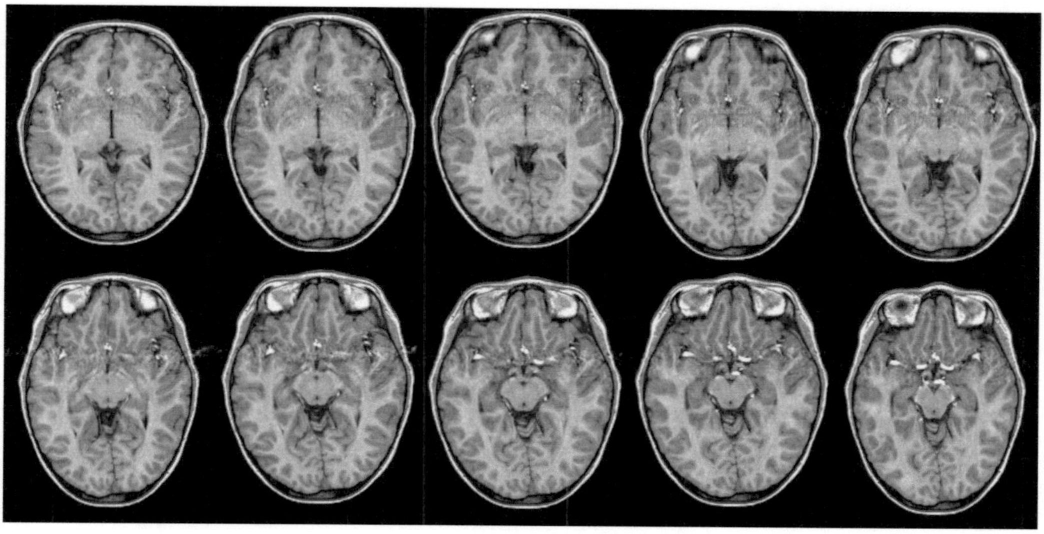

Fig. 4. High resolution axial slices taken from SSAV1

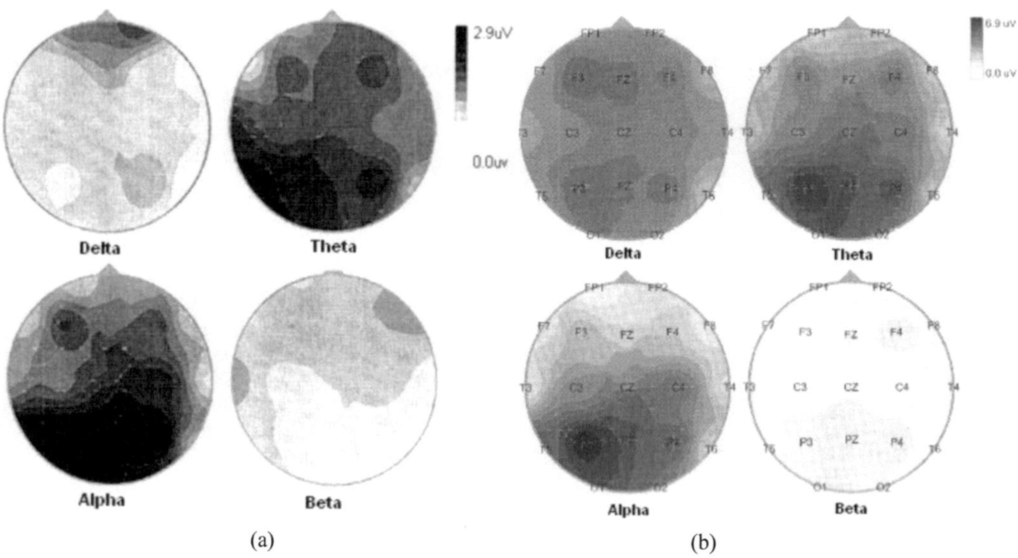

Fig. 5. DBMs showing the electrical behavior of two strabismic children. Darker regions indicate greater electrical activity. (a) Subject with DHD, (b) Subject with SSAV.

Algorithm (deskulling step):

i) Given that the interest zones are located around and within the occipital lobe, the original images located in Fig. 4 are cropped at section 160 to separate the regions of interest. This is illustrated in Fig. 6(a).

ii) Once the images are cropped, we proceed to the deskulling step. For this, the opening by reconstruction size 6 is employed (see equation (2)). The opening by reconstruction has the property of avoiding the generation of new structures. In Fig. 6(b), a set of output images is presented.

iii) Thresholding of the images in Fig. 6(b) between sections 80-255. Here the skull is eliminated and several pores appear in the binary image as a result of the thresholding procedure. The processed images are shown in Fig. 6(c).

iv) Subsequently, a closing by reconstruction size 6 is applied with the purpose of closing the pores originated by the thresholding. The output images are displayed in Fig. 6(d).

v) A mask is obtained with respect to the original image (see Fig. 4), i.e. every pixel in the images in Fig. 6(d) takes the corresponding grey level in the original image. This situation is presented in Fig. 6(e).

vi) A manual segmentation is carried out by a specialist in strabismus. Several undesired regions in the images of Fig. 6(e) are eliminated. The suppressed regions correspond mainly to dura mater and cerebellum; this can be appreciated in Fig. 6(f).

With respect to step ii) of the mentioned algorithm, an opening by reconstruction size 6 is applied. This size was elected from the graphic in Fig. 7(a). The plot was obtained by computing the volume on the image $\widetilde{\gamma}_{\mu} - \widetilde{\gamma}_{\mu+1}$. Such graphic shows the contained structures (clear regions) in the image of size μ. Observe that an important structure of white regions is found between values 1-3, where the skull information is located. To verify this, in Fig. 7(b) we have the original image, on the right we have the eroded image size 3; and this eroded image is used as marker to obtain the opening by reconstruction (last image on the right). However, given that the skull is surrounded by regions with lower intensity levels, a marker given by the morphological erosion of size $\mu = 6$ does not allow the skull reconstruction with its original intensity levels. In Fig. 7(c), the erosion size 6 for several input images is presented; these images are used as markers to obtain the opening by reconstruction. If smaller sizes of the structuring element are selected, for example $\mu = 1$, then the skull is not completely attenuated and the proposed algorithm fails in step iii). For this reason it is crucial to have this situation in mind . In Fig. 8 we illustrate the application of the opening by reconstruction size $\mu = 1$ to the images located in Fig. 6(a). Note that pixel intensity levels in the skull are hardly attenuated.

3.1 Granulometric patterns

Once the skull has been separated and the undesirable regions on the images have been suppressed, a granulometric study is carried out to determine the χ_{Clear} and ζ_{Dark} values on the segmented slices. χ_{Clear} and ζ_{Dark} quantities(see equations 3 and 4) provide information about the distribution density of the clear and dark structures within the image. In Fig. 9 we present in a general way the procedure to obtain the granulometric patterns for dark regions for both CS cases, and one SS. A similar method is applied in the case of clear structures. In

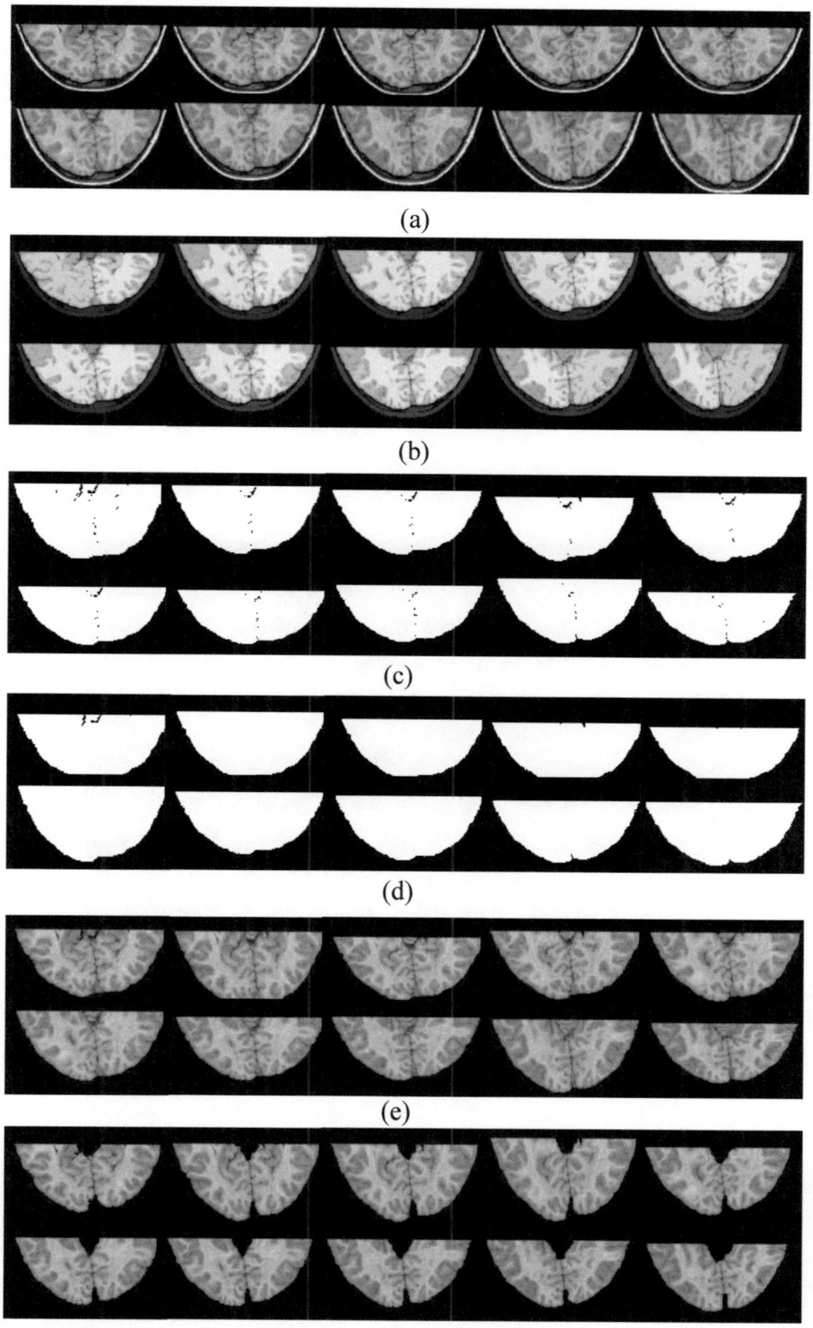

(a)

(b)

(c)

(d)

(e)

(f)

Fig. 6. Images illustrating the procedure followed for skull elimination. (a) Cropped images taken from SSAV1; (b) Opening by reconstruction; (c) Threshold; (d) Closing by reconstruction; (e) Mask; (f) Manual elimination.

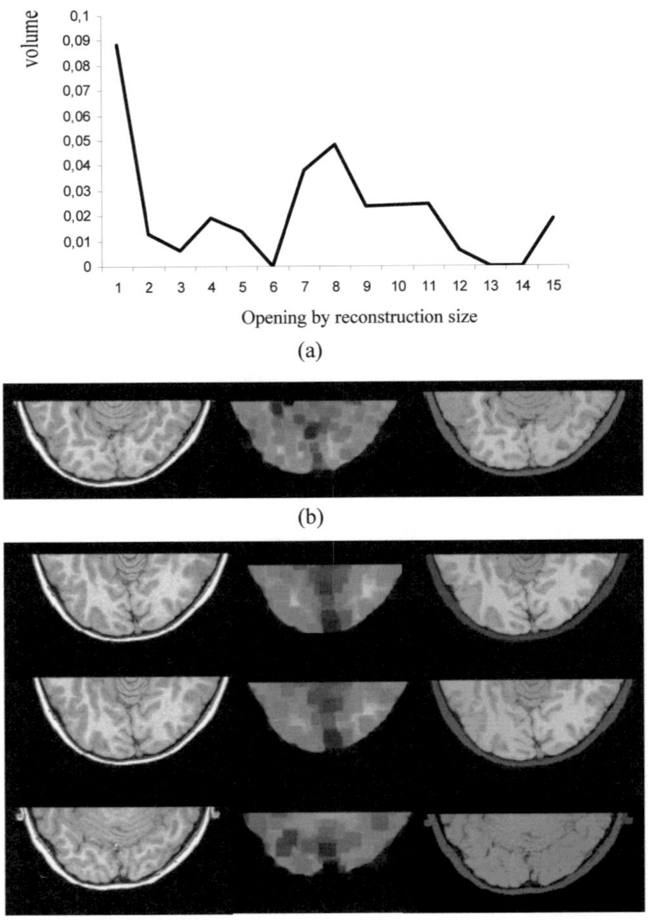

(c)

Fig. 7. Size election of structuring element to attenuate the skull. a) Graph of structures size vs volume on the image $\widetilde{\gamma}_{\mu} - \widetilde{\gamma}_{\mu+1}$, b) Original image , eroded size 3 and opening by reconstruction size 3; c) Original images, eroded size 6, and opening by reconstruction size 6

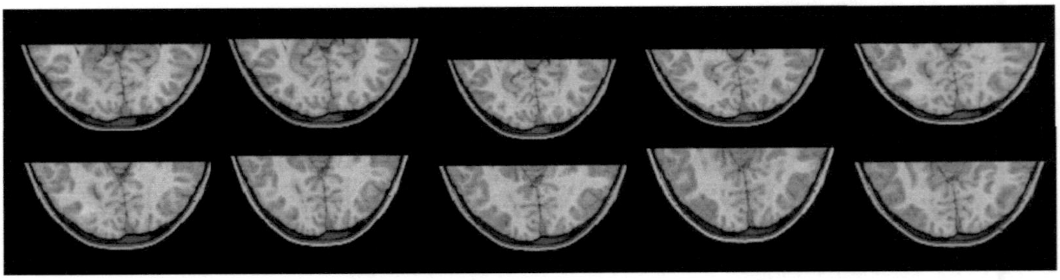

Fig. 8. Opening by reconstruction size $\mu = 1$ applied to images in Fig. 6(a).

Fig. 10, we present the granulometric patterns for the SS and the mean pattern for the CS following the procedure depicted in Fig. 9. Notice that the first two graphs of mean volume correspond to the DHD subjects and CS group; while the last two to the SSAV subjects and CS group.

The granulometric curves in Fig. 10 provide general information for the clear and dark regions detected in the whole deskulling brain. These curves have the disadvantage of being derived from non-autodual transformations, i.e. clear and dark structures are not treated in individual form. As a consequence, it is necessary to separate WM and GM to obtain the granulometric patterns of these regions. In this work, GM and WM were segmented by applying the methodology used in (20). Some output images illustrating the segmentation of such regions are presented in Fig. 11, and the granulometric patterns of WM and GM for the SS and SC are presented in Fig. 12. These graphics were obtained under the procedure depicted in Fig. 9.

4. Results

In particular, we consider three main groups of clear and dark structures. These groups take into account the size of the structuring element (the structuring element used in this paper is a square, see subsection 2.1).

Group 1(Small structures).-In this group the structures within the sizes 1 and 2 of the structuring element are comprised. *Group 2(Medium structures).*- This group contains the structures located in the size interval 3 to 6 of the structuring element. *Group 3(Large structures).*-Finally, this group comprises structure sizes 7-17 of the structuring element.

i) Clear and dark regions analysis from graphics in Fig. 10 for DHD case.-

In both clear and dark regions, a great variation in the curves of DHD subjects is observed with respect to the CS, mainly in medium and large sizes. This indicates the lack of smooth transitions between the analyzed structures.

ii) Clear and dark regions analysis from graphics in Fig. 10 for SSAV case.- Main changes in clear structures are observed in large size structures; while dark structures vary for all sizes.

Curves in Fig. 10 indicate the existence of important variations in clear and dark structures in the DHD and SSAV subjects with respect to the CS. However, clear and dark structures are mixed, and results difficult to infer, since it is not possible to determine whether the predominance or the absence of some structures sizes is due to clear or dark components. This situation occurs because WM and GM have different intensities, and the morphological transformations used to build equations 3 and 4 are not autoduals, i.e, they do not try clear and dark structures in a separate form; this causes that, some clear and dark components are mixed during the processing.

Trying to avoid this inconvenience, WM and GM will be analyzed in separate ways with the purpose of finding some morphometric differences between CS and SS.

iii) WM and GM analysis from graphics in Fig. 12 for DHD case.-

From graphs in Fig. 12, for WM and GM in the SS case, we observe the following: a) a lack of small components with respect to CS; b) the existent small components are thin; and c) medium and large structures predominate in WM and GM.

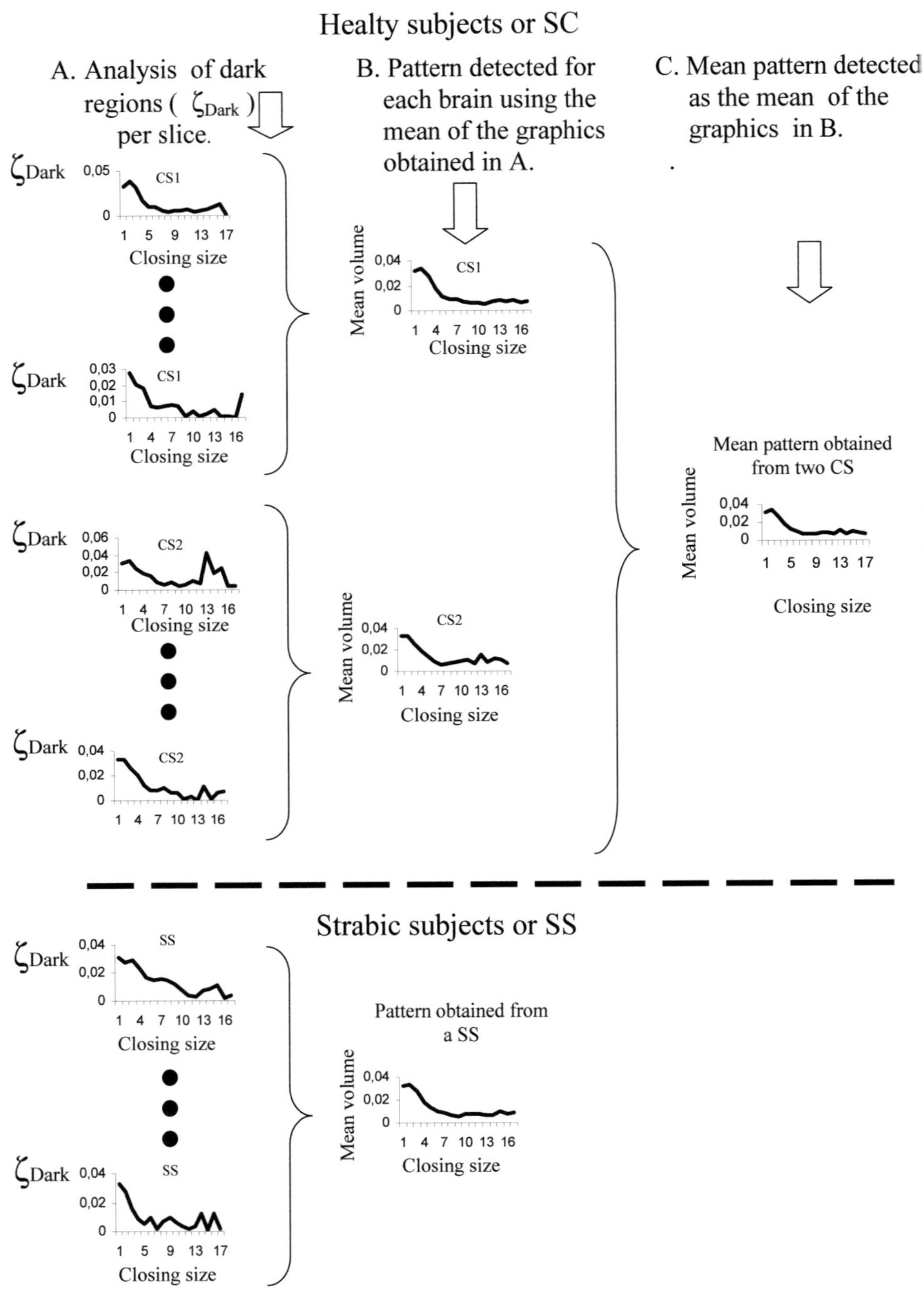

Fig. 9. Procedure to obtain granulometric patterns. In step A the graphics obtained for one slice of each of the two CS and for one SS case are illustrated. In step B, a common mean pattern is obtained for both CS and one SS. Finally, in step C, a mean pattern is obtained for the two CS.

DHD vs CS case:

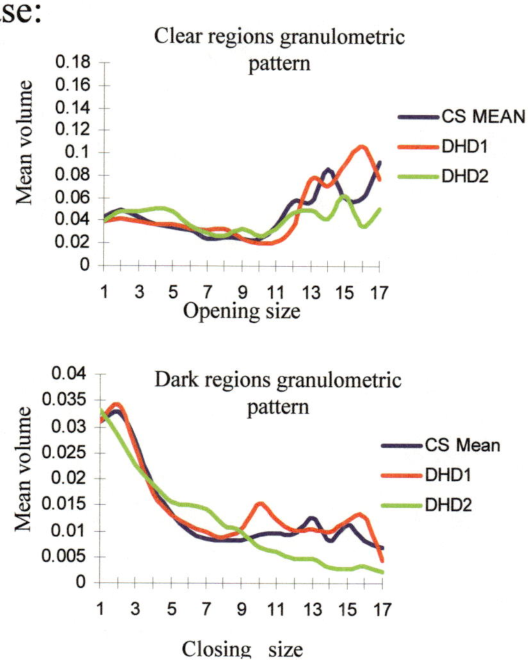

SSAV vs CS case:

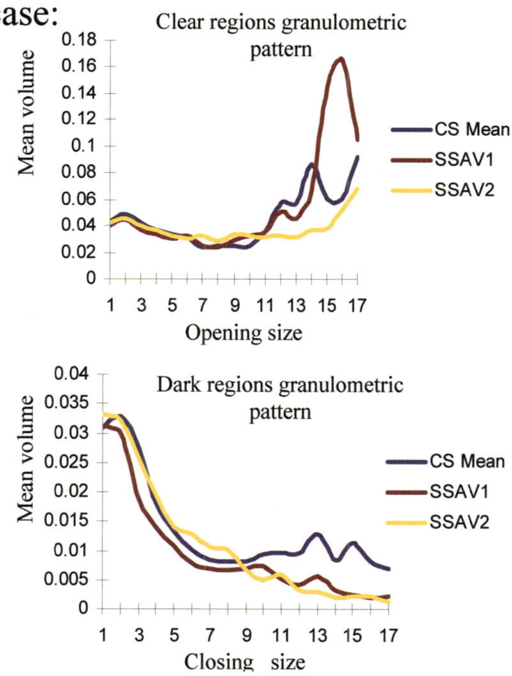

Fig. 10. Mean volume of clear and dark structures corresponding to SS and SC.

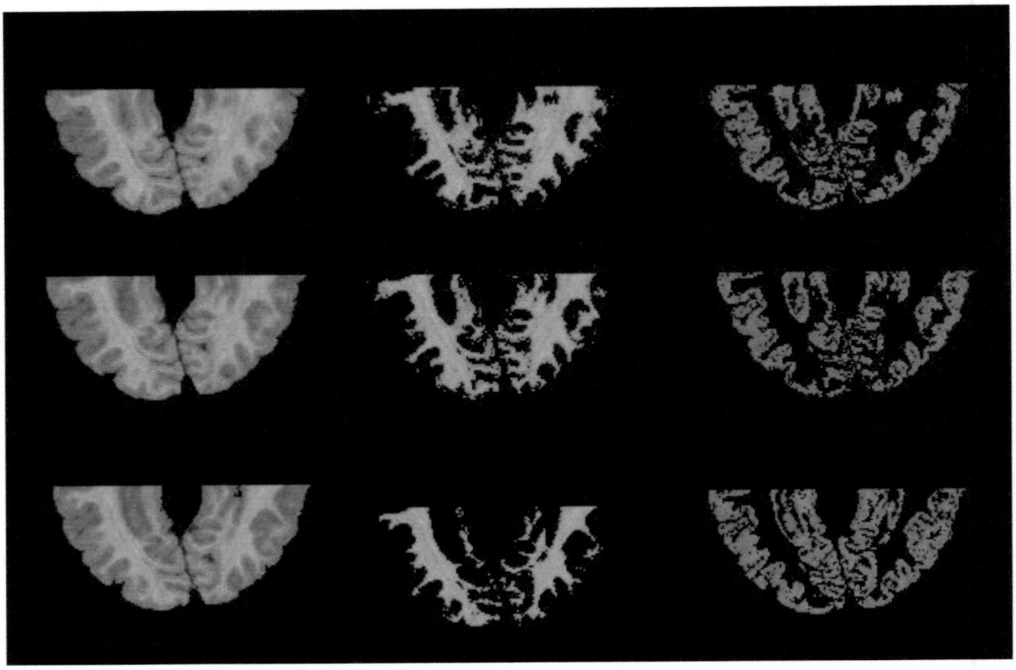

Fig. 11. Images illustrating the segmentation of WM and GM.

In order to explain this situation we divide the analysis of WM and GM as follows :

a) WM analysis.- In Fig. 13, the terms small, medium and large components are exemplified with some structures. Notice that small components in WM have the appearance of "fingers", and medium components have a characteristic neck that joins them to large structures.

The lack of small components in the SS with respect to CS group, indicates the absence of such components in the WM. Also, the graphs indicate that the existing small components are thin; therefore they are eliminated easily by small structuring elements. On the other hand, the prevalence of medium and large structures is due to absence the circumvolutions, this originates a non-smooth transition mainly between small and medium components; since medium and large components are not to much different.

In Fig. 14 small components are eliminated from slices that belong to DHD, SSAV and a CS. Notice that for DHD cases, WM has thin "fingers" which almost disappear after applying an opening of size 1; whereas for the SSAV case, "fingers" are not so thin and many of them remain after the same transformation is applied.

Note that, for the CS case, WM shows abundant appendages and coral forms. Also, observe that transitions between medium and large sizes are smooth; however for the DHD and SSAV cases, the appendages and coral forms decrease significantly.

b) GM analysis.- In the GM there is a prevalence of medium and large components. This is confirmed in the graphs of GM for DHD and SSAV cases (Fig. 12). Small, medium and large size components in GM are illustrated in Fig. 13.

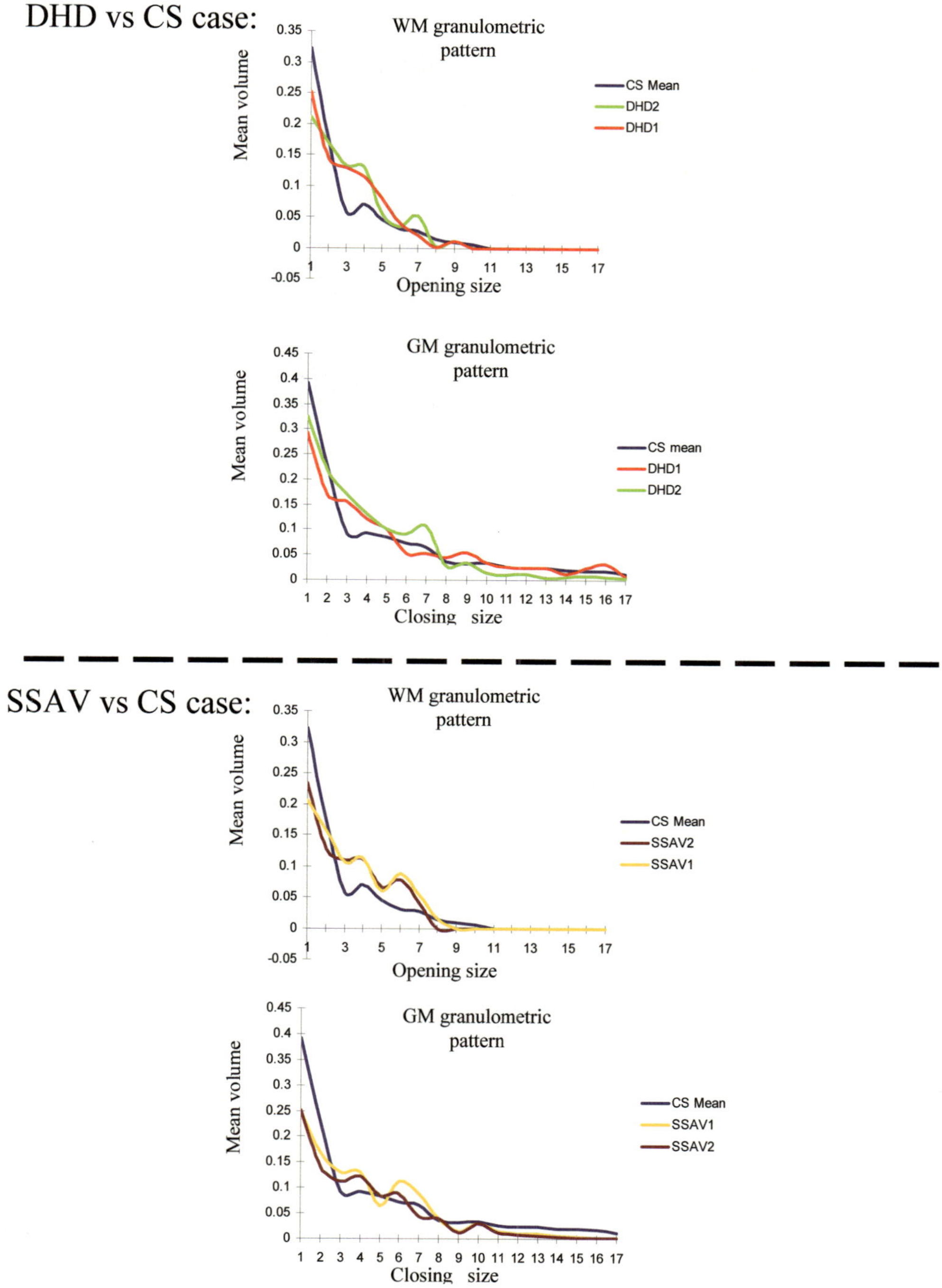

Fig. 12. WM and GM granulometric patterns for the CS and SS groups.

In trying to obtain a parameter indicating the absence, thinning, or thickening of WM or GM structures, an index is proposed. Such index is expressed as follows:

$$\iota = \frac{vol(small\ structures)}{vol(medium\ structures) + vol(large\ structures)} \tag{5}$$

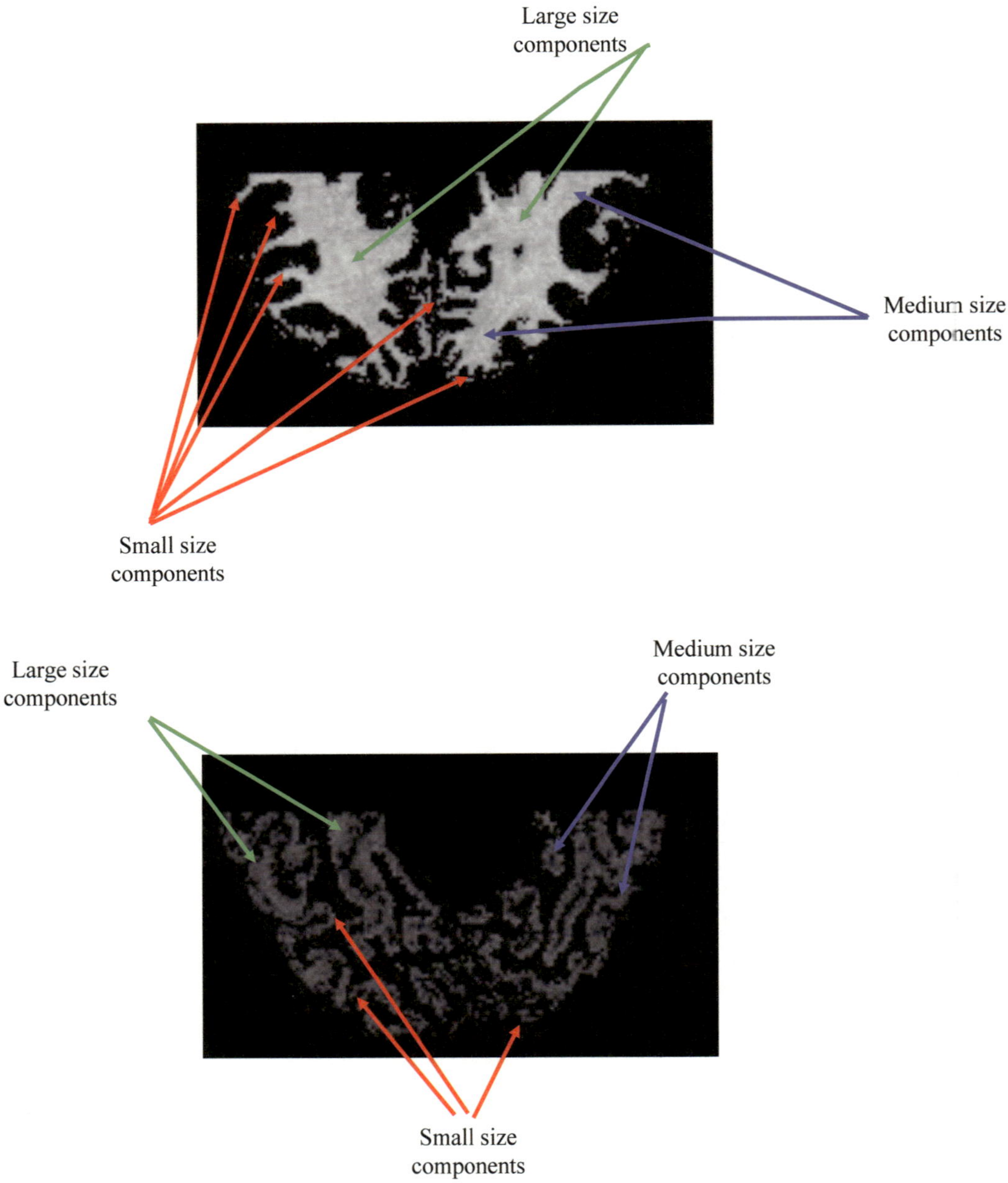

Fig. 13. Illustration of small, medium and large structures on WM and GM.

In Fig. 15, index ι was plotted for WM and GM based on the values obtained for graphs in Fig. 12. When index ι for the CS is compared with that for the SS group, significant differences are obtained, since the latter value is much smaller.

Index ι, indicates that in the WM of CS, the volume of small components is more than double that of medium and large structures together; while in GM of CS, index ι is almost equal to the unit, that is, vol(small structures) $\approx$ vol(medium structures) + vol(large structures).

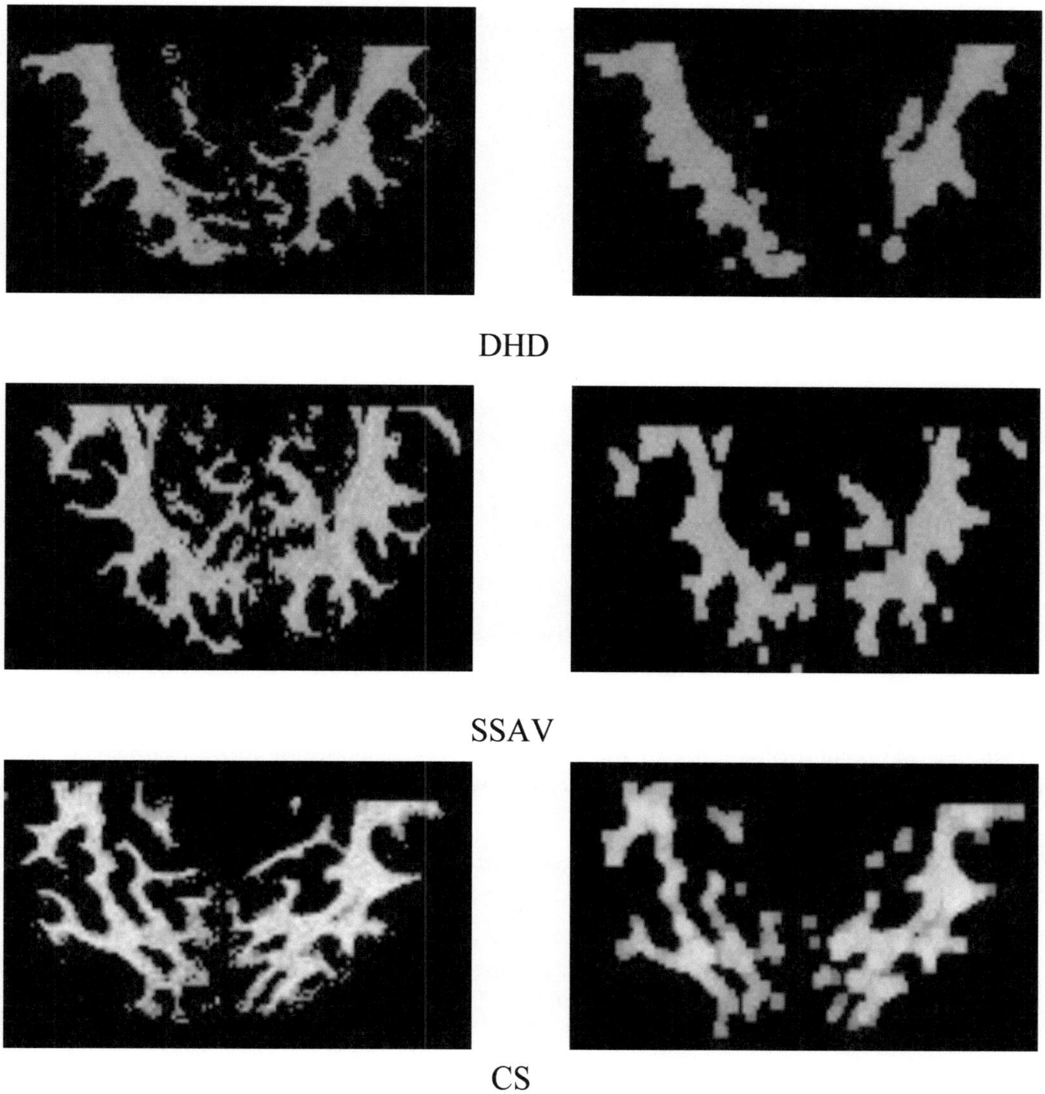

Fig. 14. Elimination of thin components.

With respect to SS, index ι presents the following behavior: a large number of medium components in WM and GM, that yields an inferior value when compared against the index for CS.

In other words, index ι for WM and GM in SS suggests: a) a lack of small components in the analyzed WM, and whenever present they are characterized by their thinness. Medium structures predominate through the analyzed WM. Given the lack of small components, and the presence of thin small structures in WM, this originates the absence of small structures in the GM, for which a predominance of medium and large structures is observed.

The absence of small components (″fingers″) in the WM may causes a lack of electrical connection among different cortical regions. As a consequence a right electrical

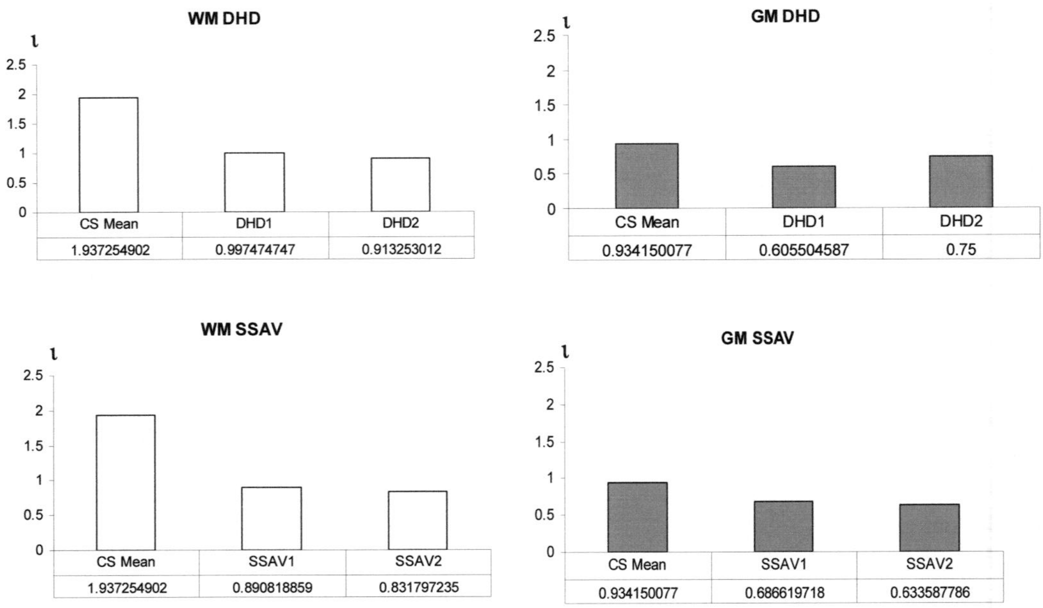

Fig. 15. Table to analyze WM and GM in all subjects through the proposed index ι. Volume values(bottom of x-axis) to evaluate the index were obtained from graphs in Fig. 12.

communication between different cortical areas is hindered. Therefore, although there are great areas of GM and WM in the SS, the lack of small components identified as fingers or thin components in the WM and GM, may cause a faulty electrical conduction and communication between these areas.

On the other side, the presence of a large volume formed of medium components in WM can be associated with a certain immaturity process, which is identified by some authors with excessive glial proliferation or abnormalities in myelin maturation or composition (27). This produces a low quality WM characterized by axons presenting certain degree of damage, with the subsequent deficiency in impulse conduction. In our case, index ι is also called immaturity index, by means of which the absence and increment of certain structures in WM or GM are measured. In this way, morphometric changes in WM and GM seem to be intimately related to the electrical and neurofunctional behavior of the analyzed SS. The granulometric study carried out in this work suggests that changes in the nerve conduction, as we have observed by means of DBM in strabismic patients (7; 8; 14; 15), could be the consequence of changes in the microstructural organization of the cerebral mass. According to this study, these alterations may be manifested as presence of immaturity of certain brain regions and lack of electrical communication between the structures conforming the WM and GM. We consider that as a result of this immaturity, alternative vias are established affecting the processes of neuronal interconnections; with the subsequent affectation, in different degrees and ways of the grey and white substance; hence different clinical expressions of the dissociated strabismus are originated.

On the other hand, studies of electrical brain function carried out by means of computed neurometry, have revealed the close correlation between the structure and cerebral function. This has been determined from the study of electrical coherence, which is a non invasive method to determine the functional relations among different brain areas. This coherence is altered when some association vias (short and large cortico-corticals, cortico-subcorticals, and short cortico-corticals), are affected structurally; this has been demonstrated in some diseases like Alzheimer's and dementia. Some aspects of the electrical behavior as in the coherence case, depend precisely on the neuro-structural substrate (28; 29). For some authors, a decrease in coherence represents a diagnostic marker. Therefore, further research is necessary on the interrelation between structure and neuronal function, to gain a better understanding into the origin of multiple diseases that have a seat in the cerebral cortex, or at least of those conditions in which the participation of the brain cortex plays a role in their physiopathology. This knowledge enable the establishment of better treatments (28).

On the other hand, during the development of the cerebral cortex or corticogenesis, there is a cellular migration of neurons that travel from periventricular regions and at the same time start maturing, until they reach more superficial regions of the brain, where their maturation culminates. During this process, interconnection vias are liable to be damaged giving place to different neurological schemes, that can affect the neuronal maturity process as well as the performance of the association routes. In the case of strabismus it is still not known, which structural alterations are the cause of this condition. (30–32). Finally, the granulometric study presented in this work, helps us understand the morphology of WM and GM at macroestructural level; however further studies are necessary to analyze the structure of the WM and GM at microestructural level.

5. Conclusions

In this work we presented a method for segmenting MRI slices, as well as the computation of two granulometric studies. The first granulometric study, analyzes clear and dark structures in the whole deskulling brain; while the second one, consists in the analysis of WM and GM separately.

Curves obtained for the whole deskulled brains were not appropriated for analyzing clear and dark regions, since WM and GM are partly composed by pixels of similar intensities.

On the other hand, important differences were found in the granulometric plots of WM and GM of the SS when compared to the graphs of CS group. Main differences consist in the lack of small components ("fingers") and predominance of medium and large structures. From this analysis, index ι was introduced, which is useful to establish an immaturity degree. In the SS, index ι results to be much smaller than that of CS; given the presence of numerous medium and large structures.

The information drawn from these results suggests that there is a faulty electrical communication among several cortical areas due to the lack of small components, and also to the thinness of these structures which are present both in WM and GM. Changes in nerve neuroconduction, similar to those observed by means of the DBM in strabismic patients (7; 8; 14; 15), could be related to the microstructural organization of the cerebral mass. Index ι values, obtained in this work from healthy and strabismic children, show significant differences in the proportion of granulometric elements in the GM and WM when healthy and SS are compared. Based on the calculated index, strabismic patients with SSAV present a greater degree of immaturity than those patients with DHD; since ι index is smaller. This can be more clearly appreciated from the graphs and derived values in Fig. 15.

On the other hand, it is rather convenient that changes consistent with the alterations in the relation volume and granulometric density can be determined in alive subjects; besides this advantage can be complemented with neurofunctional studies such as the DBM. This technique offers a high temporary resolution, though its space resolution is significantly slower. Granulometric studies offer a finest structural analysis available in vivo, that allow the interpretation of neurofunctional studies. On the one hand, granulometry is outlined as an excellent diagnosis marker for several neurologic diseases. The study carried out in this work not only suggests the neuronal immaturity associated with strabismus, but also the lack of small components("fingers") and the predominance of medium size structures mainly in the SS group. These circumstances propitiate alterations in conduction of the neuroelectrical impulses, favoring the presence of strabismus, as well as the alterations encountered in the DBM. Therefore, granulometric studies may help to gain a better insight into the origin, diagnosis and prognosis of this prevalent disease, for which so little is known. Although the amount of brains analyzed here is only six, they provide important information to establish granulometric differences between SC and SS groups. Finally, for our future research, we are considering the following things: I) Improvement of the morphologic operators involved in the obtention of granulometric curves; these operators must be autodual with the purpose of treating clear and dark components of the image separately; and II) Inclusion of a larger sample of healthy children to obtain mean patterns, as well as a larger number of patients with strabismus.

6. Acknowledgements

The authors wish to thank the Mario Moreno Reyes foundation for the financial support. Jorge D. Mendiola-Santibañez thanks to CONACyT for the financial support.

7. References

[1] Krachmer JH, Marti T.J, Corbett JJ.: Trastornos del quiasma y de las vías visuales retroquiasmáticas, En: Los requisitos en oftalmología: Neuroftalmología. Ed. Harcourt, Madrid, España. 2001; 101-108.

[2] Rakic, P; Lombroso, P.J. "Development of the cerebral cortex: I. Forming the cortical structure". J. Am Acad Child Adolesc Psychiatry 1998, 37 (1): 116-117.

[3] Zeki, SM., Watson, J.D.G, Lueck, C.J., Fristcn, K.J., Kennard, C. And Frackowiat, S.J. "A direct demostration of functional specialization in human visual cortex". J Neurosci 1991, 11(3) 641-649.

[4] Mendola JD, Conner IP, Anjali R, Chan ST, Schwartz TL, Odom JV, Kwong KK. "Voxel-based analysis of MRI detects abnormal visual cortex in children and adults with amblyopia". Human Brain Mapping 2005; 25(2) 222-236

[5] Suk-tak Ch; Kwok-win T; Kwok-cheung L; Lap-kong Ch; Mendola JD; Kwong KK. Neuroanatomy and adult strabismus: a voxel-based morphometric analisys of magnetic resonance structural scans. Neuroimage 2004 (22) 986-994.

[6] Gallegos-Duarte M. "Exploratory maneuvers in congenital endotropy ". En: Temas Selectos de Estrabismo. Centro Mexicano de Estrabismo SC. México, Composición Editorial Láser. México, D.F. 2005, 1-18.
[7] Gallegos-Duarte M; Moguel, S.; Rubín de Celis, B.; " Alterations in the cerebral mapping in the variable congenital endotropy ", Rev Mex Oftalmol; 2004; 78 (3): 122-126.
[8] Gallegos-Duarte M. " Paradoxical cortical response during the intermittent fotoestimulation in the dissociated strabismus ", Cir y Cir 2005; 73 (3): 161-165.
[9] Gallegos-Duarte M, Mendiola-Santibáñez JD, Ortiz-Retana JJ; Rubín de Celis B, Vidal-Pineda R, Sigala-Zamora. " Dissociated desviation. An strabismus of cortical origin". Cir y Cir 2007, 75 (4): (in printt).
[10] Olivares, R; Godoy,G; Adaro,L; Aboitiz, F.: "Neuronal density of the visual cortex (area 17) of two species of wild rodents". Int. J. Morphol 2004, 22 (4): 279-284.
[11] Horton, J.C., Hocking, D.R., "An adult-like pattern of ocular dominance columns in striate cortex of newborn monkeys prior to visual experience". J. Neuroscience 1996, 16:1789-1805.
[12] Horton, J.C., Hocking, D.R., Timing of the critical period for plasticity of ocular dominance columns in macaque striate cortex. J. Neuroscience 1997; 17:3684-3709,.
[13] Tychsen L; Wong AM; Burkhalter A.: Paucity of horizontal connections for binocular vision in V1 of naturally strabismic macaques: Cytochrome oxidase compartment specificity. J Com Neurol. 2004, 474 (2): 261-75
[14] Gallegos-Duarte, M, Moguel-Ancheita S: "Modifications neurologiques adaptatives après traitement médical et chirurgical du syndrome strabique avec variations des repères angulaires". En: Réunion de printemps, Association française de strabologie. 110 Congres de la société Française d´Ophtalmologie, Paris 2004. http://perso.orange.fr/hoc.lods/demo147.html.
[15] Moguel-Ancheita S, Orozco-Gómez L, Gallegos-Duarte M, Alvarado I, Montes C. " Metabolic changes in the cerebral cortex related to the strabismus treatment. Preliminary results with SPECT". Cir y Cir 2004; 72:165-170
[16] Serra, J.: Mathematical Morphology vol. I, Academic Press., London, (1982).
[17] Serra, J. y P. Salembier. "Connected operators and pyramids" ., Proc. of SPIE. Image Algebra and Mathematical Morphology'93, San Diego, July , 1993.
[18] Salembier P., and Serra J.,: Flat zones filtering, connected operators and filters by reconstruction. IEEE Transactions on Image Processing, 3(8), (1995) 1153-1160.
[19] Vincent L. and Dougherty E. R.:Morphological segmentation for textures and particles. In Digital IMage Processing Methods E.R. Dougherty, editor, . Marcel Dekker, New York, (1994) 43–102.
[20] Mendiola-Santibañez, J.D ,Terol-Villalobos, I.R., Herrera-Ruiz G. , Fernández-Bouzas, A., "Morphological contrast measure and contrast enhancement: One application to the segmentation of brain MRI", *Signal Processing*, vol. 87 , no. 9, pp. 2125-2150, 2007.
[21] Soille, P.,: Morphological image analysis: principle and applications, Springer-Verlag, 2003.
[22] Heijmans H., "Morphological Image Operators", Academic Press, USA, 1994.
[23] L. Vincent, "Morphological Grayscale Reconstruction in Image Analysis: Applications and Efficient Algorithms," *IEEE Transactions on Image Processing*, vol. 2, no. 2, pp. 176-201, Feb. 1993.
[24] Matheron G.: Eléments pour une théorie des milieux poreoux. Mason,Paris(1967).

[25] Terol-Villalobos, I.R.: Morphological Image Enhancement and Segmentation, in Advances in Imaging and Electron Physics, P. W. Hawkes Editor, Academic Press, (2001) 207–273.

[26] Mendiola-Santibañez, J.D and Terol-Villalobos, I. R. : Morphological contrast mappings on partition based on the flat zone notion. Computación y Sistemas, 6 (2002b) 25–37.

[27] M. R. Herbert, D. A. Ziegler, C. K. Deutsch,L. M. O'Brien, N. Lange, A. Bakardjiev, J. Hodgson, K. T. Adrien, S. Steele, N. Makris, D. Kennedy1, G. J. Harris and V. S. Caviness Jr ,"Dissociations of cerebral cortex, subcortical and cerebral white matter volumes in autistic boys", *Brain* , vol. 126, pp. 1182–1192, 2003.

[28] Calderón-González P.L, Parra-Rodriguez M.A., Libre-Rodríguez J.J., Gutiérrez J.V. Análisis espectral de la coherencia cerebral en la enfermedad de Alzheimer. Rev Neurol 2004; 38 (5): 422-427

[29] Dunkin JJ, Leuchter AF, Newton TF, Cook IA. Reduced EEG coherence in dementia: state or trait marker? Biol Psychiatry 1994; 35: 870-9

[30] Papovik E, Haynes, L.W Noradrenergic but not cholinergic innervation of the embryonic cortical neuroepithelium rescues germinal and postmitotic cells in heterochronic cocultures. Brain. Res 2000 (853): 227-235

[31] Chiaki Itami, Fumitaka Kimura, Tomoko Kohono, Masato Mtsuoka, Masumi Ichikawa, Tdaharu Tsumoto et Al. Brain-derived neurotrophic factor-dependen unmasking of "silent" synapses in the developing mouse barrel cortex. Neurosciencie 2003 (22) : 13069-13074.

[32] Goshima Y, Ito T, Sasaki Y, Nakamura F. Semaphorins as signals for cell repulsion and invasion. J Clin investigation 2002 (109): 993-998.

10

Intracerebral Communication Studied by Magnetoencephalography

Kuniharu Kishida
Department of Information Science, Faculty of Engineering, Gifu University
Yanagido, Gifu,
Japan

1. Introduction

Magnetoencephalography (MEG) can monitor the activation of a neuronal population with millisecond temporal resolution, and offer new noninvasive information about basic activities of the human brain. MEG is usable for the description of spontaneous brain activity and the detection of timely events such as stimulus evoked fields. The most recent advances in the field of MEG concerning cortical responses to stimulation are issued from development of multichannel recordings. We can study the temporal order of several cortical areas from averaged waveforms of MEG, e.g., auditory, visual, and somatosensory evoked responses. For three decades, dynamical information contained in MEG has been analyzed mainly in terms of averaged waveforms.

However, lots of brain activities are included in original MEG data. For spontaneous fields there are huge activities in cortical areas. Generally, it is difficult to estimate source locations of current dipole data from MEG data correctly at the present stage, if the number of current dipoles becomes large. The estimation of their locations is an underdetermined problem. In the case of spontaneous fields it is hard to obtain intracerebral communication between active cortical areas. Hence, we consider an overdetermined problem in the case of evoked fields, since their locations of active cortical areas are limited. Furthermore, we should find a possibility to obtain dynamical information by signal processing of fluctuations around concatenate average waveforms, which have been discarded without signal processing in the conventional MEG analysis. The fluctuations may be induced magnetic fields to communicate between cortical areas.

In this chapter, we will show this new direction of MEG analysis by way of example of somatosensory evoked field (SEF), and intracerebral communication between active somatosensory cortices can be expressed by system identification of fluctuations. That is, intracerebral communication between the primary somatosensory cortex in the contralateral hemisphere (cSI) and the contralateral secondary somatosensory cortex (cSII) in 2Hz median nerves stimuli will be discussed from correlation functions of SEF fluctuations by the identification method with feedback model (see Section 3.6). In this chapter, intracerebral communication between cSI and cSII will be studied not from averaged waveforms but from fluctuations around concatenate averaged waveforms by following steps:

1) Extraction of SEF fluctuations from MEG will be discussed in Section 3.3.
2) Inverse problem will be shown in Section 3.5 or 4.4.
3) Intracerebral communication will be discussed in Section 4.5 by feedback model identification.

2. Difficulties in system identification of MEG and countermeasures

2.1 Deterministic waveforms

Somatosensory activities are known as cSI, bilateral secondary somatosensory cortices (SIIs) and posterior parietal cortices in somatosensory stimuli with inter-stimulus intervals of more than one second (Kakigi et al., 2000; Wikström et al., 1996), and under more than 1 Hz periodic median nerve stimulus, the somatosensory activity is mainly observed at cSI (Wikström et al., 1996). In the previous paper (Kishida, 2009a), responses of evoked magnetic fields were studied for 5Hz periodical median nerve stimuli. In 5Hz periodic median nerve stimulus, there are the 5Hz repetitive line spectra of the somatosensory evoked field (SEF). This suggests that averaged waveforms are deterministic. Statistical properties of SEF are summarized in Kishida (2009a) as SEF includes the deterministic part of concatenate averaged waveforms and the random part of fluctuations around them.

From the Wold decomposition theorem (Mathematical Society of Japan, 1987), a stationary process is uniquely decomposed into a non-deterministic part and a deterministic part. We can define correlation functions in a stationary process, and they are described by time lag. They can be specified as two types: One type can be obtained from fluctuations and the other pseudo type is calculated from periodic functions. Under the condition of small averaged waveforms, dynamical activities of current dipoles of primary somatosensory cortexes were studied from MEG by the decorrelation method of the BSS method in Kishida (2009b). The usage of the decorrelation method can make an improvement on the signal-to-noise ratio of components of interest.

2.2 Nonlinearity

Assuming that the brain dynamics is linear, the brain functional activities can be identified by using multivariate autoregressive model. To obtain dynamical information from MEG and/or Electroencephalography data, multivariate autoregressive model has mainly been used for identification of networks or connections between cortices (Cantero et al., 2009; Florin et al., 2010; Hui et al., 2010). Furthermore, we can estimate dynamical interaction between active regions in the brain, providing their pathway is known. It means that dynamical relationship between active regions can be analyzed approximately by the multivariate autoregressive model analysis (Akaike & Nakagawa, 1988). However, the autoregressive model is all-pole type, and has no zeros. As a kind of truncated power series (Kishida, 1997b), autoregressive models are not suitable to be used for evaluating exact transfer functions between regions of cortex. To avoid this difficulty, a feedback model which has rational transfer functions with zeros and poles (Kishida, 1994; 1996) has been used for determination of impulse responses between regions of cortex.

Indeed the brain system is nonlinear. One way is to extend the identification method for a nonlinear case, while the other way is to find a linear part separated from MEG. It is difficult to extend the first approach for nonlinear cases owing to brain complexity, and by using BSS method the latter approach will be served to solve the nonlinear difficulty by elimination of concatenate averaged waveforms. In complex systems the latter approach with BSS is superior to the former approach, when the total number of data is limited. When a current dipole is usually generated by thousands of cells, we can observe its magnetic field by a superconducting quantum interference device (SQUID). Hence, SQUID data are macroscopic from the viewpoint of neuronal population activity, and the statistical nature of system size expansion can be taken as macroscopic variables of SQUID data. As pointed out in the system size expansion method developed in statistical physics (Kishida et al., 1976; Kubo et al., 1973; Tomita & Tomita, 1974; Van Kampen, 1961), the macroscopic variables have extensive property and the mean value of them obeys the nonlinear evolution equation, but their fluctuations follow the linear Gaussian equation in the normal case. This linearity of normal case is suitable for the latter approach with BSS.

In this chapter we will introduce how to separate fluctuations from evoked magnetic field data by using the decorrelation method of blind source separation (BSS). Fluctuations of MEG rather than averaged waveforms should be analyzed for the better understanding of brain functional activities as in Section 4.

2.3 Difficulties in blind source separation

In the present chapter we will study MEG data for 2Hz periodical median nerve stimuli, since activities of the secondary somatosensory cortices may be found as the somatosensory evoked field (Hamada et al., 2002; Wikström et al., 1996). If there is a current dipole in a brain region, a dipole pattern generated from it can be shown by the Biot-Savart law in SQUID channels (see Fig. 2 or 5). In the special case where there is the one-to-one correspondence between SEF current dipoles and BSS components, fluctuations of SEF can be separated easily. In general, there are no one-to-one correspondences between a current dipole and a component of BSS.

Let the dishonest BSS of Section 3.3 be a BSS processing for original MEG data with deterministic evoked waveforms. The honest BSS of Section 3.4 is defined as a BSS processing after elimination of concatenate evoked waveforms from MEG. It is difficult to select honest BSS components related to SEF from all BSS components with various dipole patterns in topographic field maps without repeated line spectrum in the power spectral density (PSD), since there are no line spectrum in PSD in honest BSS components. There remains an open problem to be solved to locate SEF fluctuations in the cases without the one-to-one correspondence. However, fluctuations of SEF can be determined from the honest BSS components, when components with nonzero waveforms of the dishonest BSS are transformed into the honest BSS components by using a transformation matrix. That is, the transformation matrix connecting two types of BSS components will be introduced for selecting the fluctuations of evoked magnetic fields (see Eq. (11)). Hence, SEF fluctuations of the somatosensory evoked field (see Eq. (13)) will be separated from MEG data by using the T/k type decorrelation method of honest BSS, after elimination of deterministic concatenate evoked waveforms. Finally, we can obtain correlation functions of SEF fluctuations from the honest BSS. Our identification method will work efficiently for SEF fluctuations in Section 4.5 and can show intracerebral communication in terms of impulse responses between cSI and cSII.

3. Methods

3.1 Magnetoencephalography (subjects and stimuli)

Five healthy subjects participated in this study. After explaining the nature of the study, informed consent was obtained. The experimental procedures were in accordance with the Declaration of Helsinki. Their median nerves were stimulated electrically with a constant voltage, square-wave pulse of 0.5 ms duration delivered at the right wrist. Stimulus frequency was periodical 2Hz or the inter-stimulus interval (ISI) was 500 ms. MEG data were recorded with a 64-channel whole-head MEG system (NeuroSQUID Model 100; CTF Systems Inc.). SQUID was the axial gradiometer type. Details were reported in Kishida (2009a).

3.2 Data analysis

MEG signals were digitized at 1250 Hz and filtered with a 300 Hz on-line low-pass filter. MEG data during 175 s per one subject were used as a single sweep for data analysis. The number of median nerve stimuli was 350. The sampling time (Δt) is 0.8 ms and let magnetic field of SQUIDs be

$$\mathbf{x}(t) = \mathbf{x}(n\Delta t) =: \mathbf{x}(n)$$

at time t or discrete time n. In periodical stimului MEG data are classified into 3 groups as

$$\mathbf{x}(n) = \mathbf{x}_s(n) + \mathbf{x}_e(n) + \mathbf{x}_a(n), \tag{1}$$

where $\mathbf{x}_s$, $\mathbf{x}_e$ and $\mathbf{x}_a$ are spontaneous and evoked magnetic fields and artifact noises. The SEF evoked magnetic field consists of a deterministic part and fluctuations around it:

$$\mathbf{x}_e(n) = L_e\mathbf{Q}_e(n) = \mathbf{u}(n) + L_e\mathbf{Q}_e^h(n), \tag{2}$$

where L_e is the lead field from the evoked current dipoles, $\mathbf{Q_e}(n)$, $\mathbf{u}(n) := r_{350}\mathbf{w}$ is defined by concatenating 350 copies of the average waveforms $\mathbf{w}$, and $\mathbf{Q}_e^h(n)$ are SEF fluctuations in the evoked magnetic field (see Eq. (16)).

3.3 Fractional type of BSS

The decorrelation method was developed by Molgedey & Schuster (1994), Ziehe et al. (2000), Murata et al. (2001) and briefly summarized in Kishida et al. (2003). However, BSS performance is strongly dependent on the choice of time lag. The temporal decorrelation method of BSS has an open problem in choice of the time lag (Hironaga & Ioannides, 2007; Kishida, 2008; Tang et al., 2005; Ziehe et al., 2000). Here it should be noted that the decorrelation method is effective for MEG data in a stationary process.

Since PSD of MEG has a line spectrum of 2Hz and those of higher harmonic modes in 2Hz periodical median nerve stimuli, improvements with the fractional type time lag τ_m defined by

$$\tau_m = \left(\frac{1250}{2}\right)/m = \frac{625}{m}, \quad m = 1, 2, \ldots, k \tag{3}$$

could be made on BSS (Kishida, 2008; 2009a). Hence, we can determine a mixing matrix $A_{(k)}$ by the blind source separation with the T/k type (fractional) time lag:

$$\mathbf{x}(n) = A_{(k)}\mathbf{s}^{(k)}(n). \tag{4}$$

In the T/k type decorrelation method, the absolute sum of off-diagonal elements of normalized correlation matrices is minimized at times corresponding to 2Hz and its higher harmonic frequencies. The main processing in the decorrelation method is removing the off-diagonal elements of the correlation matrices at fractional type time lag τ_m,

$$C_{zz}(\tau_m) = \frac{1}{N}\sum_{n=0}^{N-1} z(n)z(n+\tau_m)^T \quad m = 1,\ldots,k, \tag{5}$$

where the superscript T denotes the transposition of matrix and $z(n)$ with zero mean is orthonormalized as $\sqrt{V^{-1}}\mathbf{x}(n)$. Here V is the covariance matrix given by $E\{\mathbf{x}(n)\mathbf{x}(n)^T\}$. The Jacobi-like algorithm has been used to solve the simultaneous diagonalization problem approximately on k normalized correlation matrices (Cardoso & Souloumiac, 1996). This process is to determine a square matrix U in the problem of minimization of the cost function J,

$$J(U) = \sum_{m=1}^{k}\sum_{i\neq j}|(UC_{zz}(\tau_m)U^T)_{ij}|^2, \tag{6}$$

where $(UC_{zz}(\tau_m)U^T)_{ij}$ denotes the ij-element of matrix $UC_{zz}(\tau_m)U^T$. Finally, we have $A_{(k)}^{-1} := U\sqrt{V^{-1}}$.

For the classification of MEG we have used the T/k type of BSS with e.g. $k = 30$:

$$\mathbf{x}(n) = A_{(30)}\mathbf{s}^{(30)}(n). \tag{7}$$

Then, MEG is decomposed by the fractional BSS with $k = 30$:

$$\mathbf{x}(n) = A_{(30)}^{s}\mathbf{s}_s^{(30)}(n) + A_{(30)}^{e}\mathbf{s}_e^{(30)}(n) + A_{(30)}^{a}\mathbf{s}_a^{(30)}(n), \tag{8}$$

where $A_{(30)} = (A_{(30)}^{s}\ A_{(30)}^{e}\ A_{(30)}^{a})$ and $\mathbf{s}^{(30)}(n) = (\mathbf{s}_s^{(30)}(n)^T\ \mathbf{s}_e^{(30)}(n)^T\ \mathbf{s}_a^{(30)}(n)^T)^T$ corresponding to Eq. (1).

3.4 Honest BSS and transformation matrix

From the Wold decomposition theorem (Mathematical Society of Japan, 1987), a stationary process is uniquely decomposed into $\mathbf{x}(n) = \mathbf{u}(n) + \delta\mathbf{x}(n)$, where $\delta\mathbf{x}$(n) is non-deterministic and $\mathbf{u}(n)$ is deterministic. We can define correlation functions in a stationary process, and they are specified into two types. When concatenate averaged waveforms are very small, the decorrelation method and the identification method used in Kishida (2009b) work efficiently, since correlation functions can be described by time lag. Inversely the decorrelation method and the identification method do not work well, when concatenate averaged waveforms are not small. In the remaining part of this paper we will first eliminate concatenation of averaged waveforms from MEG data, and then apply the decorrelation method and the identification method to eliminated MEG data. Such approach was called "honest" in the (9) of discussion of Kishida (2009b).

Supposing there is a subject who has no or negligible small fluctuations of SEF, and that he has averaged waveforms of SEF. However, certain fluctuations of SEF happen to be in $\mathbf{s}_e^{(30)}(n)$ of the subject in BSS calculation of Eq. (7). Therefore BSS of Eq. (7) may be called as "dishonest", since these fictitious fluctuations cause errors in identification method. As further mentioned in Discussion, subject D corresponds to the one who has no or negligible small fluctuations of SEF. To avoid these fictitious fluctuations, we should use the honest BSS instead of the dishonest BSS of Eq. (7), since there are no deterministic parts in the honest BSS. On the other hand, it is difficult to select honest BSS components of evoked field with dipole patterns in topographic field maps, since there is no line spectrum in PSD in honest BSS components. To overcome these difficulties, a transformation matrix between components of BSS with line spectrum and those of honest BSS will be introduced.

First let us eliminate concatenation of averaged waveforms from MEG data: $\delta\mathbf{x}(n) := \mathbf{x}(n) - \mathbf{u}(n)$ where $\mathbf{u}(n) := r_{350}\mathbf{w}$. After eliminating concatenation of averaged waveforms the honest BSS and the identification algorithm can be applied. Fluctuations of MEG are decomposed by the honest BSS with e.g. $k = 25$ as the same method as in Section 3.3:

$$\begin{aligned}\delta\mathbf{x}(n) &= A^h_{(25)}\delta\mathbf{s}^{(25)}(n) \\ &= \mathbf{x}(n) - \mathbf{u}(n) \\ &= \mathbf{x}_s(n) + L_e\mathbf{Q}^h_e(n) + \mathbf{x}_a(n) \\ &= A^s_{(25)}\delta\mathbf{s}^{(25)}_s(n) + A^e_{(25)}\delta\mathbf{s}^{(25)}_e(n) + A^a_{(25)}\delta\mathbf{s}^{(25)}_a(n).\end{aligned} \tag{9}$$

In the honest BSS, there are no deterministic parts, and it would be difficult to find SEF BSS components, since there is no line spectrum of the evoked magnetic field in PSDs of honest BSS components and there were no one-to-one correspondences between dipoles and BSS components in four subjects. We must find a way to select SEF components of honest BSS.

From the two relations between Eq. (9) and Eq. (7) we can obtain approximately the next equation,

$$A_{(30)}\mathbf{s}^{(30)}(n) = A^h_{(25)}\delta\mathbf{s}^{(25)}(n), \tag{10}$$

when the amplitude of $\mathbf{u}(n)$ is negligible small in comparison with that of $\mathbf{x}(n)$. A transformation matrix is defined by

$$T := (A^h_{(25)})^{-1}A_{(30)}. \tag{11}$$

The jth column of T shows a distribution of the jth component of $\mathbf{s}^{(30)}(n)$, $s^{(30)}_j(n)$, on $\delta\mathbf{s}^{(25)}(n)$ is denoted by $T_{*,j}$:

$$\delta\mathbf{s}^{(25)}(n) = T\mathbf{s}^{(30)}(n). \tag{12}$$

That is, $T_{*,j}$ denotes the transformation from one component of $\mathbf{s}^{(30)}(n)$ to a distribution on $\delta\mathbf{s}^{(25)}(n)$. When components of honest BSS satisfy the condition that absolute value of $T_{*,j}$ is close to one, the honest BSS components can be found from the dishonest BSS components. Therefore, fluctuations of SEF are given from the fractional BSS with $k = 25$ in the honest way by

$$\mathbf{x}^h_e(n) = A^e_{(25)}\delta\mathbf{s}^{(25)}_e(n). \tag{13}$$

3.5 Estimation of SEF fluctuations of current dipoles

The problem of multi-dipole estimation can be solved efficiently by the conventional least square method (Hämäläinen et al., 1993) with the combinatory optimization problem for location of current dipoles. Estimated current dipoles were equivalently evaluated by the least mean square method with a cost function of distance between signal spaces (Yokota & Kishida, 2006). That is, the covariance matrix, $\mathbf{D} = E\{\mathbf{x}_e^h(n)\mathbf{x}_e^h(n)^T\}$, can be decomposed into eigenvectors:

$$\mathbf{D} = \sum_{k=1}^{64} \lambda_k \phi_k \phi_k^T, \tag{14}$$

where λ_k is an eigenvalue and ϕ_k is its eigenvector. Let us divide into two subspaces; one is the p dimensional signal subspace $\mathbf{V}_s$ and the other subspace is noise subspace $\mathbf{V}_n$:

$$\mathbf{V}_s = (\phi_1, \phi_2, \ldots, \phi_p), \mathbf{V}_n = (\phi_{p+1}, \phi_{p+2}, \ldots, \phi_{64}).$$

For q current dipole estimation the cost function is defined (Yokota & Kishida, 2006) by

$$J(\hat{\mathbf{r}}_1, \ldots, \hat{\mathbf{r}}_{\hat{q}}) = \det[(\mathbf{V}_s, \mathbf{L}_{\hat{\mathbf{r}}})^T (\mathbf{V}_s, \mathbf{L}_{\hat{\mathbf{r}}})], \tag{15}$$

when lead fields of evoked magnetic field are selected by

$$\mathbf{L}_{\hat{\mathbf{r}}} := (\mathbf{l}_{\hat{r}_1}, \mathbf{l}_{\hat{r}_2}, \ldots, \mathbf{l}_{\hat{r}_q}).$$

The supporting reason for cost function is that the rank of $[(\mathbf{V}_s, \mathbf{L}_{\hat{\mathbf{r}}})^T (\mathbf{V}_s, \mathbf{L}_{\hat{\mathbf{r}}})]$ becomes lower, when estimation of current dipole is true.

Hence, we can determine q current dipoles which represent dipole patterns of SEF. That is, we have from Eqs. (9) and (13)

$$L_e \mathbf{Q}_e^h(n) = A_{(25)}^e \delta \mathbf{s}_e^{(25)}(n),$$

or,

$$\mathbf{Q}_e^h(n) = L_e^\dagger A_{(25)}^e \delta \mathbf{s}_e^{(25)}(n), \tag{16}$$

where the symbol † means the Moore Penrose type of generalized inverse matrix and L_e is a lead field evaluated from q current dipoles. Equation (16) will be expressed as Eq. (23) in Section 4.4 in the case of $q = 5$, where p=4 from Eq. (22).

3.6 Identification of feedback model

The identification method mentioned in Kishida (1996; 1997a; 2009b) could be applied to evaluate dynamical properties between current dipoles in cortices. Let current diploes corresponding to cSII and cSI be $y_1(n)$ and $y_2(n)$ selected from $\mathbf{Q}_e^h(n)$. Their activities are assumed to be expressed by a feedback model defined by

$$\begin{aligned} y_1(n) &= F_{12}(z^{-1}) y_2(n) + F_1(z^{-1}) f_1(n) \\ y_2(n) &= F_{21}(z^{-1}) y_1(n) + F_2(z^{-1}) f_2(n), \end{aligned} \tag{17}$$

where z^{-1} is the time shift operator: $z^{-1}y_k(n) = y_k(n-1)$ ($k = 1$ or 2), $f_1(n)$ and $f_2(n)$ are Gaussian white random current dipoles in two regions of thalamus, $F_{12}(z^{-1})$ is an intracerebral transfer function from cSI to cSII, and $F_{21}(z^{-1})$ is a reverse intracerebral transfer function from cSII to cSI. $F_1(z^{-1})$ is a transfer function from one region of thalamus to cSII and $F_2(z^{-1})$ is that from another region of thalamus to cSI.

As mentioned in Eq. (A3) of Kishida (2009b), an innovation model of minimum phase (Kishida, 1991) can be identified from fluctuations of cSI and cSII:

$$\begin{aligned} \mathbf{x}(n|n) &= A_H\mathbf{x}(n-1|n-1) + B\gamma(n) \\ \mathbf{y}(n) &= C\mathbf{x}(n|n). \end{aligned} \tag{18}$$

Three system matrices of Eq. (18) are determined by the identification method from correlation function matrices, since correlation function matrices of Hankel matrix in Step 3 of Appendix A of Kishida (2009b) are obtained from output data of fluctuations of cSI and cSII. From Eq. (18) a closed loop transfer function matrix is

$$G(z^{-1}) = C(I - A_H z^{-1})^{-1}B. \tag{19}$$

Attention should be paid to the existence of an undetermined matrix $\mathcal{U}$ in the representation of the innovation model: $A' = \mathcal{U}^{-1}A\mathcal{U}$, $B' = \mathcal{U}^{-1}B$ and $C' = C\mathcal{U}$, although the closed loop transfer function matrix is invariant for $\mathcal{U}$, e.g., eigenvalues of A' is the same as those of A.

As in Eq. (B3) of Kishida (2009b), transfer functions between cSII and cSI are determined from Eq. (19) as

$$\begin{aligned} \hat{F}_{12}(z^{-1}) &= G_{12}(z^{-1})/G_{22}(z^{-1}) \\ \hat{F}_{21}(z^{-1}) &= G_{21}(z^{-1})/G_{11}(z^{-1}). \end{aligned} \tag{20}$$

Transfer functions of $F_{12}(z^{-1})$ and $F_{21}(z^{-1})$ of intracerebral communication between cSI and cSII can be obtained via Eqs. (19) and (20) from the feedback structure under either one of the two sufficient conditions of original feedback model (Kishida, 1994). On the other hand, transfer functions of $F_1(z^{-1})$ and $F_2(z^{-1})$ are not identified from output data of fluctuations of cSI and cSII, since input data about fluctuations of thalamus are not available.

Our algorithm to obtain transfer functions between cSI and cSII is summarized in the following flowchart:

MEG data in 2Hz median nerve stimuli	honest BSS, Eq.(9) → (dishonest BSS)	Extraction of SEF fluctuations. (see Eq. (13) or (22))
SEF fluctuations (see Eq. (13))	inverse problem, Eq. (16) →	Fluctuations of current dipoles at cSI and cSII. (see Eqs. (24) and (25))
Correlation functions of SEF fluctuations at cSI and cSII	identification method based → on feedback model, Eq. (17)	Transfer functions between cSI and cSII. (see Figs. 11 and 12)

4. Results

4.1 MEG pre-processing and SEF

After zero preset signal processing mentioned in Kishida (2009a), the average of 350 MEG responses was used. The averaged waveforms $\mathbf{w}(n)$ are obtained from SQUID time series data and shown in Fig. 1 for four subjects, where $\mathbf{w}(n)$ were defined by Eq. (1) of Kishida (2009a). Since the head of the other subject E moved during MEG measurement, the data were invalid.

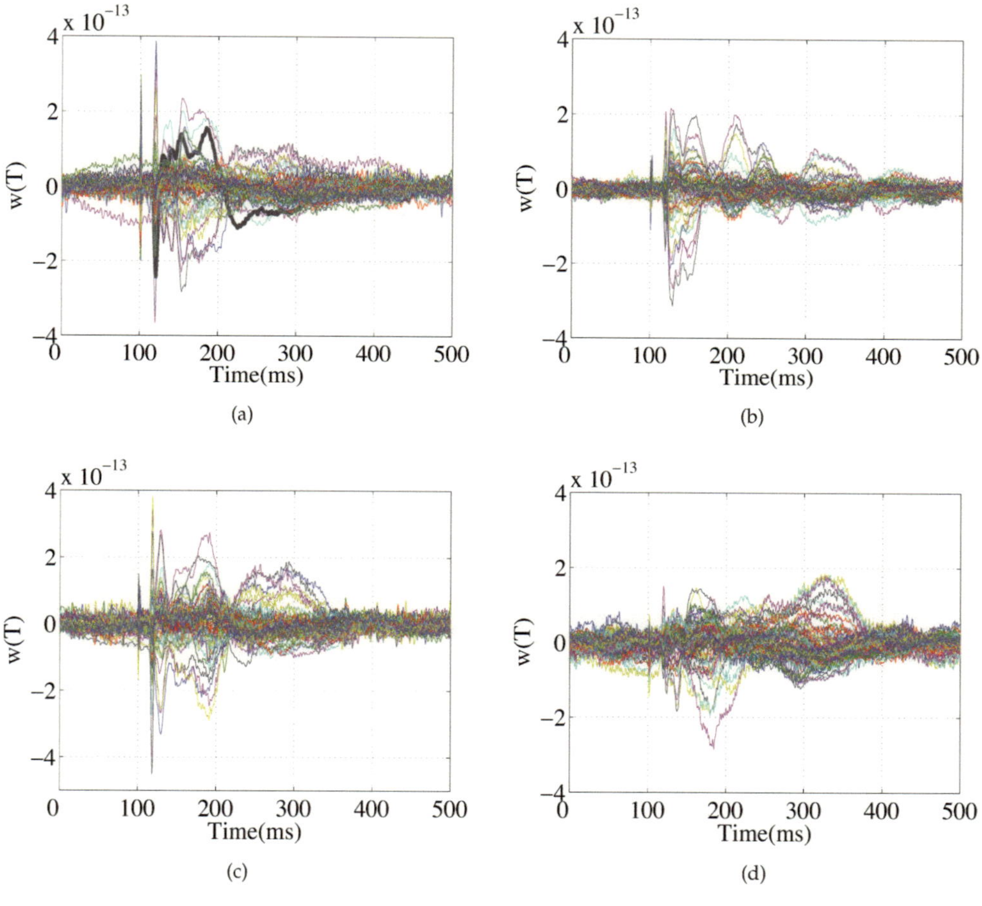

Fig. 1. Averaged waveforms of SEF. (a) subject A, (b) subject B, (c) subject C and (d) subject D.

In Fig. 1(a), electric stimulus time is at time 101.6 ms ($n = 127$) and the first peak of averaged waveforms at time 120.8 ms ($n = 151$) is known as N20 with latency 19.2 ms (Hämäläinen et al., 1993; Kakigi et al., 2000; Wikström et al., 1996). N20 has a dipole pattern of cSI in the field map of Fig. 2(a). In 2Hz median nerve stimulus, averaged waveforms usually have a dipole pattern of cSI, since activities of cSI are found in 2Hz median nerve stimulus (Wikström et al., 1996). However, a dipole pattern of SIIs was not found in averaged waveforms at a glance, even if activities of SIIs exist in 2Hz median nerve stimulus (Wikström et al., 1996). This situation is similar to the case where stars are seen in the nighttime, but not in the daytime.

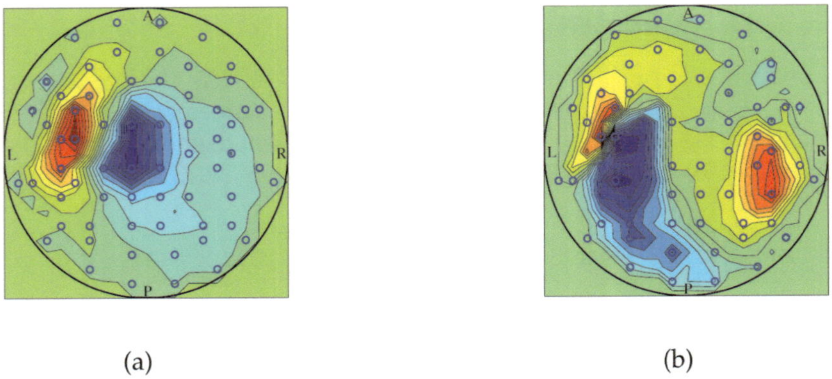

Fig. 2. Dipole pattern in the topographic field map of waveforms of subject A. (a) time 120.8ms (latency 19.2 ms), (b) time 214.4ms (latency 112.8 ms).

SIIs correspond to stars and cSI is the sun. The nighttime is a time when the sign of amplitude of cSI changes. The time is 214.4 ms corresponding to latency 112.8 ms in Fig. 1(a), and the dipole pattern of SIIs is found from $\mathbf{w}(n)$ at the time as in the field map of Fig. 2(b). From Fig. 2(b) cSII is stronger than the ipsilateral secondary somatosensory cortex (iSII). This result is consistent to that of Wikström et al. (1996).

The black bold line in Fig. 1(a) is an averaged waveform at the 14th SQUID channel, location of which will be shown by a black large circle in Fig. 10. PSD of SQUID data at the 14th channel has a line spectrum of 2Hz and those of higher harmonic modes for 2Hz periodical median nerve stimuli as in Fig. 3. The line spectrum of PSD is due to periodical structure of the somatosensory evoked magnetic field. The 2Hz repetitive line spectra of Fig. 3 show an effect of the deterministic and nonlinear part.

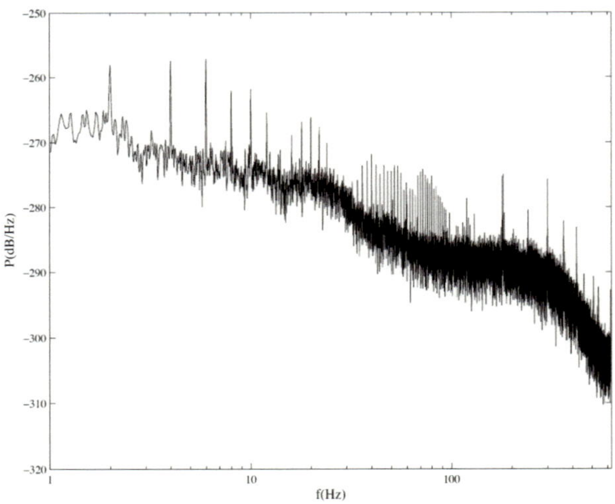

Fig. 3. PSD of the 14th SQUID channel of subject A.

We can select BSS components of the evoked magnetic field from their averaged waveforms of $\mathbf{s}^{(30)}(n)$ in Fig. 4. Averaged waveforms of BSS components were defined as $w^s(n)$ by Eq. (15) of Kishida (2009a). Cyan dotted and blue broken bold lines which have N20 peaks in Fig. 4 were the 4th and the 22nd BSS components of cSI, and yellow, red and black bold lines at time 214 ms (latency 112.4 ms) were the 13th, 17th and 35th BSS components of SIIs. The somatosensory evoked field was given by five components of BSS:

$$\mathbf{s}_e^{(30)}(n) = (s_4^{(30)}(n)\, s_{13}^{(30)}(n)\, s_{17}^{(30)}(n)\, s_{22}^{(30)}(n)\, s_{35}^{(30)}(n))^T. \tag{21}$$

Their dipole patterns of BSS components corresponding to the somatosensory evoked field are shown in the topographic field maps of Fig. 5. Here, the topographic field map of the jth component of BSS is expressed by A_j as the jth column vector of $A_{(30)}$. In subject A there were no one-to-one correspondences between two dipoles and five BSS components. There were also no one-to-one correspondences in the other subjects. It was a rare case to have the one-to-one correspondences between dipoles and BSS components.

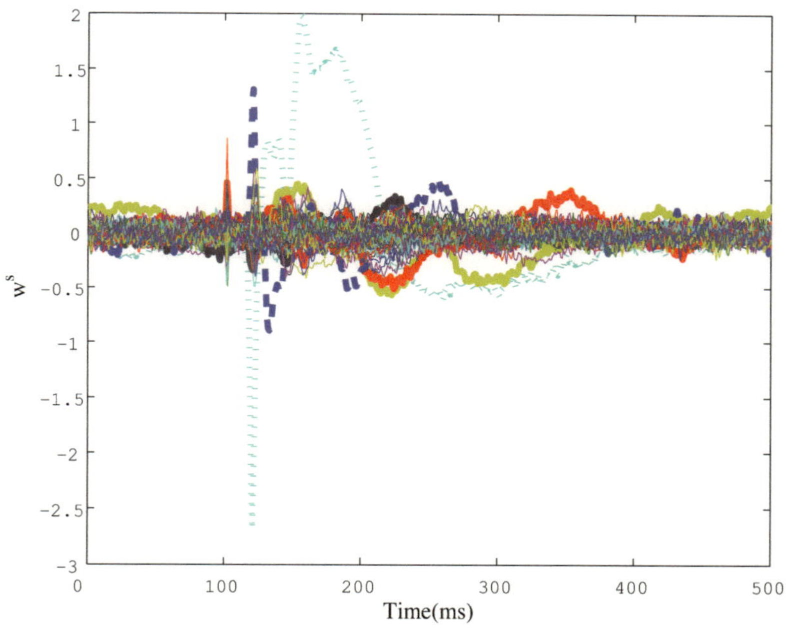

Fig. 4. BSS waveforms of subject A. Cyan bold broken and blue dotted lines are the 4th and the 22nd BSS components of cSI, and three bold lines are the 13th, 17th and 35th BSS components of SIIs.

4.2 Honest BSS

PSD of MEG with elimination of repeated waveforms has no line spectrum of 2Hz and no higher harmonic modes in Fig. 6. Here the SQUID channel of Fig. 6 is the same as that of Fig. 3. From Fig. 6 electrical power noise is clearly found in line structure at 60Hz and has higher harmonics.

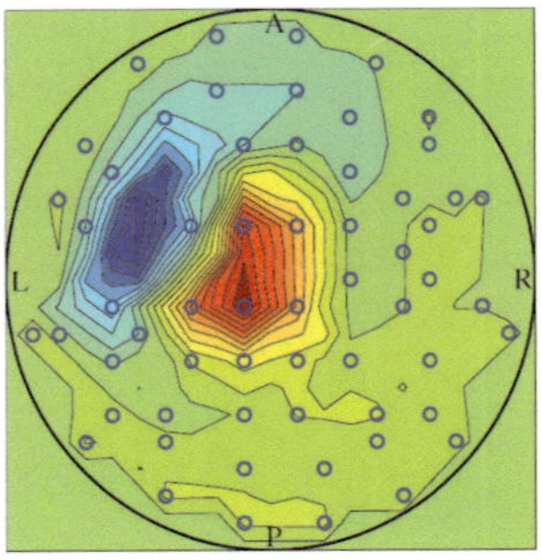

(a) A_4.

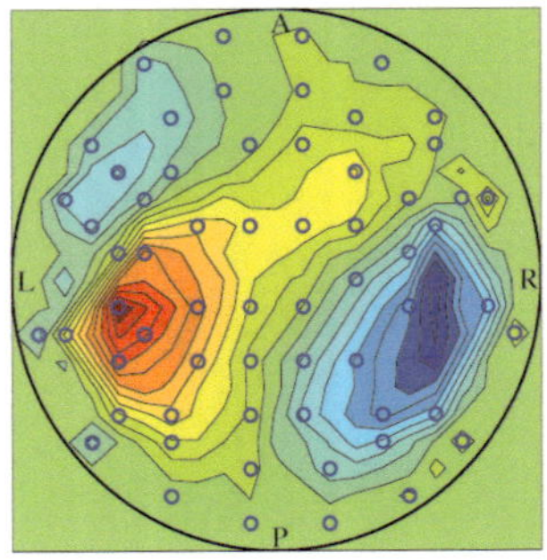

(b) A_{13}.

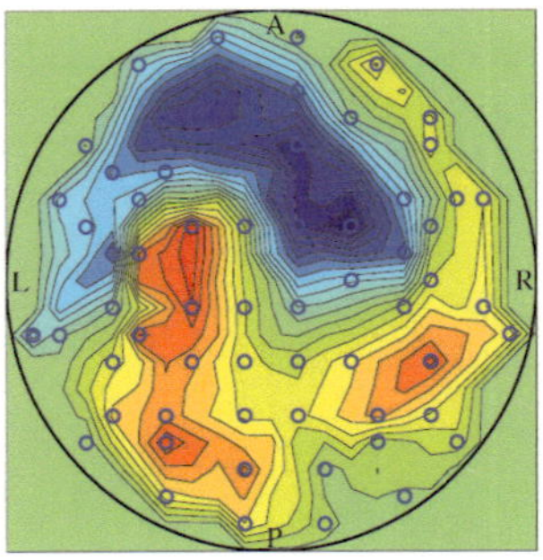

(c) A_{17}.

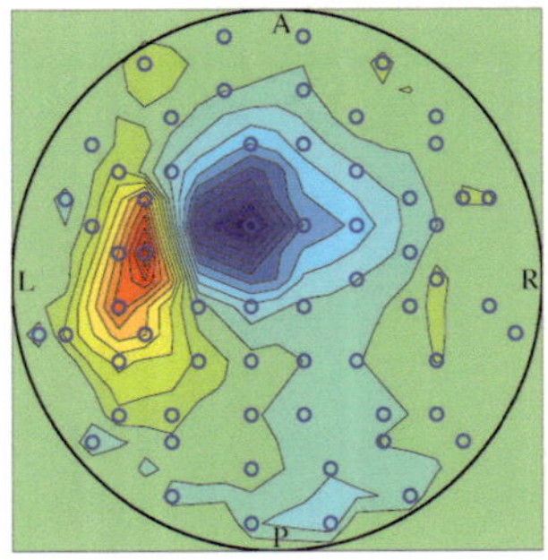

(d) A_{22}.

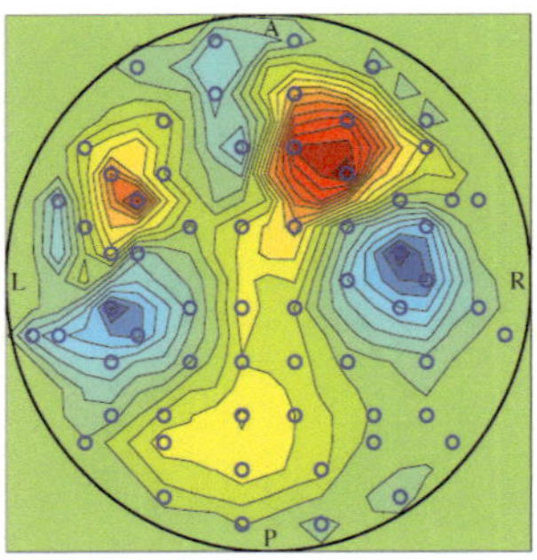

(e) A_{35}.

Fig. 5. Topographic field maps of SEF BSS components in subject A.

When components of honest BSS satisfy the condition that absolute value of $T_{*,j}$ is close to one, the dishonest BSS components are transformed into honest BSS components with similar topographic field maps. In Fig. 7 $T_{*,4}$, $T_{*,13}$, $T_{*,17}$, $T_{*,22}$ and $T_{*,35}$ of the 4th, 13rd, 17th, 22rd and 35th components of BSS with $k = 30$ are denoted by bold solid, bold 1-dot broken, bold broken, dotted and sold lines respectively. When the components of BSS with $k = 30$ satisfy

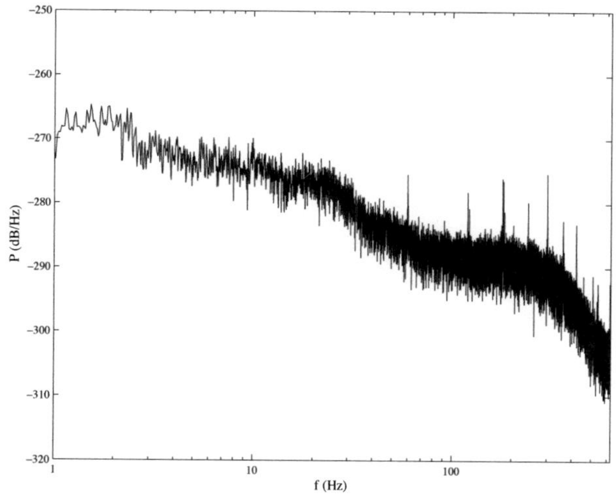

Fig. 6. PSD of the 14th SQUID channel of subject A, after elimination of concatenation of averaged waveforms from MEG.

the condition $|T_{*,j}| > 0.6$, the dishonest BSS components are transformed into those of honest BSS with $k = 25$: they are transformed into the 4th, 27th, 36th and 43rd components of honest BSS with $k = 25$.

Their topographic field maps of honest BSS components are shown in Fig. 8. Here, the topographic field map of the jth component of honest BSS is also denoted by A_j^h as the jth column vector of $A_{(25)}^h$ in the honest way. Similarities are found in patterns of dipoles between Figs. 5 and 8. If the condition $|T_{*,j}| > 0.6$ is satisfied at the least, the correspondence between the dishonest and honest BSS components is plausible. However, there was the exceptional example (see Section 5.1) that the correspondence did not hold even when the condition was satisfied.

4.3 Fluctuations of somatosensory evoked or induced field

The honest BSS is a blind source separation which relates to the block diagonal of covariance matrix. The block diagonal property is found in cross-correlation functions among honest BSS components of the evoked magnetic field. Cross-correlation functions between the 4th component of honest BSS and the other component of honest BSS are shown in Fig. 9(a), and especially those between the 4th component and the 27th, 36th and 43rd components of honest BSS are shown by yellow broken, blue 1-dot broken and blue solid bold lines in Fig. 9(b). In Fig. 9 large deviations of cross-correlation away from the time origin are found occasionally. Therefore it is concluded that there remain small correlations among honest BSS components corresponding to cSI and SIIs.

Hence, fluctuations of SEF are given from the fractional BSS with $k = 25$ in the honest way by

$$\mathbf{x}_e^h(n) = A_{(25)}^e \delta \mathbf{s}_e^{(25)}(n), \tag{22}$$

where

$$\delta \mathbf{s}_e^{(25)}(n) = (\delta s_4^{(25)}(n)\, \delta s_{27}^{(25)}(n)\, \delta s_{36}^{(25)}(n)\, \delta s_{43}^{(25)}(n))^T.$$

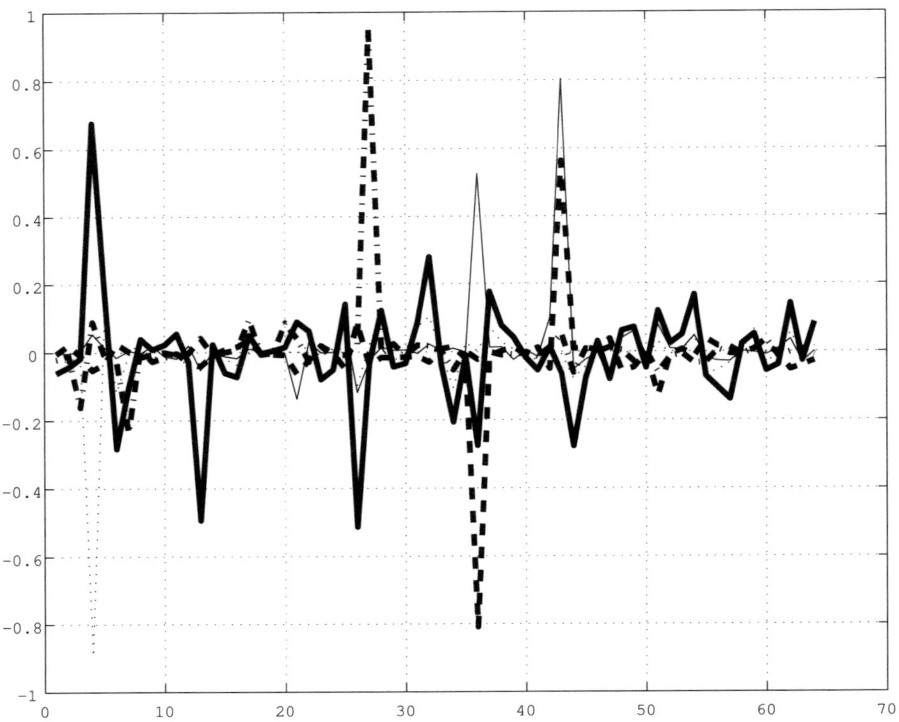

Fig. 7. Transition from dishonest SEF BSS components with $k = 30$ to honest SEF BSS components with $k = 25$.

Induced fields generated by the current dipoles at the same locations in Fig. 8 may be included in fluctuations.

4.4 Source analysis

If a brain can be approximated by a spherically symmetric model, and if the primary currents generated in the brain can be described by an equivalent current dipole, a lead field from a current dipole in the brain to SQUID channels was given by Sarvas formula (Sarvas, 1987). Current dipoles in the brain of subject A were uniformly distributed in the sphere with a radius 0.07 m at a center (0, 0, 0.045) [meter] in the MEG head coordinates. They are expressed by tiny symbol of square in Fig. 10. The number of them was 9081. Large circles in Fig. 10 are 64 SQUIDs. Here the black large circle in Fig. 10 is the 14th SQUID channel mentioned in Figs. 3 and 6.

Five current dipoles were estimated by applying the method of dipole current estimation (see Section 3.5). 66.8 % of the covariance matrix of $\mathbf{D} = E\{\mathbf{x}_e^h(n)\mathbf{x}_e^h(n)^T\}$ could be expressed by five current dipoles. Five current dipoles at position 7706 with angle 9.06 degrees, position 1835 with angle 100.27 degrees, position 1210 with angle 108.72 degrees, position 363 with angle 130.26 degrees and position 62 with 36.98 degrees are shown by symbols □ with magenta, yellow, blue, green and red respectively in Fig. 10. That is, we have

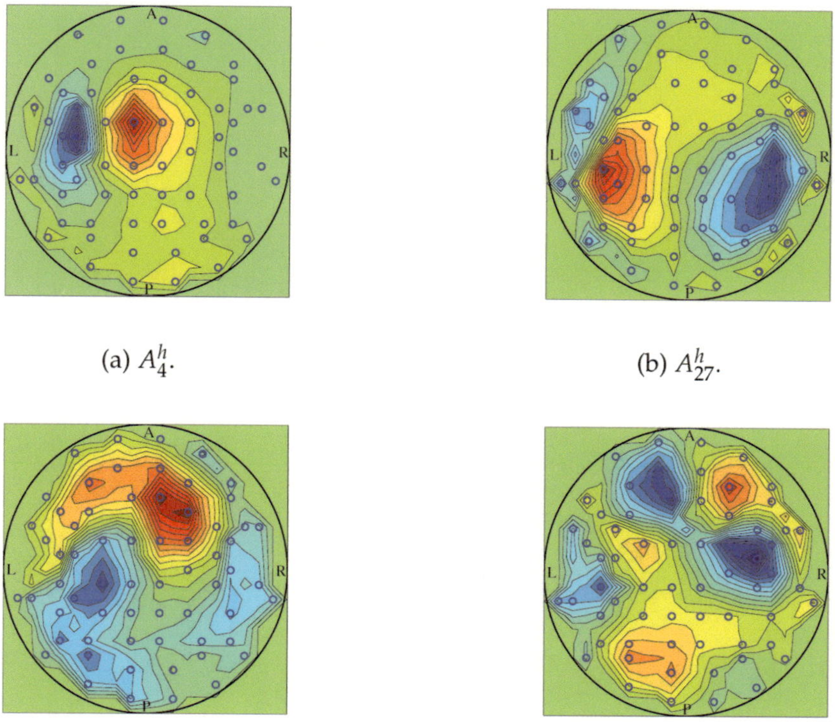

(a) A_4^h. (b) A_{27}^h.

(c) A_{36}^h. (d) A_{43}^h.

Fig. 8. Topographic field maps of honest SEF BSS components in subject A.

$$\mathbf{Q}_e^h(n) = L_e^{\dagger} A_{(25)}^e \delta \mathbf{s}_e^{(25)}(n), \tag{23}$$

where

$$\mathbf{Q}_e^h(n) := \begin{pmatrix} Q_{62}^h(n) \\ Q_{363}^h(n) \\ Q_{1210}^h(n) \\ Q_{1835}^h(n) \\ Q_{7706}^h(n) \end{pmatrix},$$

$$\mathbf{L}_e = (\underline{l}_{62}, \underline{l}_{363}, \underline{l}_{1210}, \underline{l}_{1835}, \underline{l}_{7706}),$$

$$\text{with } \underline{l}_* := \begin{pmatrix} l_1(*,x)\cos\theta_* + l_1(*,y)\sin\theta_* \\ l_2(*,x)\cos\theta_* + l_2(*,y)\sin\theta_* \\ \vdots \\ l_{64}(*,x)\cos\theta_* + l_{64}(*,y)\sin\theta_* \end{pmatrix}.$$

Here, notations of the above equation were reported in Kishida (2009b).

From location of current dipoles in Fig. 10 cSII corresponds to the current dipole at position 1835: fluctuation $y_1(n)$ of cSII with yellow symbol □ in Fig.10 is mixed by a matrix $L_e^{\dagger} A_{(25)}^e$

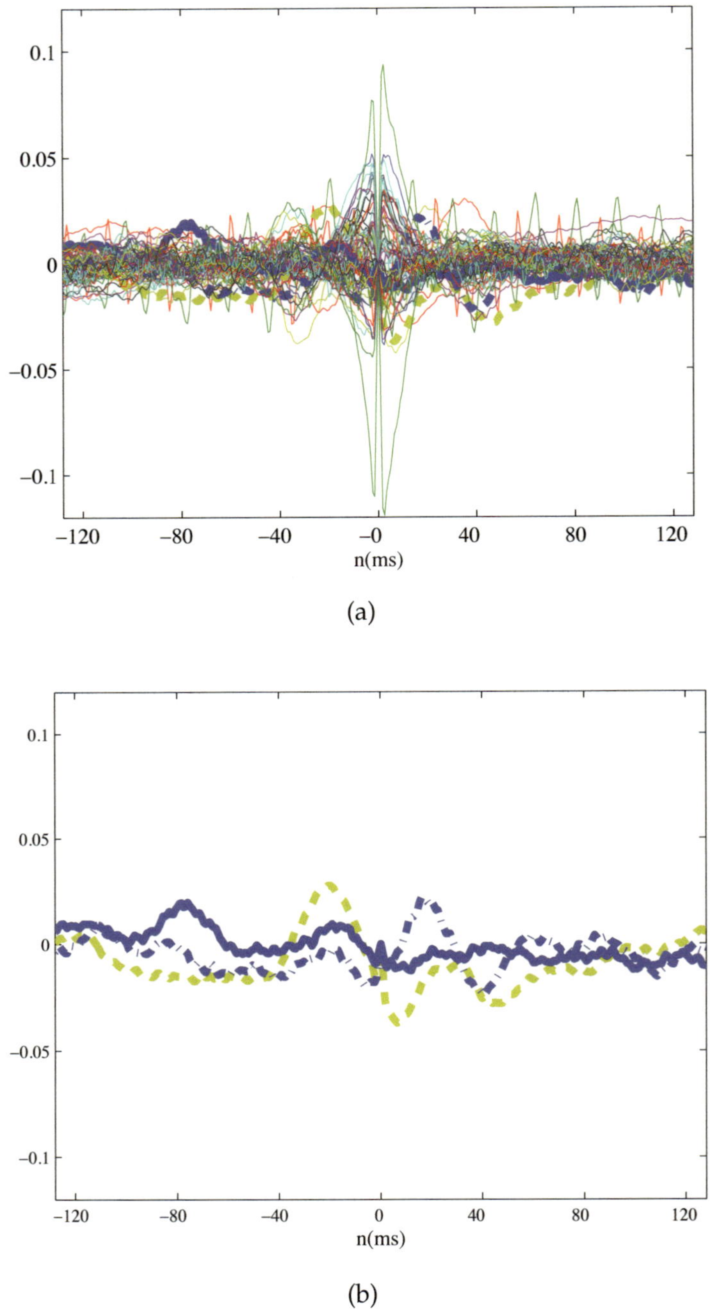

Fig. 9. Cross-correlation functions between the 4th honest BSS and the other honest BSS of subject A in the honest way. (a) All cross-correlation functions. (b) Three cross-correlation functions.

from $\delta \mathbf{s}_e^{(25)}(n)$, and is evaluated from Eq. (16) or (23) as

$$y_1(n) = Q^h_{1835}(n). \tag{24}$$

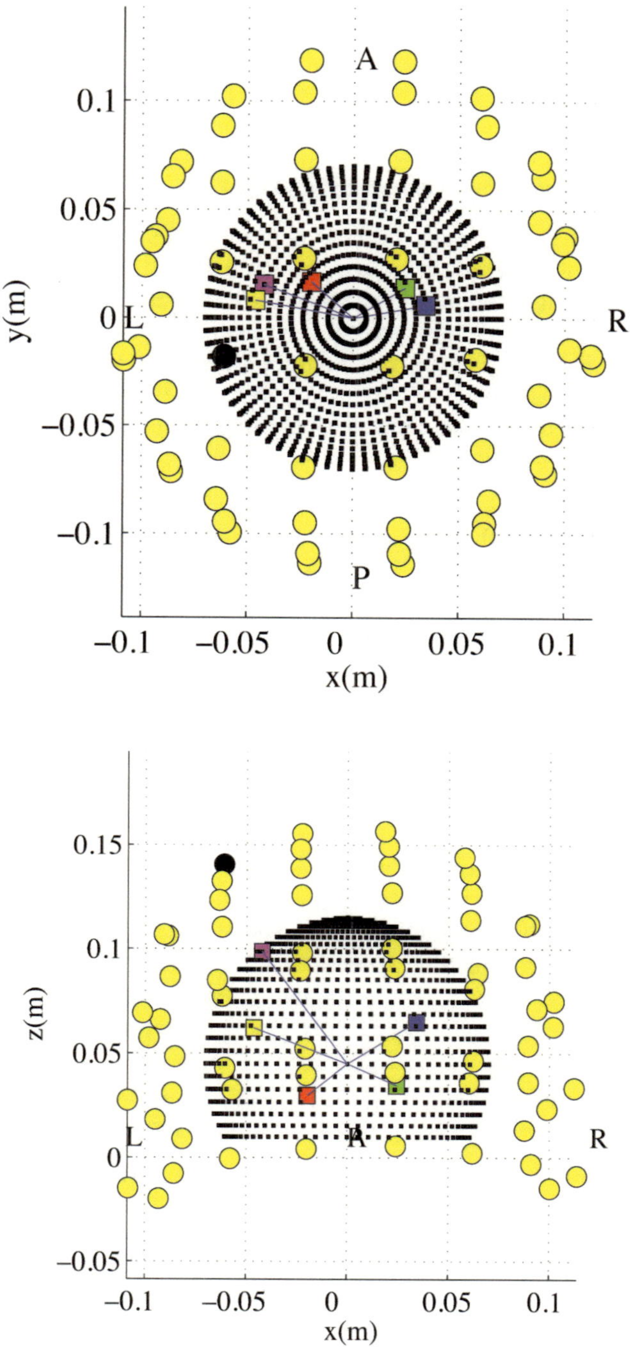

Fig. 10. Location of SQUIDs and current dipoles of subject A in the MEG head coordinates. (top) Axial view (bottom) Coronal view.

Fluctuation $y_2(n)$ of cSI with magenta symbol □ in Fig.10 corresponds to the current dipole at position 7706 is also expressed by

$$y_2(n) = Q^h_{7706}(n). \tag{25}$$

Finally, fluctuations of cSI and cSII of feedback model were given by

$$\mathbf{y}(n) = \begin{pmatrix} y_1(n) \\ y_2(n) \end{pmatrix}.$$

4.5 Intracerebral communication between cSI and cSII

Coefficient matrices of the data-oriented innovation model of Eq. (18) must satisfy the minimum phase properties which are the pole stability and the zero invertibility (Kishida, 1991; 1996). Otherwise, the data-oriented innovation model cannot produce correct results theoretically. Pole stability and zero invertibility mean that roots of $|I - A_H z^{-1}| = 0$ and those of $|I - A_H(I - BC)z^{-1}| = 0$ are outside the unit circle in the complex plane of z^{-1}. Or Eigenvalues of matrices A_H and $A_H(I - BC)$ are inside the unit circle in the complex plane. The feedback model of Eq. (17) has excellent advantages for identification of MEG (Kishida, 2005; 2009b).

The number of singular values of Hankel matrix was 10, when the data-oriented innovation model was determined under the condition of minimum phase properties. Transfer functions of $F_{12}(z^{-1})$ and $F_{21}(z^{-1})$ of intracerebral communication between cSI and cSII could be obtained via Eqs. (19) and (20) from the feedback structure under the condition that a sufficient condition was satisfied in original feedback model (Kishida, 1994; 1996). The bode diagrams of $\hat{F}_{12}(z^{-1})$, $\hat{F}_{21}(z^{-1})$ and their impulse responses are shown in Figs. 11 and 12. The top and middle panel of figure is the magnitude and the phase of Bode diagram of each transfer function, and the bottom panel of figure is the impulse response. There are two modes from cSI to cSII found in Fig. 11. One is a rapid mode which is within about 5ms and the other is a slow mode with about 30ms order. On the other hand a rapid mode from cSII to cSI within about 5 ms is found in Fig. 12.

The reproducibility of the modes in impulse responses of intracerebral communication between cSI and cSII are now examined. In subject B, cSI and SIIs were represented by the 2nd, 4th, 14th, 19th and 20th components of dishonest BSS from the fractional BSS with $k = 30$. They were transformed into the 2nd, 22nd, 40th, 42nd and 57th components of honest BSS with $k = 25$. Six current dipoles were estimated from the same method of dipole current estimation. 76.2 % of the covariance matrix of D of subject B could be expressed by six current dipoles. The number of singular values of Hankel matrix was 9, when the data-oriented innovation model was determined. In Fig. 13, obtained impulse responses are shown by bold dotted lines, while bold solid lines indicate impulse responses of subject A in Fig. 13.

In subject C, cSI and SIIs were represented by the 4th, 12th, 14th, 33rd and 35th components of dishonest BSS from the fractional BSS with $k = 30$. They were transformed into the 10th, 13th, 14th, 35th and 36th components of honest BSS with $k = 25$. Seven current dipoles were also estimated. 75.7 % of the covariance matrix of D of subject C could be expressed by seven current dipoles. The number of singular values of Hankel matrix was 10, when the data-oriented innovation model was determined. The impulse responses are shown by bold broken lines in Fig. 13.

In Fig. 13, impulse responses of three subjects are summarized for clarifying the intracerebral communication between cSI and cSII. Two modes from cSI to cSII were found in Fig. 13(a). One rapid mode from cSII to cSI within 5 ms was mainly found in Fig. 13(b).

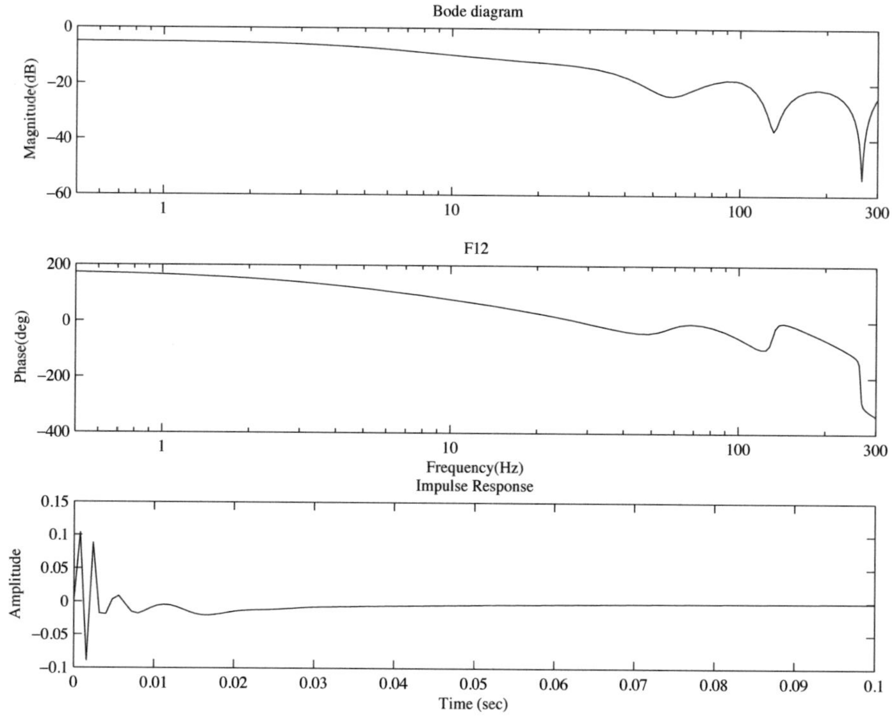

Fig. 11. Bode diagram of F_{12} from cSI to cSII and its impulse response of subject A.

Since no suitable component of cSI in the honest BSS of subject D could be found, there are no impulse responses in subject D. This will be explained in Discussion 5.1.

5. Discussion

5.1 Separation of fluctuations of SEF

From averaged waveforms of subject D shown in Fig. 1(d), dipole patterns at time 120 and 180 ms are shown in the field maps of Figs. 14(a) and 14(b). The dipole pattern at time 120 or 180 ms was that of cSI. In 2Hz median nerve stimulus waveforms, it corresponds to what usually have a dipole pattern of cSI (Wikström et al., 1996). Then the fourth BSS component with the dipole pattern similar to that of cSI could be produced, as shown in Fig. 15(a). Transformation matrix from the fourth BSS component to components of honest BSS is given by $T_{*,4}$ in Fig. 15(c). $T_{*,4}$ denotes the 32nd component of honest BSS with $k = 25$ corresponding to the fourth component of BSS with $k = 30$. However, there is no similarity between dipole pattern of A_4 in the topographic field map in Fig. 15(a) and that of A^h_{32} in Fig. 15(b). Separating the fluctuations of cSI in subject D does not succeed. This means that fluctuations of SEF in subject D were small and they have not been separated from MEG data by the honest BSS. Hence we have no impulse responses of subject D.

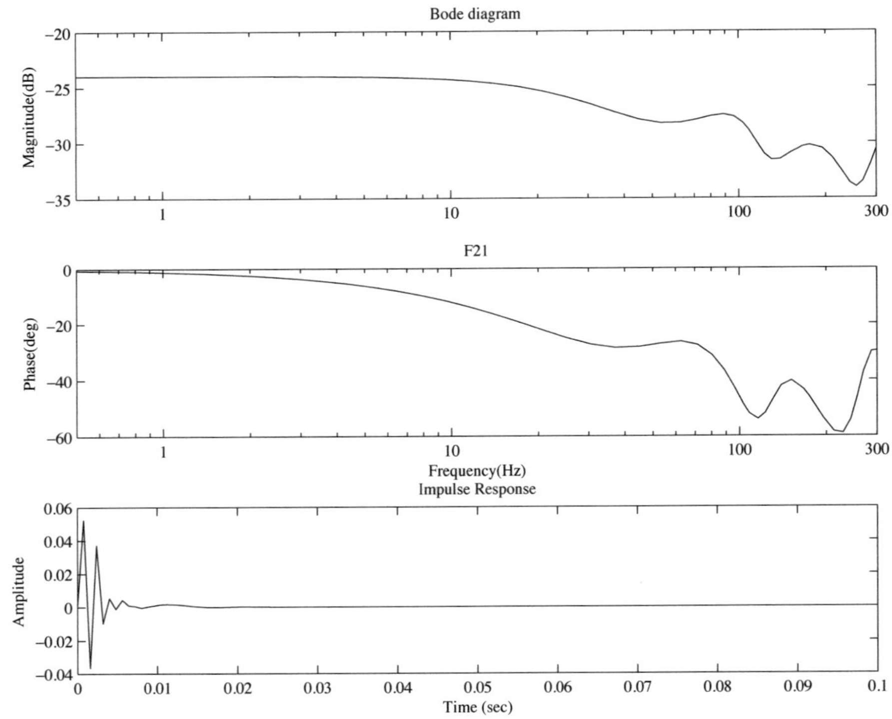

Fig. 12. Bode diagram of F_{21} from cSII to cSI and its impulse response of subject A.

5.2 Comparison between dishonest BSS and honest BSS

In our research, honest BSS was used after elimination of concatenate averaged waveforms, and impulse responses from fluctuations of SEF were identified.

There is another way to determine impulse responses: If the dishonest BSS is used first, SEF data can be selected and then it is possible to eliminate concatenate averaged waveforms from SEF data before identification of impulse responses. Two ways are summarized as

$$\begin{array}{ccc} \mathbf{x}(n) & \Longrightarrow & \begin{array}{c}\mathbf{x}_e(n) \\ \text{(see Eq.(2))}\end{array} \\ \downarrow_E & & \downarrow_E \\ \begin{array}{c}\delta\mathbf{x}(n) \\ \text{(see Eq. (9))}\end{array} & \Longrightarrow & A_h^e\mathbf{s}_e^h(n) \neq A_d^e\mathbf{s}_e^d(n) - \mathbf{u}(n). \end{array} \tag{26}$$

Here A_d^e is defined by $A_{(30)}^e$ in Eq. (8) and $\mathbf{s}_e^h$ corresponds to $\delta\mathbf{s}_e^{(25)}$ in Eq. (9). In Eq. (26), the symbol "$\Longrightarrow$" means application of BSS and selection of SEF components, and the symbol "$\downarrow_E$" is elimination of concatenate averaged waveforms.

In comparison with Fig. 13, Fig. 16 shows impulse responses in the dishonest way. When calculating SEF fluctuations in the dishonest way, the same positions of dipole currents have been used. Robustness of impulse responses of Fig. 16 is lower in comparison with Fig. 13.

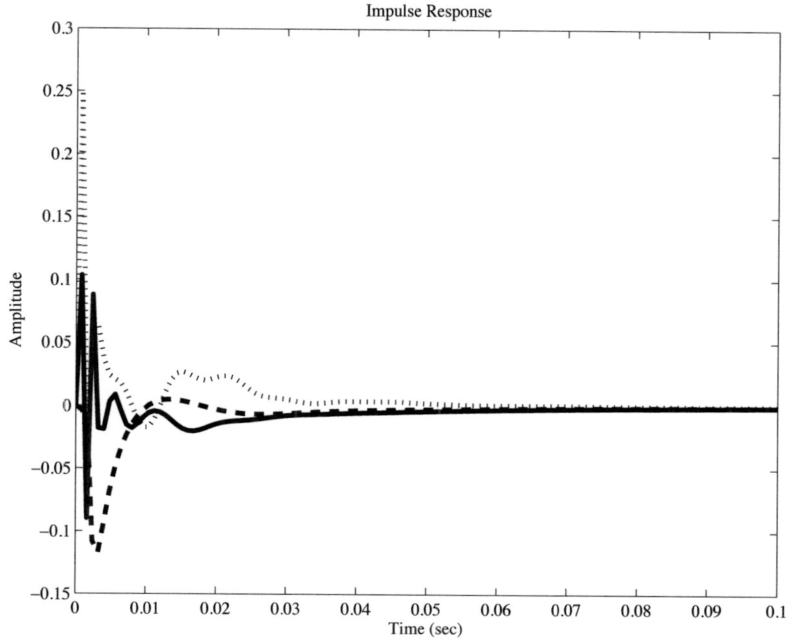

(a)

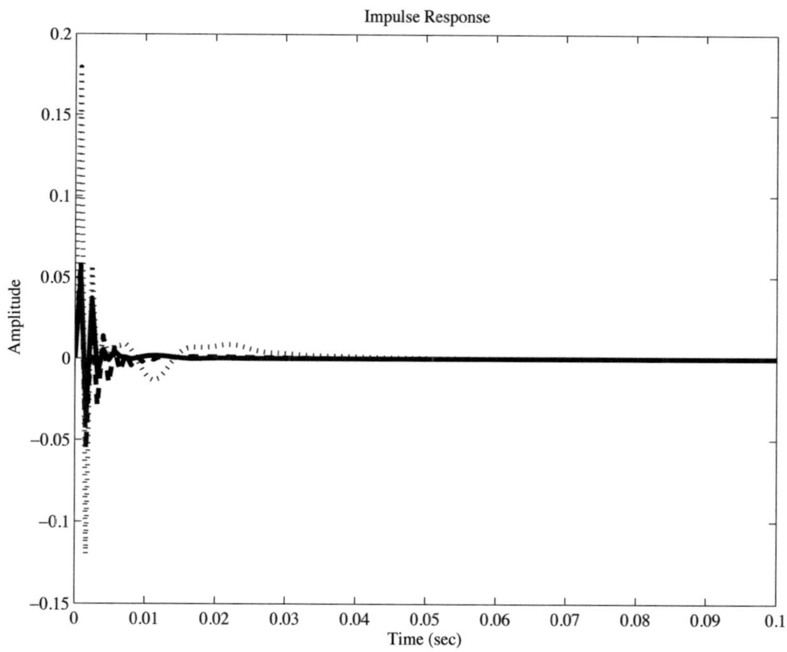

(b)

Fig. 13. Impulse responses between cSI and cSII by using the honest BSS (Kishida, 2011). (a) Impulse responses from cSI to cSII (F_{12}). (b) Impulse responses from cSII to cSI (F_{21}).

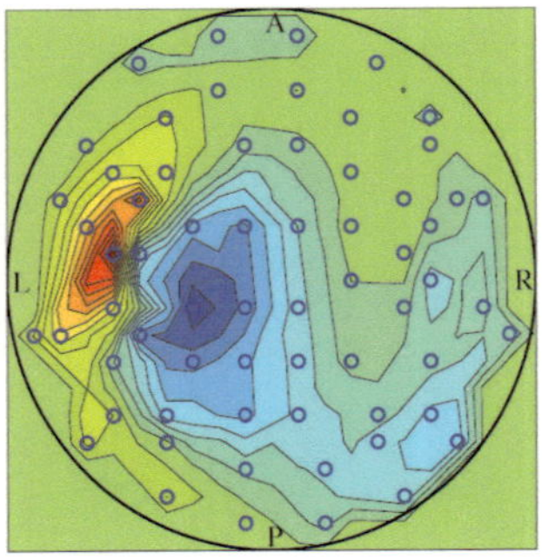

(a)

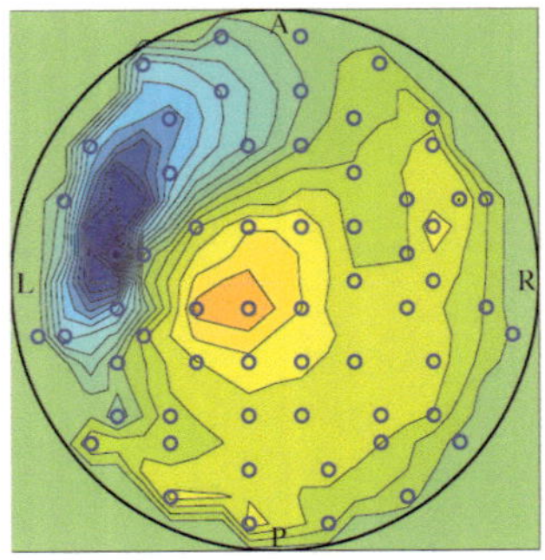

(b)

Fig. 14. Dipole patterns in the topographic field map of averaged waveforms of subject D in Fig. 1(d). (a) Time 120ms. (b) Time 180ms.

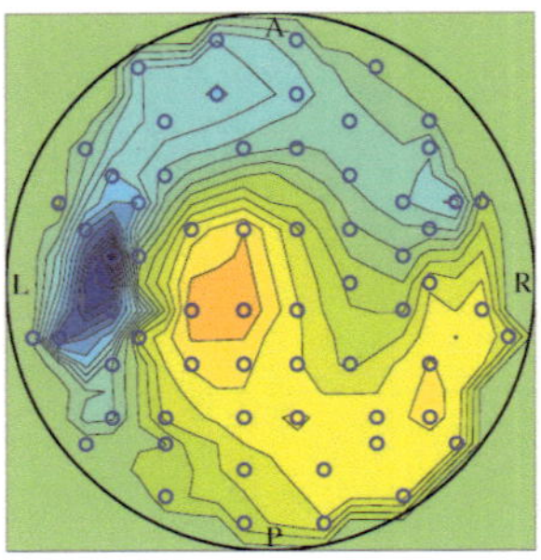

(a) A_4.

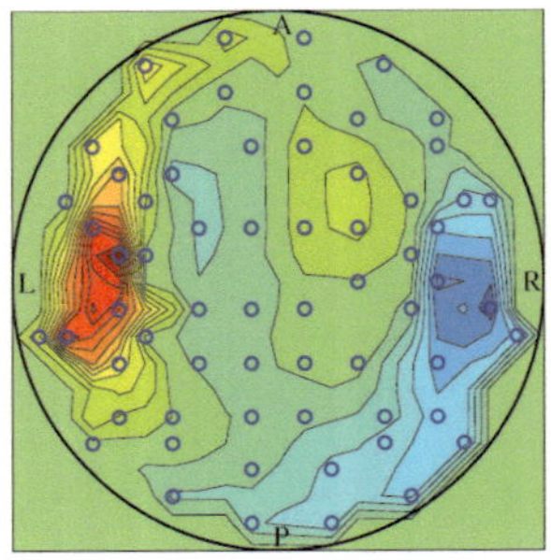

(b) A^h_{32}.

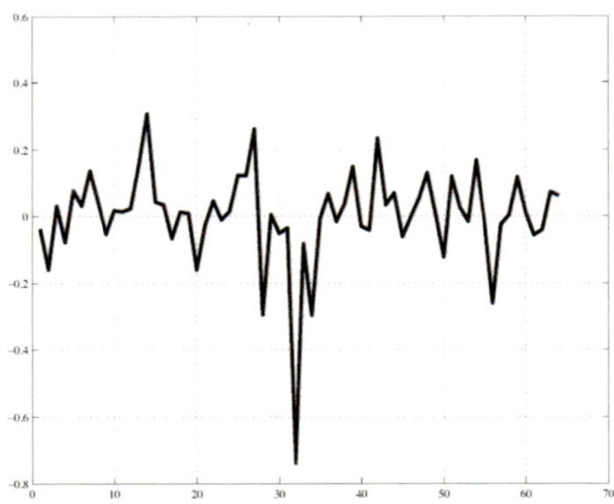

(c)

Fig. 15. Dipole pattern of BSS component corresponding to cSI and its transformation. (a) Topographic field map of dishonest BSS, (b) Topographic field map of honest BSS, (c) Transformation from the fourth BSS to components of honest BSS.

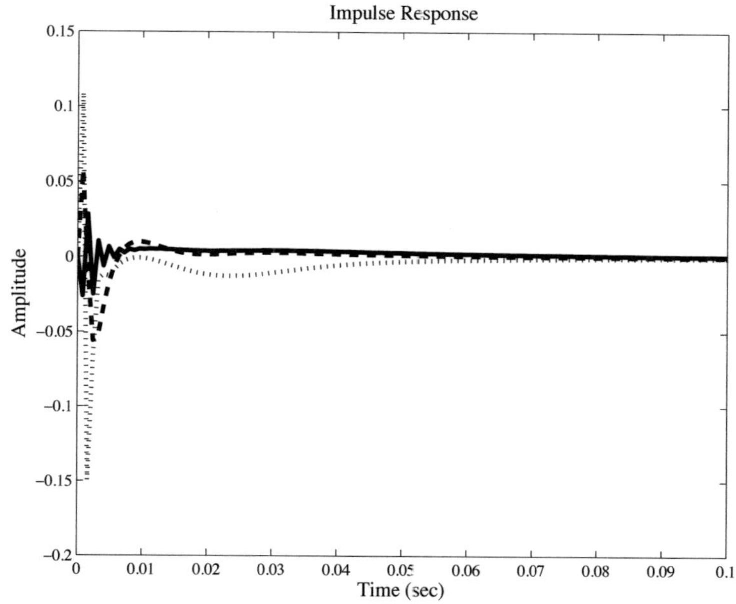

(a)

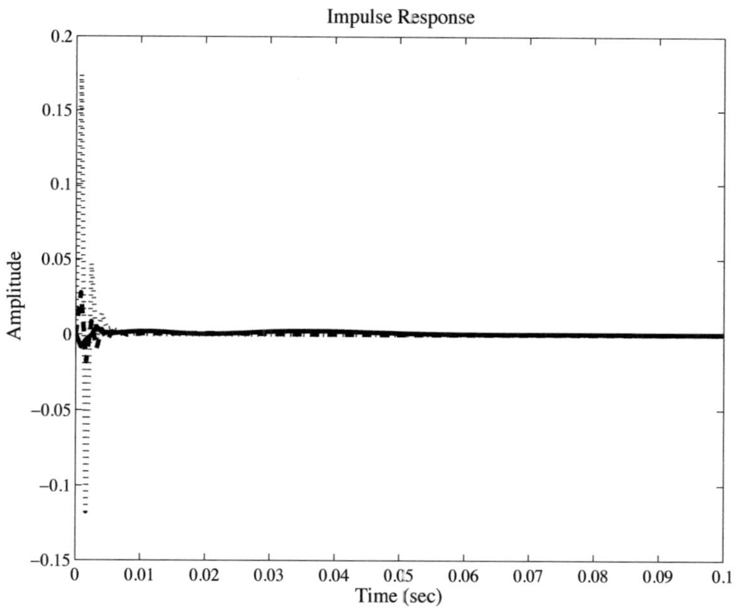

(b)

Fig. 16. Impulse responses between cSI and cSII by using the dishonest BSS. (a) Impulse responses from cSI to cSII (F_{12}). (b) Impulse responses from cSII to cSI (F_{21}).

5.3 SEF with steady state responses

Although separate fluctuations of SEF in subject D could not be separated, the other three subjects could be separated, and the intracerebral communication between cSI and cSII was identified. Our method is applicable to the normal case, in which there are line spectrum of fundamental frequency of SEF and higher harmonic ones. In the case of more than 20Hz ISI, steady state responses were observed for the somatosensory evoked potentials (Snyder, 1992; Tobimatsu et al., 1999). Their mechanism is different from transient responses of SEF. Supposing the normal scaling does not hold in the case, a new identification formalism is needed for nonlinear model, instead of linear feedback model in Eq. (17).

6. Conclusion

Intracerebral communication between cSI and cSII of human brain in 2Hz median nerves stimuli was studied by MEG. The honest type of blind source separation was used for identification of feedback model between cSI and cSII, current dipole data of which were in a stationary process.

In the special case where there was the one-to-one correspondence between current dipoles and BSS components (Kishida, 2009b), fluctuations of SEF could be separated after selection of BSS components with nonzero waveforms in the dishonest BSS. In general, there are no one-to-one correspondences between them. However, fluctuations of SEF could be determined from the honest BSS components as in Eq. (22), when more than three components of the dishonest BSS with nonzero waveforms were transformed into the honest BSS components by using the transformation matrix. That is, the transformation matrix between components of two types of BSS, Eq. (11), was introduced for selecting the fluctuations of evoked magnetic fields from MEG.

The identification method based on feedback system theory applied to fluctuations of evoked magnetic fields demonstrated two transit modes between cSI and cSII in impulse responses of transfer functions: One was a slow mode of order 30ms and the other was rapid one within 5 ms. It should be noted that the transfer functions are not necessarily elementary but overall process between active regions. If fluctuations generated by more than three current dipoles, we must use a multi-feedback model (Kishida, 1999) to obtain elemental transfer functions. Furthermore, physiological meanings of two modes in impulse responses will be future problems.

7. Acknowledgment

The author would like to thank Prof. K. Shinosaki for providing MEG data. This research was supported by Grant-in-Aid for Scientific Research (No.22500254) of Japan society for the Promotion of Science.

8. References

Akaike, H. & Nakagawa, T. (1988). Statistical Analysis and Control of Dynamic Systems, KTK Scientific Pub., originally published (in Japanese) by Saiensusya, 1972.

Cantero, J.L., Atienza, M., Cruz-Vadell, A., Suarez-Gonzalez, A. & Gil-Neciga, E. (2009). Increased synchronization and decreased neural complexity underlie thalamocortical oscillatory dynamics in mid cognitive impairment, NeuroImage, 46, 938-948.

Cardoso J. F. & Souloumiac, A. (1996). Jacobi angles for simultaneous diagonalization, SIAM J. Mat. Anal. Aplpl., 17, 161-163.

Florin, E., Gross, J., Pfeifer, J., Fink, G. R. & Timmermann, L. (2010). The effect of filtering on Granger causality based multivariate causality measures, NeuroImage, 50, 577-588.

Hamada Y., Otsuka, S., Okamoto, T. & Suzuki, R. (2002). The profile of the recovery cycle in human primary and secondary somatosensory cortex: a magnetoencephalography study, Clin. Neurophysiol., 113, 1787-1793.

Hämäläinen, M., Hari, R., Ilmoniemi, R. J., Knuutila, J. & Lounasmaa, O. V. (1993). Magnetoencephalography - theory, instrumentation, and applications to noninvasive studies of the working human brain, Rev. Mod. Phys., 65, 413-497.

Hironaga N. & Ioannides, A. A. (2007). Localization of individual area neuronal activity, NeuroImage, 34, 1519-1534.

Hui, H. B., Pantazis, D., Bressler, S. L. & Leahy, R. M. (2010). Identifying true cortical interactions in MEG using the nulling beamformer, NeuroImage, 49, 3161-3174.

Kakigi R., Hoshiyama, M., Shimoto, M., Naka, D., Yamasaki, H., Watanabe, S., Xiang, J., Maeda, K., Lam, K., Itomi, K. & Nakamura, A. (2000). The somatosensory evoked magnetic fields, Prog. Neurobiology, 61, 495-523.

Kishida, K., Kanemoto, S. & Sekiya, T. (1976). Reactor noise theory based on system size expansion, J. Nucl. Sci. Technol., 13, 19-29.

Kishida, K. (1991). Contraction of information in systems far from equilibrium, J. Math. Phys., 32, 92-98.

Kishida, K. (1994). A theory of reactor diagnosis in feedback systems, J. Nucl. Sci. Technol., 31, 526-538.

Kishida, K. (1996). Contraction of information and its inverse problem in reactor system identification, in Advances in Nuclear Science and Technology, edited by Lewins and Becker, Plenum Press, 23, 1-68.

Kishida, K. (1997a). Numerical study on identification of transfer functions in a feedback system and model reduction, J. Nucl. Sci. Technol., 34, 1115-1120.

Kishida, K. (1997b). Identification of transfer function in a feedback system and autoregressive analysis, Proc. 11th IFAC symposium on system identification (SYSID' 97), 3, 1437-1442.

Kishida, K. (1999). Identification of transfer functions in a feedback system and stochastic inverse problem. Proc. 31st ISCIE International Symposium on Stochastic Systems Theory and its Applications, Yokohama, Nov., 25-30.

Kishida, K., Fukai, H., Hara, T. & Shinosaki, K. (2003). A new approach to blind system identification in MEG data. IEICE Trans. Fundamentals, E86-A, 611-619.

Kishida, K. (2005). Blind identification of brain mechanism in MEG. Proc. IEEE International Symposium on Circuits and Systems (ISCAS), Kobe, May, 5694-5697.

Kishida, K. (2008). Classification of activities related to 5Hz periodical median nerve stimuli by using the temporal decorrelation method of BSS, in Biomagnetism - Interdisciplinary Research and Exploration, R. Kakigi, K Yokosawa and S. Kuriki Eds. Sapporo; Hokkaido University Press, 124-126.

Kishida K. (2009a). Evoked magnetic fields of magnetoencephalogrphy and their statistical property, Phys. Rev. E, 79, 011922(1-7).

Kishida, K. (2009b). Dynamical activities of primary somatosensory cortices studied by magnetoencephalography. Phys. Rev. E, 80, 051906(1-13).

Kishida, K. (2011). Intracerebral communication in 2 Hz periodical median nerve stimuli. J. Japan Biomag. Bioelectromag. 24 (in Japanese), 212-213.

Kubo, R., Matsuo, K. & Kitahara, K. (1973). Fluctuations and relaxation of macrovariables, J. Stat. Phys. 9, 51-96.

Mathematical Society of Japan, (1987). Encyclopedic Dictionary of Mathematics. (2nd edition) K. Ito Eds., vol. III; MIT Press, p.1463.

Molgedey L. & Schuster, H. G. (1994). Separation of a mixture of independent signals using time delayed correlations, Phys. Rev. Lett., 72, 3634-3637.

Murata, N., Ikeda, S. & Ziehe, A. (2001). An approach to blind source separation based on temporal structure of speech signals, Neurocomputing, 41, 1-24.

Sarvas, J. (1987). Basic mathematical and electromagnetic concepts of the biomagnetic inverse problem, Phys. Med. Biol., 32, 11-22.

Snyder, A. Z. (1992). Steady-state vibration evoked potentials: description of technique and characterization of responses. Electroencephalogr. Clin. Neurophysiol., 84, 257-268.

Tang, A. C., Sutherland, M. T. & McKinney, C. J. (2005). Validation of SOBI components from high-density EEG, NeuroImage, 25, 539-553.

Tobimasu, S., Zhang, Y. M. & Kato, M. (1999). Steady-state vibration somatosensory evoked potentials: physiological characteristics and tuning function, Clin. Neurophysiol., 110, 1953-1958.

Tomita K. & Tomita, H. (1974). Irreversible circulation of fluctuation, Prog. Theor. Phys., 51, 1731-1749.

Van Kampen, N. G. (1961). A power series expansion of the master equation, Can. J. Phys. 39, 551-567.

Wikström, H., Huttunen, J., Korvenoja, A., Virtanen, J., Salonen, O., Aronen, H. & Ilmoniemi, R. J. (1996). Effects of interstimulus interval on somatosensory evoked magnetic fields (SEFs): a hypothesis concerning SEF generation at the primary sensorimotor cortex. Electroencephalogr. Clin. Neurophysiol., 100, 479-487.

Yokota, Y. & Kishida, K. (2006). Signal source search method using a distance between signal spaces as an evaluation function, IEICE Trans. Fundamentals, J89-A (in Japanese), 1108-1118.

Ziehe, A., Müller, K. R., Nolte, G., Mackert, B. M. & Curio, G. (2000). Artifact reduction in magnetoneurography based on time-delayed second-order correlations, IEEE Trans. Biomed. Eng., 47, 75-87.

11

Pre-Attentive Processing of Sound Duration Changes: Low Resolution Brain Electromagnetic Tomography Study

Wichian Sittiprapaporn
Department of Educational Psychology and Guidance, Faculty of Education, Mahasarakham University, Maha Sarakham, Thailand

1. Introduction

The human central auditory system has a remarkable ability to establish memory traces for invariant features in the acoustic environments in order to correct the interpretation of natural acoustic sound heard. Even when no conscious attention is paid to the surrounding sounds, changes in their regularity can cause the listener to redirect his or her attention toward the sound heard (Tervaniemi *et al.,* 2001). When engaged in a conversation, listeners tune in to the relevant stream of speech and filter out irrelevant speech input that may be present in the same environment. Nonetheless, attention might be involuntarily diverted to meaningful items coming from an ignored stream, like in the well-known own-name effect (Moray, 1959). This brings up the question of to what extent speech is processed in the ignored streams. In the past decade, there have witnessed a resurgence in the electrophysiological literature of attempts to understand how the brain processes the speech signal (Kraus *et al.,* 1993, 1996; Molfese, 1985). One of the most used and well known paradigms in electrosphysiological research is the so-called oddball paradigm, in which typically two stimuli are presented, in random order. One of the stimuli occurs less frequently than the other and the subject is required to discriminate the infrequent stimulus (deviant, target or oddball) from the frequent one (standard). Two main types of ERPs have been described in the literature as a response to the detection of the deviant: P300 and the MMN (Aaltonen *et al.,* 1994; Kraus *et al.,* 1993, 1996). If the subject is required to respond overtly --- for example, by pressing a button – each time he/she detects the deviant, a positive wave peaking approximately 300 ms after deviant onset is elicited. This wave is called P300 and it is largest over electrode sites in normal adults. Such positivity is thought to reflect voluntary focused attention (context updating, response selection). However, if the subject is not required to respond overtly, and one subtracts the event-related potentials (ERPs) obtained in response to the standard, from the ERPs obtained for the deviant, so-called mismatch negativity (MMN) may be observed, usually peaking between 100 and 300 ms after stimulus onset depending on the characteristics of the difference between standard and deviant stimuli. This component is thought to reflect a pre-attentional detection of deviation, a mismatch between the deviant and the memory trace formed by the standard.

Event-related potentials (ERPs) recordings have bought new insight to the neuronal events behind auditory change detection in audition. ERPs components reflect the conscious detection of a physical, semantic, or syntactic deviation from the expected sounds (Tervaniemi *et al.*, 2001). The ERPs recordings thus allow one to probe the neural processes preceding the involvement of the attentional mechanisms. For instances, ERPs have been recorded that reflect memory traces representing sounds composed of several simultaneous or successive tonal elements (Schröger *et al.*, 1996; Alain *et al.*, 1994; Alho *et al.*, 1996). In auditory perception, the occurrence of the deviant (infrequent) stimulus after a sequence of the standard (Frequent) stimuli tends to elicit MMN in event-related potentials (ERPs) and its magnetic equivalent called the magnetic mismatch field (MMF) in magnetoencephalography (MEG). The MMN/MMF component may be considered to reflect the pre-attentive auditory memory processes and represents neuronal correlates of change detection and sound discrimination (Näätänen, 1992). Previous studies showed that for sinusoidal tones, the MMF is sensitive to the direction of a change within the stimulus, being more robustly activated for duration shortening or pitch falling as opposed to lengthening or leveling (Inouchi *et al.*, 2002). These studies also revealed no significant differences between subjects who spoke a pitch-accent language (Japanese) and those who did not (English). It has been reported that MMN/MMF is indeed sensitive to cross-linguistic relevance. Unlike short-to-long vowel duration and falling-to-level pitch changes, long-to-short duration and level-to-falling pitch changes elicited a prominent MMF bilaterally for both groups, peaking at around 100 ms after change onset for duration and 200 ms for pitch. The MMF component is sensitive is sensitive to vowel shortening rather than lengthening and to pitch falling rather than leveling (Inouchi *et al.*, 2002, 2003).

2. Neurophysiological features of mismatch negativity

The search for an objective index of change detection in the human brain can be traced back to 1975, with the proposition that stimulus deviation per se (irrespective of, e.g., stimulus significance, attentional mechanisms) should produce a measurable brain response (Näätänen, 1992). Experimental evidence for this suggestion was obtained in experiments conducted by Näätänen, Gaillard, and Mäntysalo in 1975 (subsequently reported in 1978). In this dichotic listening study, the subject's task was to detect occasional deviant stimuli in the stimulus sequence presented to a designated ear while ignoring the concurrent sequence presented to the opposite ear. The irrelevant stimulus sequence included deviant stimuli that were physically equivalent to the deviant stimuli (targets) of the attended input sequence. The deviant stimuli were either tones of a slightly higher frequency or tones of a slightly greater intensity than the standard tones. A neurophysiological paradigm well suited to examine pre-attentive and automatic central auditory processing is the mismatch negativity (MMN). This is a negative component of the event-related brain potential (ERP), elicited when a detectable change occurs in repetitive homogeneous auditory stimuli (Näätänen, 1992). The most commonly described MMN occurs at 100-300 ms post-stimulus onset although other studies have found later MMNs between 300 and 600 ms (Kraus *et al.*, 1996). The MMN is elicited by any change in frequency, intensity or duration of tone stimuli, as well as by changes in complex stimuli such as phonetic stimuli (Näätänen, 1992). It is assumed to arise as a result of a mechanism that compares each current auditory input with a trace of recent auditory input stored in the auditory memory. The MMN usually reaches its amplitude maximum over the fronto-central scalp (Näätänen, 1992).

The deviant stimuli both in the attended and unattended stimulus sequence elicited negativity in the 100-200 ms latency range, which could not be seen in response to the standard stimuli. This negativity, usually described by the deviant-minus-standard difference wave, was very similar for the attended and ignored input sequences, suggesting that attention was not required. Näätänen *et al.* (1978) proposed that it may well be that a physiological mismatch process caused by a sensory input deviating from the memory trace formed by a frequent background stimulus is such an automatic basic process that it takes place irrespective of the intentions of the experimenter and the subject, perhaps even unmodified by the latter. On the basis of the relatively large MMN amplitudes above the temporal areas, the authors further suggested that the mismatch negativity reflects specific auditory stimulus discrimination processes taking place in the auditory primary and association areas. The latter processes are suggested to be largely automatic, beyond the control of will, instructions, etc. This finding, suggesting the existence of an automatic memory mechanism subsequently paved the way for a series of new experiments where changes in basic stimulus features (frequency, intensity, and duration) and the elicitation of the MMN were addressed in more detail. It was established that the MMN is elicited by both increments and decrements in basic stimulus features. The MMN, however, is not elicited when a stimulus sequence begins or, similarly, when stimuli are presented with very long interstimulus intervals (ISIs). Thus, it was concluded that no stimulus per se is an adequate stimulus for the MMN generator mechanism, as the system responds to the difference between the consecutive stimuli. This response pattern is clearly separable from the behavior of N1 response; the N1 amplitude is largest in response to the first stimulus of a series, strongly attenuating thereafter and showing only partial recovery to a subsequent different stimulus.

Mismatch negativity (MMN), an index of preattentive processing of perceived sounds, is an Event-related Potential (ERP) component elicited by rare deviant stimuli within a sequence of repetitive auditory stimuli. Mismatch negativity component of ERP is theoretically elicited in the auditory cortex when incoming sounds are detected as deviating from a neural representation of acoustic regularities. The mismatch negativity (Näätänen *et al.*, 1978) and its magnetic equivalent (MMNm) are elicited by any discriminable change in some repetitive aspect of auditory stimulation, irrespective of the direction of the subject's attention. It is mainly generated in the auditory cortex (Scherg *et al.*, 1989) occurring between 100 to 250 ms and thus long been regarded as specific to the auditory modality (Näätänen, 1992; Nyman *et al.*, 1990). Additionally, this negative component of the auditory event-related potential (ERPs), usually peaking 100-300 ms from change onset, is based on, and reflects, neural traces by which the auditory cortex models the repetitive aspects of the acoustic past (Näätänen and Winkler 1999). These traces might contain sensory information on sound frequency, duration and inter-stimulus interval (ISI), but also on more complex aspects of auditory stimulation, such as rhythmic patterns or speech sounds (Näätänen and Winkler 1999). The properties of these traces (which usually last several seconds, although even permanent traces can be reflected (Näätänen and Winkler 1999)) can be probed by presenting infrequent deviant events in the sequence of repetitive events ('standard') (Näätänen and Winkler 1999). MMN is elicited even in the absence of attention, for example, in individuals in a coma a few days before the recovery of consciousness (Kane *et al.*, 1993), which indicates that MMN indexes pre-attentive (attention-independent) auditory processing. The automatic change-detection system in the human brain as reflected by the

MMN thus requires the storage of the previous state of the acoustic environment for detecting an incoming deviating sound (Näätänen, 1992; Brattico *et al.*, 2002). Furthermore, MMN implies the existence of an auditory sensory memory that stores a neural representation of a standard against which any incoming auditory input is compared (Ritter et al., 1995). In the auditory modality, MMN is an automatic process which occurs even when the subject's attention is focused away from the evoking stimuli (Näätänen, 1992). Its onset normally begins before the N2b-P3 complex which occurs when attention is directed to the stimuli. The duration of MMN varies with the nature of the stimulus deviance but it invariably overlaps N2b when the latter is present (Tales *et al.*, 1999)

The main neural generators of MMN are bilaterally located in the supratemporal plane (Alho, 1995), which is indicated by dipole modeling (Scherg *et al.*, 1989) and scalp current density map (Giard *et al.*, 1990) of scalp-recorded event-related potentials, as well as by magnetic recordings, intracranial MMN recordings in cats, monkeys and humans, and by positron emission tomography, functional magnetic resonance imaging, and optical imaging data. Furthermore, the exact locus of MMN in auditory cortex depends on the attribute (Giad *et al.*, 1995) (and even on the complexity of stimulus configuration (Alho *et al.*, 1996)) in which the change occurred. Therefore, one can conclude that the auditory processes that generate MMN originate, in the first place, in the auditory cortex. In addition, MMN also receives a contribution from a (mainly right hemispheric) frontal generator that appears to be triggered by this auditory-cortex change-detection process and be associated with the initiation of attention switch to the change (Escera *et al.*, 2000).

The present study compared preattentive brain processes during the discrimination of the different synthesized sounds duration. A single pair of the synthesized long and short sounds selected to represent ideal exemplars. This study chose to record and compared the MMN elicited by these synthesized sounds, hoping to find evidence for specific brain signatures of both synthesized long and short sounds processing in the human auditory cortex. Two questions were examined using this approach: (1) whether the MMN would index differences in the brain's discrimination of this different synthesized sounds duration; and (2) whether the MMN amplitude and/or latency would reflect acoustic differences between the rare deviant and the frequent standard stimuli. Additionally, the low-resolution electromagnetic tomography (LORETA) analysis were used to locate multiple non-dipolar sources particularly involved in the discrimination of these different synthesized sounds duration within the MMN paradigm.

3. Participants, handedness and ethical consideration

EEG recordings were collected from eleven healthy young, Thai-speaking adults (eight female) and their age range: 23-29 years. All participants were right-handedness assessed according to Oldfield (Oldfield, 1971). They had normal hearing, corrected to normal vision and had no history of neurological or psychiatric history. The mean (±sd) age was 25.73 (±3.1) years. The Ethics committees of the involved institutions accepted the study. The concept was explained to the participants, and written informed consent was obtained. All participants gave their written informed consent to participate in the experiments and were paid for their participation. The experiments were performed in accordance with the Helsinki Declaration. Ethical permission for the experiments was issued by the Committee on Human Rights Related to Human experimentation.

The handedness of the participants was assessed with the Edinburgh Handedness Inventory (Oldfield, 1971). The degree of the right handedness of the subjects was assessed based upon ten items; writing; drawing; throwing; scissors; toothbrush; knife (without fork); spoon; broom; striking a match; and open box lid. The participant was instructed to make a "+" on which hand he/she would prefer to use for each action. They were instructed to mark a "++" when the preference was so strong that he/she never used the other hand unassisted. If, in any case, the participant did not have any preference, he/she was instructed to mark a "+" for both hands. The numbers of "+" marked for each hand were totaled. Then, a handedness index was calculated to be the difference of the numbers of "+"'s between the right and left hands divided by the total number of "+"'s for both hands. A handedness index of 1.0 indicated completely right handed, -1.0 corresponded to completely left handed, and 0 suggested ambidextrous. The participant was also asked which foot was preferred for kicking, which eye was preferred when only using one eye, and whether both parents were right handed.

4. General electrophysiological procedures

Two different sounds duration were synthetically generated with short and long sounds. All of the stimuli were digitally edited to have an equal maximum energy level in dB SPL with the remaining intensity level within each of the stimuli scaled accordingly. The stimuli were digitally edited using the Cool Edit Pro v. 2.0 (Syntrillium Software Cooperation) with 500 ms duration (long sound) and 300 ms duration (short sound). All sounds were identical at their frequencies, thus eliminating any effect due to differences in frequency of occurrence of sound. The sounds were presented binaurally via headphones at a comfortable listening level of ~85 dB. The sound pressure levels of stimulus pairs were then measured at the output of headphones using a Brüel and Kjaer 2230 sound level meter. The standard (S)/deviant (D) pairs for each condition were [Condition 1: long-to-short sounds change] Standard/S-(2), Deviant/D-(1), [Condition 2: short-tolong sounds change] S-(1), D-(2). Thus, in both conditions pairs were designed to contrast short and long sounds. The stimuli were presented in a passive oddball paradigm. Deviant stimuli appeared randomly among the standards at 10% probability. Each condition included 125 deviants. The stimuli were binaurally delivered using SuperLab software (Cedrus Corporation, San Pedro, CA, USA) via headphones (Telephonic TDH-39-P). The inter-stimulus interval (ISI) was 1.25 second (offset-onset). EEG signal recording was time-locked to the onset of the sound. Participants were instructed not to pay attention to the stimuli presented via headphones, but rather to concentrate on a self-selected silent movie. Afterwards, they reported the impression of the movie.

Participants are instructed to sit relaxing in comfortable reclining chair in an electrically and acoustically dampened room. They were told that they would participate in the experiment and that the experimenter would be recording their brain electrical activity. They were given written instructions and provided with a grid for their judgements and a pen. They silently read the instructions and at the end the experimenter verifies that everything was clear. Their histories were taken, including age, educational level, handedness, occupation, current medications, medical history (which included past illness, surgical history, head trauma or accident) and history of alcohol consumption or smoking. If there was any significant history of neurological problems, psychiatric problems or head trauma, that participant was excluded. For the Mismatch Negativity (MMN) study, all participants were instructed to ignore the stimuli by watching a silent, subtitled video of their choice (ignore condition). They were asked to avoid body and eye movements and to keep alert. Before the recording session, the task was explained and a practice block of 50 tones (50 deviants) was presented to the participant to ensure a good level performance. In order to avoid alpha rhythm synchronization during the recording session, participants were instructed to remain with their eyes open while watching a silent, subtitled video of their choice and were instructed to avoid eye movement and blinking. The total experimental session was 1-2 h, including approximately 0.20 h. for electrode placement. During the experimental session, participants took a rest breaks (one 15-min break occurring halfway through the recording session and shorter 5-min breaks as needed). Participants were tested in all experimental conditions on the same day.

5. Electroencephalographic processing

EEG data were collected with a Quick-Cap equipped with 64 channels according to the international 10-20 system using Scan system (Scan 4.3, Neurosoft, Inc. Sterling, USA). Reference electrode was at both ear lobes. The signals were bandpass filtered at 0.05-100 Hz and digitized at 1000 Hz. The impedance of the electrode was below 5 kΩ. Eye movements were monitored with two EOG electrodes. Four electrodes monitored horizontal and vertical eye movements for off-line artifact rejection. Vertical and horizontal electro-oculogram (EOG) was recorded by electrodes situated above and below the left eye, and on the outer canthi of both eyes, respectively. Epochs with EEG or EOG with a large (>100 μV) amplitude were automatically rejected. The artifact-free epochs were filtered at 0.1-15 Hz, baseline corrected and averaged. EEG was segmented into 1000 ms epochs, including the 100 ms pre-stimulus period. The average waveforms obtained from the standard and deviant were digitally filtered by a 0.1 - 15 Hz band-pass filter and finally baseline-corrected. Grand-averaged difference waveforms were calculated by subtracting the standard from the deviant waveforms. For each condition, presence of a prominent MMN was identified by measuring the integrated power amplitudes over the 40-ms time window centered on the MMN peak in the difference waveform. An MMN component was judged prominent if the amplitude difference between standard and deviant within predefined the window was statistically significant. For each participant, the averaged MMN responses contained 125 accepted deviants.

6. Intracerebral distribution of differences in brain electrical activity

In order to visualize and to measure the MMN (deviant-tone ERP-minus-standard-tone ERP difference), after the recording, differences were calculated by subtracting the ERP elicited by the standard tones from that elicited by the corresponding deviant tones of the same stimulus class. The MMN was quantified by first determining the MMN peak latency from the frontal (Fz) grand-average difference waves separately for each deviant. The latency windows for picking up the MMN peaks were predefined on the basis of the across-participants peak latency distribution, determined by visual inspection. The MMN component was defined as the most prominent negative peak within the time windows between 100 and 300 ms. Latency and amplitude figures for waveforms were picked at their point of maximal deflection, as seen at their electrode site of maximal voltage distribution of frontal (Fz) electrode site. Peak-picking of the prominent peak (MMN) was accomplished by means of moving an 'enhanced point' cursor through the waveforms displayed on the computer screen, while simultaneously paying attention to the resultant changes in the topographic maps. The mean MMN amplitudes at the frontal (Fz) electrode site were calculated as a mean voltage of the 40 ms intervals (so the peak plus minus 20 ms), centered at the corresponding peak latencies of the left and right frontal electrodes in the grand-averaged waveforms, separately for each stimulus type. The amplitudes were determined by using the 100 ms pre-stimulus baseline. When the participants were watching a silent, subtitled video, MMN to spatial acoustic changes was observed as a significant difference between ERPs to the deviant tones and those to the standard tones. It was at its maximum at the frontal (Fz) electrode site consisting of a negative deflection (note that analyses are based on averaged 40-ms blocks of sample points). MMN amplitudes were measured as the mean amplitude over the 100-300 ms period after the stimulus-onset from the deviant-tone ERP-minus-standard-tone ERP differences.

The average MMN latency was defined as a moment of the global field power with an epoch of 40-ms time window related stable scalp-potential topography (Pascual-Marqui, 1994). In the next step, low-resolution electromagnetic tomography (LORETA) was applied to estimate the current source density distribution in the brain, which contributes to the electrical scalp field (Pascual-Marqui *et al.,* 1994). Maps were computed with the Low Resolution Electromagnetic Tomography. Two radically oriented point sources (dipoles) in the brain were selected and computed the 21 channels forward solution electric potential map using a 3-shell unit radius spherical head model. The forward solution maps were then used as input for the LORETA computation in order to test the location precision and the ability of the method to separate the two known dipole locations. Scalp potentials re-referenced to the average reference, excluding the EOG electrodes, were interpolated for mapping using the surface spline method. The CSD maps were computed with the spherical spline interpolated data. The maps were computed at a single time point where the component in question was largest in the grand mean waveforms of each stimulus type and condition separately. LORETA computed the smoothest of all possible source configurations throughout the brain volume by minimizing the total squared Laplacian of source strengths.

Low-resolution Electromagnetic Tomography (LORETA) is the new implementation of LORETA in the Talairach brain. LORETA makes use of the three-shell spherical head model registered to the Talairach human brain atlas (Talairach and Tournoux, 1988), available as a digitized MRI from the Brain Imaging Center, Montreal Neurologic Institute. Registration between spherical and realistic head geometry use EEG electrode coordinates reported by Towle et al. (1993). The solution space is restricted to cortical gray matter and hippocampus, as determined by the corresponding digitized Probability Atlas also available from Brain Imaging Center, Montreal Neurologic Institute. A voxel is labeled as gray matter if it meet the following three conditions: its probability of being gray matter is higher than that of being white matter, its probability of being gray matter is higher than that of being cerebrospinal fluid, and its probability of being gray matter is higher than 33%. Only gray matter voxels at 7-mm spatial resolution are produced under these neuroanatomical constraints. LORETA computations use the exact head model determined from each individual subject's MRI. The final step in any analysis procedure would be to cross-register the individual's anatomical and functional image to the standard Talairach atlas.

The individual momentary potential measures from 21 electrodes at the MMN latency were analyzed with LORETA to determine the MMN source loci (Pascual-Marqui, 1994). These latencies were between 100-140 ms for long- and short-sound duration changes. LORETA calculated the current source density distribution in the brain, which contributed to the electrical scalp field, at each of 2395 voxels in the gray matter and the hippocampus of a reference brain (MNI 305, Brain Imaging Centre, Montreal Neurological Institute) based on the linear weighted sum of the scalp electric potentials (Pascual-Marqui, 1994). LORETA chooses the smoothest of all possible current density configurations throughout the brain volume by minimizing the total squared Laplacian of source strengths. This procedure only implicates that neighboring voxels should have a maximally similar electrical activity, no other assumptions were made. The applied version of LORETA used a three-shell spherical head model registered to the Talairach space and calculated the three-dimensional localization of the electrical sources contributing to the electrical scalp filed for all subjects and conditions, defining the regions of interest on the basis of local maxima of the LORETA distribution. Stereotaxic coordinates of the voxels of the local maxima were determined within areas of significant relative change associated with the tasks. The anatomical localization of these local maxima was assessed with reference to the standard Stereotaxic atlas, and validation of this method of localization was obtained by superimposition of the SPM maps on a standard MRI brain provided by the SPM99. Peaks located within superior temporal gyrus was also identified by using published probability maps following a correction for the differences in the coordinate systems between the Talairach and Tournoux atlas and the Stereotaxic space employed by SPM99.

Regarding to the Brodmann areas(s) and brain regions localization, the Talairach Daemon (TD) will be taken into consideration. The Talairach Daemon (TD) is a high-speed database server for querying and retrieving data about human brain structure over the Internet (http://ric.uthscsa.edu/td_applet/). The TD server data is searched using x-y-z coordinates resolved to 1x1x1 mm volume elements within a standardized stereotaxic space. An array, indexed by x-y-z coordinates, that spans 170 mm (x), 210 mm (y) and 200 mm (z), provides high-speed access to data. Array dimensions are selected to be approximately 25% larger than those of the Co-planar Stereotaxic Atlas of the Human Brain (Talairach and Tournoux, 1988). Coordinates tracked by the TD server are spatially consistent with the Talairach Atlas. Each array location stores a pointer to a relation record that holds data describing what is present at the corresponding coordinate. Presently, the data in relation records are either Structure Probability Maps (SP Maps) or Talairach Atlas Labels, though others can be easily added. The relation records are implemented as linked lists to names and values for brain structures. The TD server is run on a Sun SPARCstation 20 with 200 Mbytes of memory. Intention is to provide 24-hour access to the data using a variety of client applications, as well as continue to add more brain structure information to the database.

7. Statistical evaluation

The statistical significance of MMN (deviant-minus-standard difference) was tested with one-sample *t*-tests by comparing the mean MMN amplitude at the frontal (Fz) electrode site, where the MMN was most prominent. The MMN was measured using the mean frontal (Fz) amplitude in the 100 - 300 ms interval of the deviant-minus-standard difference curves. This interval included the grand mean MMN peak latencies in those conditions where MMN was elicited. One-sample t- tests were used to verify the presence of the MMN component, by comparing the mean amplitude of the 100 - 300 ms interval against a hypothetical zero, separately in each condition. The MMN latency values was also compared. Repeated measure ANOVA was carried out on the topographic descriptors of the MMN. In order to gather information on cortical sources specifically involved in the MMN generation, LORETA images for deviant sounds were compared with those for standard sounds using paired t-test statistics, after logarithmic transformation of the data. All results were expressed as mean ± S.D and all significant

For the LORETA analyses, the average LORETA images were constructed across participants: the brain electric activity during the ERPs amplitude waveforms for each condition and the voxel-by-voxel t test differences between conditions. The voxel-by-voxel paired t tests were run to assess in which cortical regions the conditions differed. The t maps were threshold at $p < 0.0001$. As pointed out above, reliable differences in the scalp ERP field configuration can unambiguously be interpreted as suggesting that at least partially different neuronal populations are active during the conditions. LORETA assesses in which brain regions the conditions differed. The Structure-Probability Maps Atlas (Lancaster *et al.*, 1997a; 1997b) was also used to determine which brain regions were involved in differences between conditions. Brodmann area(s) (BA) and brain regions closet to the observed locations identified by the Tarairach coordinates were reported. Overall, one sample *P*-values were reported.

8. Pre-attentive processing and lateralization of sound duration changes

The finding indicated that the prominent response to both sounds elicited MMN peaking at 128 to 212 ms from stimulus onset. The grand-averaged ERPs showed that the MMN mean amplitude of both sounds was statistically significant (t-test). The paired sample t-test revealed a significant difference between conditions (t (10) = 73.00; $p < 0.0001$) showing that both sounds equally elicited a MMN. The magnitude of the acoustic difference between the stimulus pairs was reflected by the MMN amplitude, showing larger MMN amplitudes in long sound compared to the short one. The difference in MMN latencies to both sounds might reflect differential processing of the human auditory cortex. The delay in the MMN to the long sound might reflect additional time required to process sound perception. This processing apparently involves activation of a memory trace, or cell assembly, which possibly represents and the processes the sounds.

Estimated source localization of the average MMN responses evoked by both sounds was clearly identified. The current source density values in the time frame 128-212 ms post-stimulus were calculated with LORETA. Stronger activation for long sound was found at 212 ms in the left middle temporal gyrus (MTG) (-59, -32, 1; t-value, 1.81), while the short sound most strongly activated at 128 ms in the left superior temporal gyrus (STG) (-59, -39, 8; t-value, 1.03) (see Figure 1). Analysis of the MMN responses indicated left-hemispheric laterality in both sound durations (F (3,30) = 47.02; $p < 0.0001$). The source analysis indicated strongest MMN response tentatively originating in the left hemisphere and possibly involving the perisylvian area in both sounds, with a more superior distribution for the long sound and a more medial distribution for the short one.

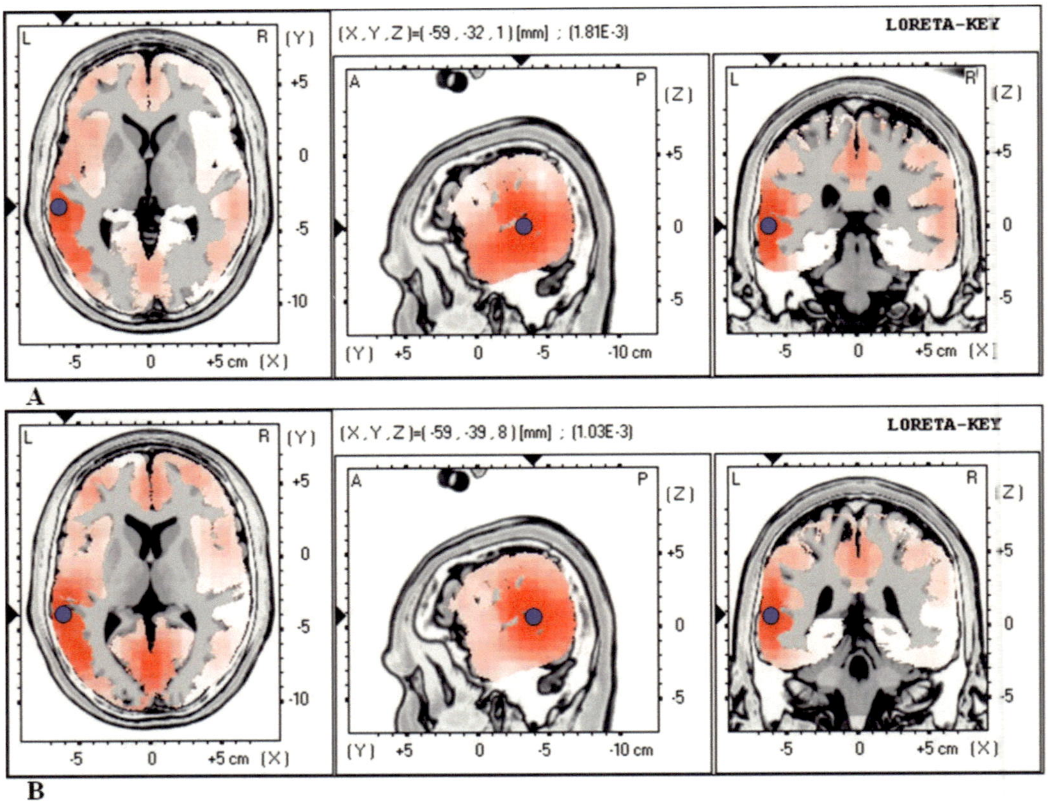

Fig. 1. Graphical representation of the low-resolution electromagnetic tomography (LORETA *t*-statistic comparing the event-related potentials for mismatch negativity (MMN) responses at the time point of the individual peak over Fz for the long sound (A) and short sound (B) activated in the left hemisphere. Red color indicates local maxima of increased electrical activity for both sounds responses in an axial, a saggital and a coronal slice through the reference brain. Blue dots mark the center of significantly increased electric activity.

As it was well established that the MMN amplitude indexes the change detection accuracy (Näätänen, 1999), the MMN to short sound was significantly smaller than those for the long one. The source analysis for the long sound revealed that the source for long sound was located significantly more superior than for short sound in the left hemisphere. In addition, the estimated source strength was not difference between long and short sounds. It is thus the source location rather than its signal strength that might be a primary reason for the reduced responses for short with long sounds. These results may be comparable to those of a previous report by Tiitinen *et al.* (1993) indicating that the MMN sources as well as N100m have a frequency-dependant tonotopy.

Additionally, source analysis suggested MMN sources to be in the vicinity of the left perisylvian area with a more medial distribution for the long deviant and more superior distribution for the short one. It may be that these similar topographies of the neurophysiological brain response do not reflect differential cortical distributions of the underlying neuronal assemblies. The finding of a significantly left-lateralized electric MMN in the present study supports to the previous study indicating a particularly strong asymmetry between the activated neuronal generators in the two hemispheres. There are two possible interpretations for this laterality. First, the functional information tied to the sound no matter of the type of the sounds underlies this laterality. As a second possibility, it may be that it is the functional information related to the stimulus contrasts that is crucial for the strong involvement of left hemispheric processes. Therefore, the MMN response topography and latency in the present study may reveal cortical distribution and activity dynamics of these memory traces. One possible explanation of this hemispheric discrepancy in the MMN effect is that the temporal window of integration (Näätänen and Winkler, 1999; Sussman *et al.*, 1999) differs between two hemispheres. The left hemisphere is suggested to be more sensitive than the right hemisphere to high-frequency temporal patterns of sounds including the stimulus duration. In fact, the perceptual right-ear advantage, regarded as an index of the left hemisphere dominance, can be observed for high-frequency sounds and this advantage is reversed for low-frequency sounds. This may relate to the lack of frequency and duration effect in the right hemisphere, since the long and short distinction mainly rests on the difference of the relatively high frequencies for each of the stimuli. Additionally, the sources for the short stimuli were located more posterior and superior in the left hemisphere than in the right hemisphere. The results replicated previous studies (Alho *et al.*, 1998; Rinne *et al.*, 1999; Tervaniemi *et al.*, 1999). For the source strength of the long and short stimuli, no hemispheric difference was observed. It should be also noted that MMN to short and long sounds showed significant left hemisphere dominance. These results might be in accordance with the findings of Mathiak et al. (1999) rather than studies reporting the left lateralized MMN for speech sounds (Näätänen *et al.*, 1992; Tervaniemi *et al.*, 1999). However, the present study used only one single pair of sounds (i.e., long and short) as an exemplar, which imposes certain limitations on generalization of the current results to all other long and short sounds. Studying this issue using different long and short sounds thus appears to be a fruitful target for further experiments.

9. Conclusion

The prominent MMN component was elicited and more sensitive to the long sound than the short one. The MMN presumably reflect the early stage of processing of different sound duration in the human brain. So, from the known early auditory-cortex responses to sounds, the MMN reflects an early, pre-attentive, automatic processing of diferent sound duration. The MMN is therefore a potential interest as a technique of evaluating duration of different sounds lateralization, since its measurement is non-invasive, relatively inexpensive (especially in case of the EEG), and applicable to any subjects or patients. The present study has added physiological evidence to earlier psychological and clinico-anatomical evidence that functional characteristics of auditory stimuli differentially influence the brain circuits used at higher cortical stages for processing of different sound duration. Automatic detection of long sound may be a useful index of auditory memory traces of sound perception in the human auditory perception.

10. References

Aaltonen, O.; Eerola, O.; Lang, A.H.; Uusipaikka, E. & Tuomainen, J. (1994). Automatic discrimination of phonetically relevant and irrelevant vowel parameters as reflected by mismatch negativity. *J. Acoust. Soc. Am.*, Vol. 96, pp.1489-1493.

Alain, C.; Woods, D.L. & Ogawa, K.H. (1994). Brain indices of automatic pattern processing. *NeuroReport*, Vol. 6, pp. 140-144.

Alho, K. (1995). Cerebral generators of mismatch negativity (MMN) and its magnetic counterpart (MMNm) elicited by sound changes. *Ear Hear.*, Vol. 16, pp. 38-51.

Alho, K.; Tervaniemi, M.; Huotilainen, M.; Lavikainen, J.; Tiitinen, H.; Ilmoniemi, R.J.; Knuutila, J. & Näätänen, R. (1996). Processing of complex sounds in the human auditory cortex as revealed by magnetic brain responses. *Psychophysiol.*, Vol. 33, pp. 396-375.

Brattico, E.; Winkler, I.; Näätänen, R.; Paavilainen, P. & Tervaniemi, M. (2002). Simultaneous storage of two complex temporal sound patterns in auditory sensory memory. *NeuroReport*, Vol. 13, pp. 1747-1751.

Escera, C. (2000). Involuntary attention and distractibilioty as evaluated with event-related brain potentials Audiol. *Neuro-Otol.*, Vol. 5, pp. 151-166.

Giard, M.H.; Perrin, F.; Pernier, J. & Bouchet, P. (1990). Brain generators implicated in processing of auditory stimulus deviance: a topographic event-related potential study. *Psychophysiol.*, Vol. 27, pp. 627-640.

Giard, M.H.; Lavikainen, J.; Reinikainen, K.; Perrin, F.; Bertrand, O.; Thevenet, M.; Pernier, J. & Näätänen, R. (1995). Separate representation of stimulus frequency intensity and duration in auditory sensory memory: An event-related potential and dipole-model analysis. *J. Cogn. Neurosci.*, Vol. 7, pp. 133-143.

Kane, N.M.; Curry, S.H.; Butler, S.R. & Gummins, B.H. (1993). Electrophysiological indicator of awaking from coma. *The Lancet*, Vol. 341, pp. 688.

Kraus, N.; Micco, A.G. & Koch, D.B. (1993). The mismatch negativity cortical evoked potential elicited by speech in cochlear-implant users. *Hear Res.*, Vol. 65, pp. 118-124.

Kraus, N.; McGee, T.; Carell, T.; Zecker, S; Nicol, T. & Koch, D. (1996). Auditory neuro physiologic response and discrimination deficits in children with learning problems. *Science*, Vol. 273, pp. 971-973.

Lancaster, J.L.; Summerln, J.L.; Rainey, L.; Freitas, C.S. & Fox, P.T. (1997). The Talairach Daemon, a database server for Talairach Atlas Labels. *Neuroimage,* Vol. 5 (4), pp. S633.

Lancaster, J.L.; Rainey, L.H.; Summerlin, J.L.; Freitas, C.S.; Fox, P.T.; Evans, A.E.; Toga, A.W. & Mazziotta, J.C. (1997). Automated Labeling of the Human Brain: A Preliminary Report on the Development and Evaluation of a Forward-Transform Method. *Hum. Brain Mapp.,* Vol. 5, pp. 238-242.

Molfese, D.L.; Linnville, S.E. & Wetzel, W.F. (1985). Electrophysiological correlates of handedness and speech perception contrasts. *Neuropsychologia,* Vol. 23, pp. 77-86.

Näätänen, R.; Gaillard, A.W.K. & Mantysaalo, S. (1978). Early selective effect on evoked potential reinterpreted. *Acta Psychologia,* Vol. 42, pp. 313-329.

Näätänen, R. & Winkler, I. (1999). The concept of auditory stimulus representation in cognitive neuroscience. *Psychol. Bull.,* Vol. 125, pp. 826-859.

Näätänen, R. (1992). *Attention and Brain Function.* Erlbaum, Hillsdale, NJ.

Nyman, G.; Alho, K.; Iaurinen, P.; Paavilainen, P.; Radil, T. & Rainikainen, K. (1990). Mismatch negativity (MMN) for sequences of auditory and visual stimuli: evidence for a mechanism specific to the auditory modality" *Electroenceph. Clin. Neurophysiol.,* Vol. 77, pp. 436-444.

Pascal-Marqui, R.D.; Michel, C.M. & Lehmann, D. (1994). Low resolution electromagnetic tomography: a new method for localizing electrical activity in the brain. *Int. J. Psychophy.,* Vol. 18, pp. 49-65.

Pascual-Marqui, R.D. (1999). Review of Methods for Solving the EEG Inverse Problem. *Int. J. Bioelectromag.,* Vol. 1, pp. 75-86.

Oldfield, R. (1971). The Assessment and Analysis of Handedness: The Edinburgh Inventory. *Neuropsychologia,* Vol. 9, pp. 97-113.

Ritter, W.; Deacon, D; Gomes, H.; Javitt, D.C. & Vaughan, H.G. Jr. (1995) The mismatch negativity of event- elated potentials as a probe of transient auditory memory: a review. *Ear Hear.,* Vol. 16, pp. 52-67.

Scherg, M.; Vajsar, J. & Picton, T.W. (1989). A source analysis of the late human auditory evoked potentials. *J. Cogn. Neurosci.,* Vol. 5, pp. 363-370.

Schröger, E.; Tervaniemi, M.; Wolff, C. & Näätänen, R. (1996). Preattentive periodicity detection in auditory patterns as governed by time and intensity information. *Brain Res. Cogn. Brain Res.,* Vol. 4, pp. 145-148.

Sussman, E. (1999). An investigations of the auditory streaming effect using event-related brain potentials. *Psychophysiol.,* Vol. 36, pp. 22-34.

Talairach, J. & Tournoux, P. (1988). *Co-planar stereotaxic atlas of the human brain.* Stuttgart: Thieme.

Tales, A.; Newton, P.; Troscianko, T. & Butler, S. (1999). Mismatch negativity in the visual modality. *NeuroReport,* Vol. 10, pp. 3363-3367.

Tervaniemi, M.; Kujala, A.; Alho, K.; Virtanen, J.; Ilmoniemi, R.J. & Näätänen, R. (1999). Functional specialization of the human auditory cortex in processing phonetic and musical sounds: A magnetoencephalographic (MEG) study. *Neuroimage,* Vol. 9, pp. 330-336.

Tervaniemi, M.; Rytkonen, M.; Schröger, E.; Ilmoniemi, R. & Näätänen, R. (2001). Superior formation of cortical memory traces for melodic patterns in musicians. *Learn. & Mem.*, Vol. 8, pp. 295-300

Towle, V.L.; Bolanos, J.; Suarez, D.; Tan, K.; Grzesczuk, R.; Levin, D.N.; Cakmur, R.; Frank, S.A. & Spire, J.P. (1993). The spatial location of EEG electrodes: locating the best-fitting sphere relative to cortical anatomy. *Electroenceph. Clin. Neurophysiol.*, Vol. 86, pp. 861-866.

12

White Matter Changes in Cerebrovascular Disease: Leukoaraiosis

Anca Hâncu, Irene Răşanu and Gabriela Butoi
County Emergency Clinical Hospital Constanta, Romania

1. Introduction

The term 'leukoaraiosis', derived from the Greek 'leuko' meaning white and 'araios' meaning rarefied, was introduced in 1987, as a "neutral term, exact enough to define white-matter changes in the elderly or the demented, general enough that it serves as a description and a label, and demanding enough that it calls for a precise clinical and imaging description accompanied when possible by pathologic correlations" (Hachinski et al., 1987).

When the term leukoaraiosis (LA) was introduced, only CT imaging was widely available. Similar appearance is conspicuous, and more florid on T2-weighted magnetic resonance imaging (MRI), particularly on fluid attenuated inversion recovery (FLAIR) images. Leukoaraiosis is currently defined as diffuse, confluent white matter abnormality (low density on CT, hyperintensity on T2-weighted or FLAIR MRI), often with irregular margins, commonly seen in the normal elderly and in association with vascular risk factors such as hypertension, or in context of cognitive impairment. The term was introduced to avoid confusing an imaging appearance with a specific pathology (O'Sullivan, 2008). Leukoaraiosis can be focal, patchy or diffuse area in the white matter and it is located periventricularly or deeper in the white matter.

Leukoaraiosis severity has traditionally been graded by visual scales. Simples scales like that of van Swieten divide the appearances into only two grades of severity; more complex scales like the Fazekas scale discriminates "punctate", "early confluent" and "confluent" white matter lesions, while the Sheltens scale adopts a 0-6 scale in multiple anatomical regions (including periventricular and nonperiventricular white matter lesions - WML; periventricular hyperintensities are further separated into frontal, occipital, and lateral aspects) (O' Sullivan, 2008; Scheltens et al., 1993, as cited by Bohnen et al., 2009). Other rating scales of WML are the Brant-Zawadzki Scale and the Cardiovascular Health Study Scale both of which place relatively more emphasis on periventricular WML (Bohnen et al., 2009). However, even fully quantitative volumetric measurements of leukoaraiosis correlate weakly with cognitive and physical function, suggesting that T2-weighted MRI provides only a rough impression of the severity of the underlying pathology (O' Sullivan, 2008).

T2-weighted imaging is sensitive to liquid, gliosis and the effects of demyelination. FLAIR images are heavily T2-weigtened with cerebrospinal fluid suppression. This makes it possible to detect also leukoaraiotic lesions situated close to the cerebrospinal fluid and to differentiate Virchow-Robin spaces from leukoaraiosis. The decline in cerebral blood flow in areas with leukoaraiosis can be detected with imaging techniques such as average apparent diffusion coefficient (ADCav) where tissues with faster diffusion appear bright and tissues with slower diffusion dark. Normally axons produce significant hindrance to water diffusion but leukoaraiosis causes axonal loss and furthermore leads to an increase in water content of the tissue which can be detected with these imaging techniques. DWI (diffusion weighted MRI) makes it possible to differentiate acute and chronic ischemic stroke lesions from leukoaraiosis. In DW images, tissues with faster diffusion appear dark and tissues with slower diffusion bright (Helenius et al., 2002, as cited by Kurkinen, 2009).

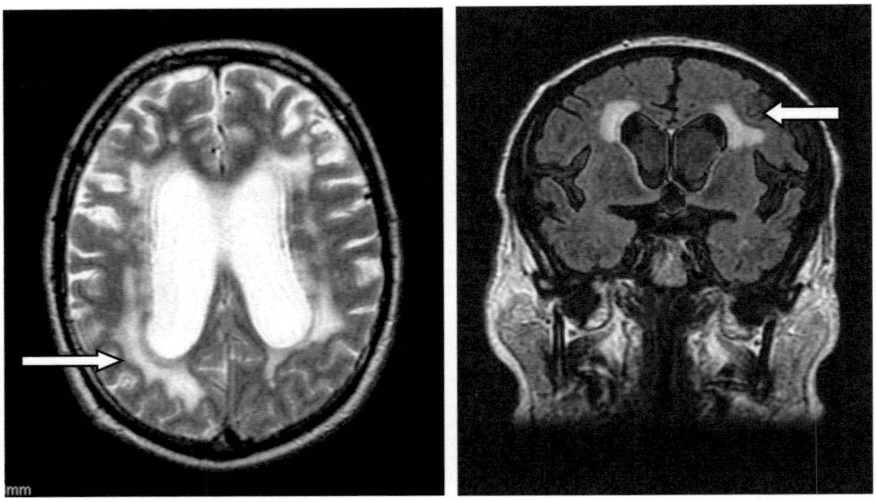

Fig. 1. Cerebral MRI scan showing leukoaraiosis (arrows); left: axial T2 weighted; right: coronal FLAIR sequence.

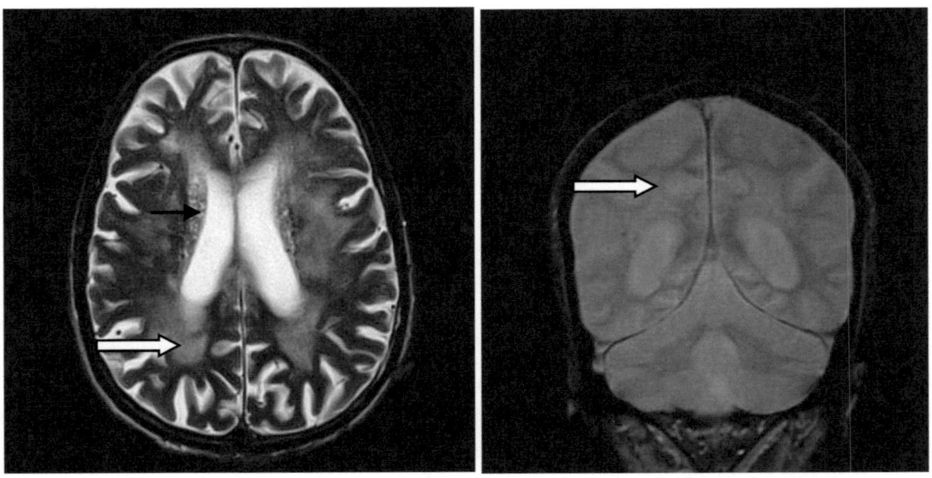

Fig. 2. MR images from a 76-year old patient; left: T2- weighted sequence showing leukoaraiosis (white arrow) and perivascular dilated spaces (black arrow); right: Proton density sequence showing leukoaraiosis (white arrow).

Newer MRI sequences can provide useful additional information. Diffusion-weighted imaging, for example, allows the distinction of new lacunar infarcts from background leukoaraiosis. In patients who presents with intracerebral haemorrhage, especially lobar haemorrhage, gradient acho (T2*-weighted) images should be performed to look for evidence of previous haemorrhages or microbleeds. In terms of quantifying white matter damage, several techniques (such as diffusion tensor MRI) are proving superior to T2-weighting imaging. Diffusion tensor MRI provides a much better index of white matter damage, and simple whole-brain measurements, such as diffusion histograms, can help track disease progression. Diffusion tensor MRI also demonstrates the variability in the extent of white matter disruption both within lesions and in normal-appearing white matter (O' Sullivan, 2008).

2. Epidemiology of leukoaraiosis

Several studies have described the prevalence of leukoaraiosis in different population groups, but there is considerable variability in the published figures. This variability can be attributed to the heterogeneity of age and vascular risk factors of patients with different imaging modalities used and differences in the scales used to define the leukoaraiosis. Often, when first discovered, white matter hyperintensities occur in the context of relatively normal brain function. But these lesions are not normal as they indicate an increased risk for stroke, cognitive decline, dementia, and death, as reported by Debette and Markus (2010) at the end of their metanalysis of the existing literature through November 2009. They examined 46 prospective longitudinal studies and found that white matter hyperintensities predict an increased risk of stroke (hazard ratio 3.3), dementia (hazard ratio 1.9) and death 2.0 (hazard ratio 2.0).

Roppele et al. (2010) performed magnetization transfer imaging in 328 neurologically asymptomatic Austrian Stroke Prevention Study participants (age range, 52–87 years). FLAIR was used to delineate white matter hyperintensities and to define normal-appearing brain tissue. The magnetization transfer ratio was measured globally in normal-appearing brain tissue by using a histogram analysis technique and focally in white matter hyperintensities. Associations of magnetization transfer ratio metrics with sex and a large battery of different cerebrovascular risk factors (age, arterial hypertension, diabetes mellitus, smoking, body mass index, cholesterol and triglyceride levels, glycated hemoglobin, and the presence of cardiac disease) were assessed with univariate and multiple regression analysis.

Age was seen to affect all magnetization transfer ratio histogram metrics of normal-appearing brain tissue, and a faster decrease of the magnetization transfer ratio peak height occurred in men. Independent associations with magnetization transfer ratio metrics were found for arterial hypertension and diabetes mellitus. Besides lesion grade, arterial hypertension was also significantly associated with a lower magnetization transfer ratio in white matter hyperintensities.

3. Pathophysiology of leukoaraiosis

The pathogenesis of leukoaraiosis remains controversial. It is unclear whether the mechanisms are the same for large and small punctate foci and for extensive diffuse leukoaraiosis. Moreover, pathological changes could be consequences of reaching the white matter rather than causes of it.

It has been assumed that the ischemic insult, responsible for LA, results from the vulnerable nature of the long penetrating end-arteries that feed the deep white matter. The deep brain structures (white matter and deep gray nuclei) are supplied by perforating arteries that are end-arteries with no collateral supply. These penetrating arteries do not arborise but give off perpendicularly oriented short branches that irrigate the white matter, each of which provides the blood supply to a cylindrically shaped metabolic unit. In the region between the cortical and ventricular surfaces, centripetal and centrifugal penetrating arteries from an internal watershed area lacking anastomoses is particularly susceptible to being injured as a result of systemic or focal decreases in cerebral blood flow (Rowbotham et al., 1965, De Reuck, 1971, as cited by Birns & Kalra, 2008).

At the vascular level, the continuum extends from the findings of hyaline thickening of the walls of small arteries to the lipohyalinosis (a major disruption in wall with infiltration of macrophages and luminal narrowing). At the level of the parenchyma, there is a loss of myelin and axons with a glial reaction and even areas of infarction (Fazekas et al., 1993, Lotz et al., 1986).

The main pathogenic hypotheses involve:

3.1 Ischemia, cerebral vasoreactivity and autoregulation

The pathological studies suggest that leukoaraiosis is one manifestation of cerebral small vessel disease. This is supported by strong pathological and clinical associations with the other major manifestation of small vessel disease—lacunar stroke. The pathogenesis of cerebral small vessels disease is still a matter of investigation but both clinical and pathological studies support the most popular hypothesis that acute disruption of blood supply in one arterial territory results in lacunar infarction while a more chronic and widespread reduction in perfusion causes leukoaraiosis. This is consistent with the spatial pattern and distribution of leukoaraiosis, which arises first in those areas furthest from the origin of the arterioles in the periventricular and deep white matter regions (Hassan et al., 2003, Pantoni, 2002, as cited by Birns & Kalra, 2008).

Reductions in white matter perfusion in leukoaraiosis have been demonstrated using xenon-CT, MRI, PET and SPECT and in some studies, the degree of hypoperfusion has been found to correlate with the severity of leukoaraiosis (Oishi et al., 1999, Miyazawa et al., 1997, as cited by Birns & Kalra, 2008). Furthermore, quantitative perfusion and diffusion tensor MRI studies have revealed reduced cerebral blood flow in normal appearing white matter in periventricular regions in patients with leukoaraiosis, suggesting that areas are "at risk." (O' Sullivan, 2001, 2002). Two studies on the relationship between cerebrovascular reactivity and cerebral small vessels disease (which excluded patients with carotid artery stenoses or those undertoken soon after an acute ischaemic event, knowing the effect of these comorbidities on cerebrovascular reactivity) demonstrated impaired reactivity in patients with multiple lacunar infarctions but no association between cerebrovascular reactivity and the severity of leukoaraiosis on brain MRI (Molina et al., 1999, Cupini et al., 2001 as cited by Birns & Kalra, 2008).

Supporting the role of ischemia in the pathogenesis of leukoaraiosis, the results of a study showed a statistically significant correlation between the presence and severity of leukoaraiosis and degree of carotid stenosis. A trend toward increased risk of development of leukoaraiosis in carotids with fatty plaques also was observed. The data confirmed that the development of leukoaraiosis is strongly correlated with age (Saba et al., 2009). A further study showed a statistically significant correlation between increased carotid artery wall thickness and LA (and its severity) (Saba et al., 2011).

3.2 Endothelial dysfunction/blood-brain barrier abnormalities

Histopathological evidence of endothelial cells activation and retraction with increased vascular permeability, increased circulating levels of leukocyte adhesion molecules such as ICAM1 (intercellular adhesion molecule-1) and E selectin (shed from the surface of activated endothelial cells) and a rise in the markers of coagulation activation (including thrombin-antithrombin complex and prothrombin fragments $_{1+2}$) have been reported in patients with small vessels desease compared with controls (Lin et al., 2000, Hassan et al., 2003, Fassbender et al., 1999, Tomimoto et al., 1999, as cited by Birns & Kalra, 2008). In addition, serum concentration of thrombomodulin and von Willebrand factor, which are both molecular markers of endothelial cell damage, have been shown to correlate with MRI evidence of small vessels disease (Ishii et al., 1991, Kohriyama et al., 1996 as cited by Birns & Kalra, 2008).

A number of studies have shown that chronic hypertension predisposed to impaired blood-brain barrier function, with endothelial cell retraction, increased vascular permeability and greater susceptibility to white matter injury for relatively small insults (Tomimoto et al., 1996, Lin et al., 2000, Pantoni, 2002, Wardlaw et al., 2003, Birns et al., 2005, as cited by Birns & Kalra, 2008).

In patients with subcortical white matter disease, plasma proteins have been found in the tissue around perforating arteries and increased concentrations of a number of proteins in the cerebro-spinal fluid have been found compared with controls, supporting the idea that the proteins reached the cerebro-spinal fluid via leakage from small perforating arteries (Akiguchi et al., 1998., Pantoni et al., 1993, as cited by Birns & Kalra, 2008).

One study has demonstrated intravenously injected contrast agent to leak into the brain, particularly in the territory of the perforating arteries, more in those with leukoaraiosis than in controls (Starr et al., 2003, as cited by Birns & Kalra, 2008).

3.3 Disturbances in cerebro-spinal fluid circulation

Murata et al (1981) hypothesized that disturbances in cerebro-spinal fluid circulation may play a role in the pathogenesis of leukoaraiosis. Roman suggested that increased accumulation of cerebro-spinal fluid in the ventricules raises the interstitial pressure in the periventricular parenchyma, thus causing ischaemia to the white matter (Roman, 1991, Kimura et al., 1992, as cited by Birns & Kalra, 2008).

3.4 Plasma viscosity

Schneider et al (1997) showed plasma viscosity to be elevated in patients with leukoaraiosis and lacunar infarction and considered that it may alter cerebro-spinal fluid properties and favour chronic ischaemic white matter damage.

3.5 Platelet hyperaggregability and other coagulation abnormalities

Fujita et al (2011) demonstrated a significantly increased incidence of platelet hyperaggregability in 73 patients with leukoaraiosis compared with 102 controls. Twenty-one patients with leukoaraiosis and uncorrected platelet hyper-aggregability were compared with 21 controls matched for age, grade of leukoaraiosis and observation period whose platelet hyper-aggregability was corrected. The results of their study showed that the progress of leukoaraiosis is significantly inhibited by long-term correction of platelet hyper-aggregability, suggesting platelet hyper-aggregability as a risk factor for leukoaraiosis

Martí-Fàbregas et al. (2002) investigated whether there is a direct correlation between plasma fibrinogen levels and the amount of leukoaraiosis in 28 patients with symptomatic small-vessel disease. They found a significant correlation between plasma fibrinogen levels and the amount of leukoaraiosis in patients with symptomatic cerebral small-vessel disease. This result suggests that fibrinogen may be involved in the pathophysiology of leukoaraiosis in these patients.

Hassan et al showed that while tissue factor and the ratio of tissue factor to TFPI (tissue factor pathway inhibitor) did not differ significantly between patients with small vessel disease and controls, the tissue factor/TFPI ratio was higher in small vessel disease patients with leukoaraiosis compared with isolated lacunar infarction (Hassan et al., 2003, as cited by Birns & Kalra, 2008).

3.6 Cerebral venous circulation impairment

Some authors found an age-related gradual increase in the thickness of the walls of veins and venules near the lateral ventricles and a striking degree of vessels wall thickening, resulting in narrowed lumina and even occlusion, in patients with leukoaraiosis. The thickened vascular walls stained strongly for collagens I and III. In the studied cases, the degree of venous collagenosis statistically correlated with the severity of leukoaraiosis. The authors questioned whether increased resistance to venous blood flow resulting from the venous stenosis, might induce chronic ischaemia and/or oedema in the deep white matter, perhaps somehow leading to leukoaraiosis, or indeed whether the collagenosis itself occurs as a result of ischaemia (Moody et al., 1995, Brown et al., 2002, as cited by Birns & Kalra, 2008).

More recently, Chung & Hu (2010) hypothesed that chronic cerebral hypoperfusion associated with vasogenic edema, microbleeding or/and endothelial dysfunction found in leukoaraiosis favors venous ischemia, in stead of arterial ischemia, as its pathogenesis. Given that the involved regions in leukoaraiosis (periventricular and subcortical regions) are the drainage territory of deep cerebral venous system and the watershed region between the superficial and deep cerebral venous system respectively, and adding the facts that periventricular venule collagenosis, and retinal and intraparenchymal venules dilatation are related to the severity of leukoaraiosis, the authors suggested that cerebral venous hypertension caused by downstream venous outflow impairment might play a major role in the pathogenesis of leukoaraiosis. Jugular venous reflux is therefore suggested to play a key role in the pathogenesis of leukoaraiosis through a sustained or long-term repetitive retrograde-transmitted cerebral venous pressure and venous outflow insufficiency, which might lead to chronic cerebral venous hypertensions, abnormal cerebral venules structural changes, decreased cerebral blood flow, endothelial dysfunction, and vasogenic edema in cerebral white matters.

3.7 Others hypothesis

It has been also demonstrated homocysteine (which is toxic to the endothelium) to be a strong risk factor for small-vessel disease on 90 patients with leukoaraiosis and lacunar infarction compared to 52 patients with isolated lacunar infarction after controlling for both conventional risk factors and age (Hassan at al., 2004, Khan et al., 2007, as cited by Birns & Kalra, 2008).

Matrix metalloproteinases are neutral proteases that disrupt the blood-brain barrier and degrade myelin basic protein under conditions of neuroinflammation. Candelario-Jalil et al., studied 60 patients with suspected vascular cognitive impairment due to small vessel disease (twenty-five of which were classified as subcortical ischemic vascular disease, whereas other groups included mixed Alzheimer disease and vascular cognitive impairment, multiple strokes, and leukoaraiosis when white matter lesions were present and the diagnosis of vascular cognitive impairment was uncertain) by measuring metalloproteinase-2, metalloproteinase-3 and metalloproteinase-9 activity as well as the albumin level in the cerebrospinal fluid. They found that increased levels of metalloproteinases are associated with increased cerebrospinal fluid albumin and suggest that they may contribute to the pathophysiology of subcortical ischemic vascular disease.

Since necrosis is not obvious in LA lesions, Brown et al. investigated the occurrence of apoptosis. They obtained 1.5-cm-thick coronal brain slices at autopsy from two patients with LA. MRI was performed on the brain slices. Sections were stained by several methods including the terminal deoxynucleotidyl transferase dUTP (uridine 5'-triphosphate) nick end labeling (TUNEL) method for DNA fragmentation. The presence of numerous scattered cells in the LA lesions showing DNA fragmentation suggests that those cells are damaged and dying, at least some by apoptosis. The apoptosis in the white matter adjacent to the LA lesions suggests progressive cell loss and expansion of the LA lesions (Brown et al., 2002).

3.8 Genetic factors

RNA expression was assessed in the blood of individuals with and without extensive white matter hyperintensities (WMH) to search for evidence of oxidative stress, inflammation, and other abnormalities described in WMH lesions in brain. Cluster and principal components analyses showed that the expression profiles for almost 300 genes distinguished WMH+ from WMH− subjects. Function analyses suggested that WMH-specific genes were associated with oxidative stress, inflammation, detoxification, and hormone signaling, and included genes associated with oligodendrocyte proliferation, axon repair, long-term potentiation, and neurotransmission (Xu et al., 2010).

Fernandez-Cadenas et al. analyzed 212 single nucleotide polymorphisms (SNPs) in 142 patients with ischaemic stroke, generating a total of 30104 genotypes. Seventy-nine subjects (55.6%) presented leukoaraiosis measured by the Fazekas scale and 69 (48.6%) by age-related white matter changes (ARWMC) scale. This study revealed that the genes associated with leukoaraiosis were involved in blood-brain barrier (BBB) homeostasis (Fernandez-Cadenas et al., 2010).

4. Specific features of LA in the main types of cerebrovascular diseases

4.1 Stroke

Although patients with cerebrovascular disease may have white matter abnormalities related to large-vessel, embolic or ischemic-hypoxic etiologies, by far small-vessel disease is believed to be the most common substrate in case of diffuse, bilateral, preferential white matter involvement (Gomes & Caplan, 2008).

Leukoaraiosis (LA) is a common finding in stroke (particularly ischemic) and shares similar risk factors and pathophysiologic mechanisms with both ischemic and hemorrhagic stroke. LA may also be an independent predictor of stroke outcomes.

After an acute ischemic stroke LA is associated with an increased risk of death or dependency, recurrent stroke, intracerebral hemorrhage under anticoagulation, myocardial infarction, and poststroke dementia. There is increasing evidence from neuroimaging studies to support the concept that some cases of LA are caused by white matter infarcts, which may be particularly frequent in patients with widespread small vessel disease. Th e relatively similar distribution of LA regardless of the distribution of vascular pathology suggests a conserved vulnerability to white matter injury across various vascular diseases, possibly related to the resting patterns of blood fl ow (Mijajlovic et al., 2011).

LA is frequently observed in patients with acute stroke, ischemic as well as hemorrhagic. Previous studies indicated that LA was strongly associated with lacunar strokes rather than non-lacunar, territorial strokes. Stroke and LA are likely two related diseases. In many aspects, LA is an ischemic disease, as is ischemic stroke. Also, intracerebral hemorrhage (ICH) and LA share a common cause, that of arterial hypertension. If LA shares with stroke (ischemic and hemorrhagic) common mechanisms, and the appearance of LA on imaging predicts stroke, then, according to the current terminology, LA can be regarded as an intermediate surrogate of stroke. (Jimenez-Conde et al., 2010, Pu et al., 2009, Lee et al., 2008, Inzitari, 2003, as cited by Mijajlovic et al., 2011)

Putaala et al. hypothesized that risk factors, neuroimaging characteristics, and associations with the overt clinical stroke may be diff erent in young patients with ischemic stroke with or without silent brain infarcts (SBIs) and LA. Of the 669 patients included, 86 (13%) had SBIs, 50 (7%) had LA, 17 (3%) had both, and 550 served as controls. Most SBIs were located in basal ganglia (39%) or subcortical regions (21%), but cerebellar SBIs also were rather frequent (15%). LA was mainly mild to moderate. Silent cardioembolism may in part explain the frequency of cerebellar SBIs in younger patients. As observed, younger stroke patients tend to have more frequently overt posterior territory ischemia and cerebellar infarcts. Th is observation, jointly with the frequency of cerebellar SBIs, might reflect the same, yet unclear, pathophysiologic mechanisms. Independent risk factors for SBIs in younger adults were type 1 diabetes, obesity, smoking, and increasing age. Risk factors for LA were type 1 diabetes, obesity, female sex, and increasing age. Small-vessel disease was the predominant cause of stroke in both those with SBIs (31%) and LA (44%) (Putaala et al., 2009, as cited by Mijajlovic et al., 2011).

Prospective observations further corroborated the relationship between LA and stroke and the distinct role of lacunar infarcts. The presence of LA on CT scan predicted subsequent stroke in patients with first-ever lacunar stroke, in those with lacunar or cortical infarction, in elderly patients with gait problems and LA on CT scan, and in patients with lacunar stroke or trivial neurological symptoms. Recurrent stroke was predominantly of the lacunar type. When studies took into account the severity of LA the risk of recurrence proved to be proportional to the extent of LA (Miyao et al., 1992, van Zagten et al., 1996, Inzitari et al., 1995, Yamauchi et al., 2002, as cited by Inzitari, 2003).

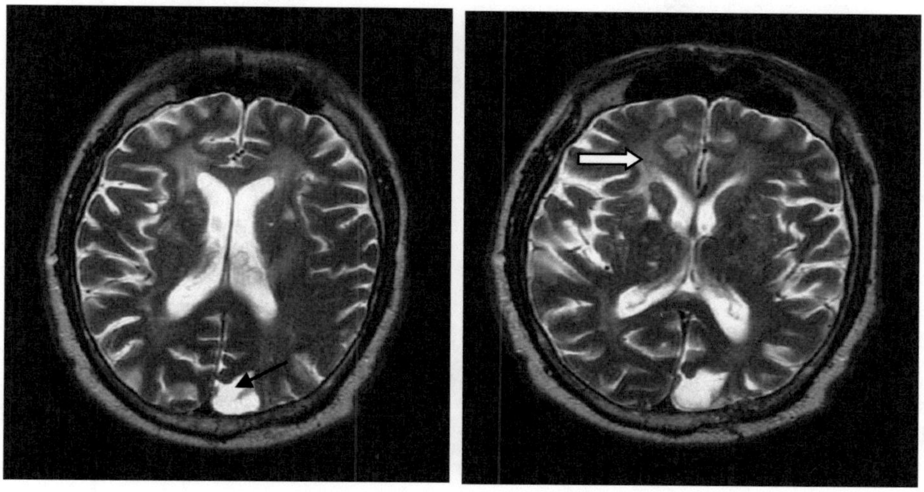

Fig. 3. Cerebral MRI (axial T2 weighted sequences) of a 70 years old male, known with arterial hypertension, diabetes mellitus, and a left posterior cerebral arterial ischemic stroke 3 years ago, admitted for right hemiparesis and mixed aphasia; an old stroke in the left posterior cerebral artery territory (black arrow) and leukoaraiosis (white arrow) can be seen.

In 2008 we attempted to assess the correlation between leukoaraiosis and associated vascular pathologies in a group of 50 hospitalized patients whose cerebral MRI revealed leukoaraiosis. The study revealed that:

- Stage II leukoaraiosis (Brant-Zawadzki scale) was present frequently in patients with acute stroke.
- Stage III leukoaraiosis (Brant-Zawadzki scale) predominated in patients with chronic vascular lesions.
- Stage IV (Brant-Zawadzki scale) in our studied group was found in those with Binswanger disease.
- Severity of leukoaraiosis increased with age.
- Severity of neurologic symptoms was in direct proportion with severity of leukoaraiosis.
- Leukoaraiosis associated cognitive decline and brain atrophy in 66% of cases.
- Presence of leukoaraiosis was associated with increased risk of stroke recurrence (almost half of the cases) (Hâncu et al., 2009).

4.2 Large arteries stroke

In most of the studies, cortical territorial infarct was largely less probable than lacunar or hemorrhagic stroke as recurrent stroke. The main causes of cortical infarcts are large-artery disease and cardioembolism.

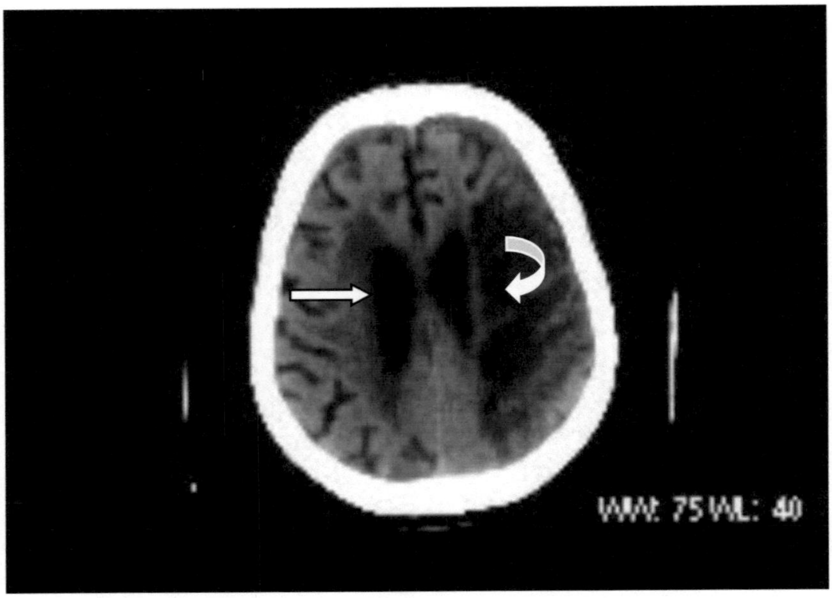

Fig. 4. Cerebral CT scan showing leukoaraiosis (white arrow) in a pacient with an old ischemic stroke in the left middle cerebral artery territory (white curved arrow).

In regard to the first mechanism, while cross-sectional data from the patients randomized in the North American Symptomatic Carotid Endarterectomy Trial (NASCET) showed an inverse relationship between the degree of carotid stenosis and presence of LA, a few population studies have consistently reported an association between intima-media thickness or the presence of carotid plaques and white matter hyperintensities on MRI, even after adjustment for other vascular risk factors. Atrial fibrillation, a major cause of cardioembolic stroke, was found to be negatively associated with LA in 1 study and positively associated in 2 other studies. These conflicting results are likely justified by the variable impact of age and other age-related vascular risk factors as confounders for these associations (Brun & Englund, 1986, Pico et al., 2002, Bots et al., 1993, Manolio et al., 1999, Henon et al, 1996, Raiha et al., 1993, as cited by Inzitari 2003).

In a Korean study, a significant association between leukoaraiosis and the stroke subtypeswas found. The large-artery-disease group had a higher prevalence of leukoaraiosis than did the other groups (55.4% in the large-artery-disease group, 30.3% in the lacunar group and 14.3% in the cardioembolic group, P = 0.016 by chi-square test). On the multivariate linear regression analysis, age, the presence of hypertension, previous stroke and stroke subtype were independently associated with the presence of leukoaraiosis. In the sub analysis of the large-artery-disease group, the leukoaraiosis had a tendency to be more prevalent in the mixed and intracranial stenosis group than did the extracranial stenosis group (45.5% in the mixed group, 40.3% in the intracranial group and 26.9% in the extracranial group, P = 0.08 by chi-square test). The association of leukoaraiosis with large-artery disease in this study might be due to the relatively high prevalence of intracranial occlusive lesions in Korean stroke patients compared to other ethnic groups (Lee et al., 2008).

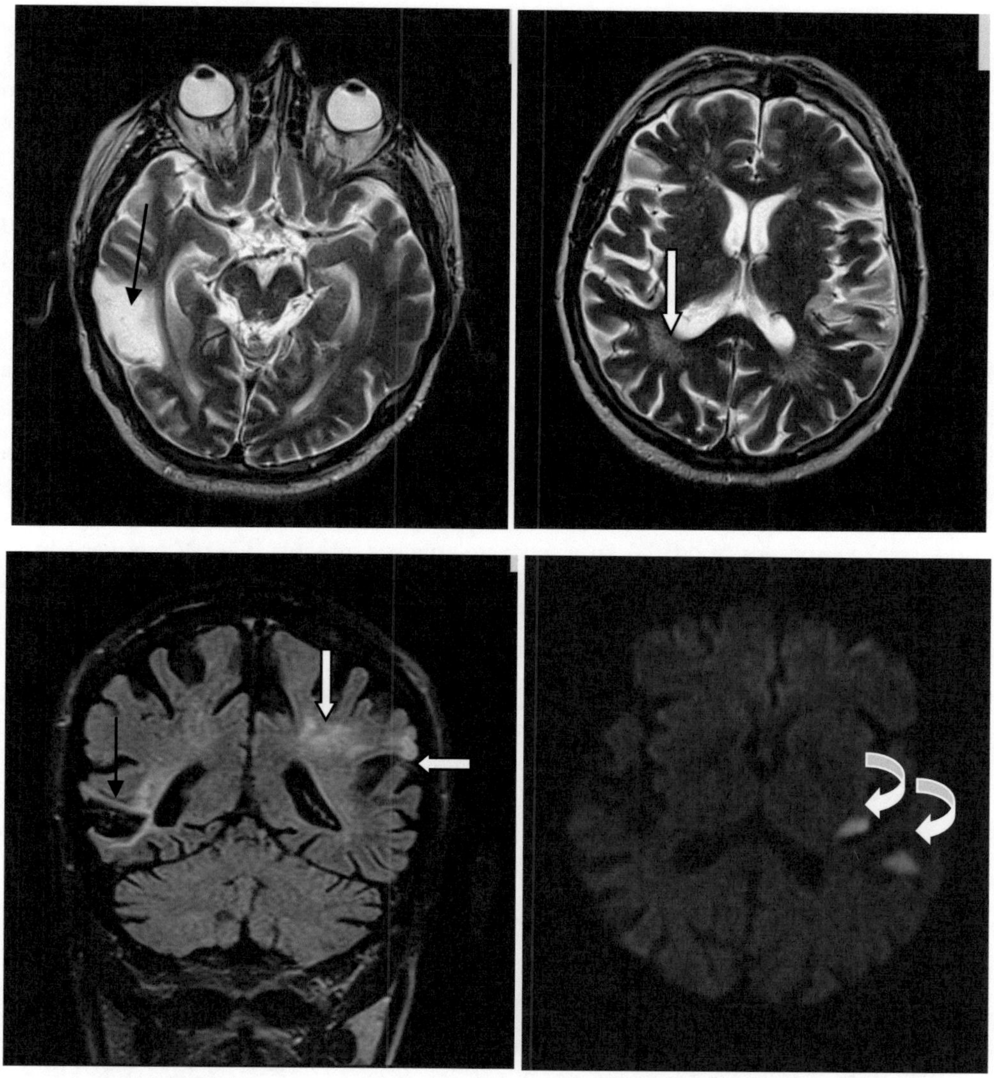

Fig. 5. Cerebral MRI (above: axial T2 weighted sequences, left-below: coronal FLAIR sequence, right-below: diffusion-weighted sequence) showing an old right temporal lobe ischemic stroke (black arrow), acute left temporo-frontal ischemic stroke (white horizontal arrow), leukoaraiosis (white vertical arrow) and diffusion – hypersignal spots in left temporal lobe (curved white arrows).

4.3 Lacunar stroke

Although leukoaraiosis and lacunar infarcts are often found together, in individual patients one type of imaging appearance may predominate, leading to the notion of subtypes of diffuse small vessel disease; either what has been labelled as ischaemic leukoaraiosis (defined by the combination of leukoaraiosis with a history of a clinical lacunar syndrome), or isolated lacunar infarction (in which a similar clinical presentation is accompanied by multiple lacunar lesions but no leukoaraiosis on imaging). These two imaging types have recently been shown to differ in their risk factor profile; age and hypertension are most strongly associated with ischaemic leukoaraiosis while hypercholesterolaemia, diabetes mellitus and myocardial infarction are more associated with isolated lacunar infarction. These findings suggest some differences in pathogenesis, with leukoaraiosis, perhaps reflecting a non-atheromatous pathology of smaller calibre vessels than those implicated in lacunar infarcts. A better appreciation of distinct subtypes may explain conflicting results about the association of certain novel risk factors with stroke; for example, although homocysteine is a risk factor for both types of manifestation, it has a much stronger association with ischaemic leukoaraiosis than with isolated lacunar infarction (Khan et al., 2007, Hassan at al., 2004, as cited by O' Sullivan, 2008).

White matter hyperintensities on magnetic resonance imaging can be used as surrogate markers of small vessel disease (Wallin & Fladby, 2010).

Rost et al. measured WMH volume (WMHV) in cohorts of prospectively ascertained patients with acute ischemic stroke (AIS) (n = 891) and ICH (n = 122). Patients with larger WMHV were more likely to have lacunar stroke compared with cardioembolic, large artery, or other stroke subtypes ($p < 0.03$). In a separate analysis, greater WMHV was seen in ICH compared with lacunar stroke and in ICH compared with all ischemic stroke subtypes combined ($p < 0.007$). These data support the model that increasing WMHV is a marker of more severe cerebral small-vessel disease (Rost et al., 2010).

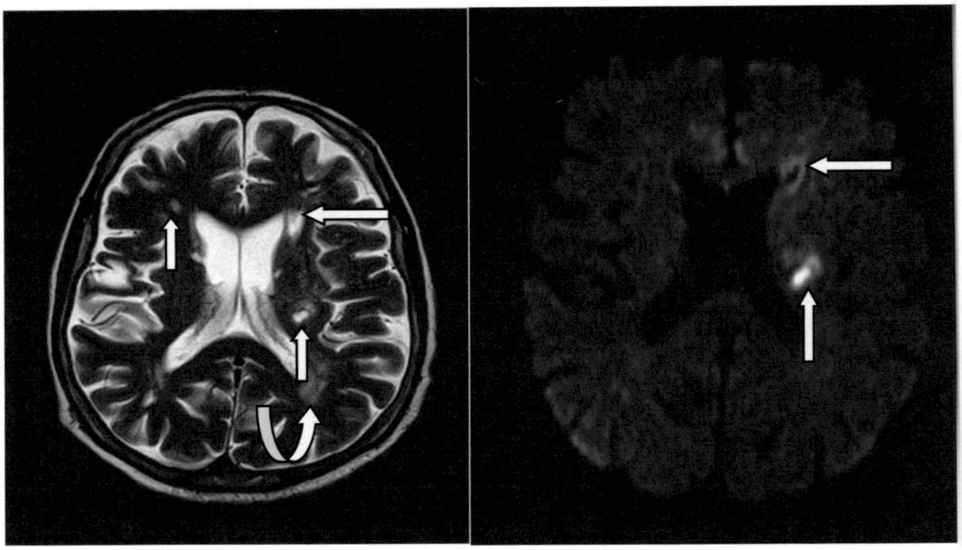

Fig. 6. Cerebral MR scan of a 60 years old female (left: T2 weighted sequence; right: diffusion weighted sequence) showing an old microbleeding (horizontal arrow), lacunar ischemic strokes (vertical arrow) and leukoaraiosis (curved arrow).

4.4 Hemorrhagic stroke

2 cross-sectional studies of hospitalized stroke patients reported in 1989 and 1990, for the first time, the association between LA and ICH. The latter of the 2 studies also examined the possible confounders for this association. In this study extensive LA was over twice more

prevalent among 116 patients with ICH than among 155 control patients without ICH. In an analysis with a multivariate adjustment for other vascular risk factors, the association was almost fully explained by the higher prevalence of arterial hypertension and lacunar infarcts on CT scan (Selekler & Erzen, 1989, Inzitari et al., 1990, as cited by Inzitari, 2002).

The Stroke Prevention in Reversible Ischemia Trial (SPIRIT), a prospective trial of secondary prevention with anticoagulation and target international normalized ratio (INR) values of 3.0 to 4.5 in patients with cerebral ischemia of presumed arterial origin, revealed the independent role of LA as a risk factor for major bleeding during anticoagulation after cerebral ischemia (Gorter, 1999). This was confirmed by a recent study which investigated radiographic and clinical characteristics of patients with warfarin-related ICH following ischemic stroke. The 26 eligible ICH cases and 56 controls were compared for vascular risk factors, stroke characteristics, and extent of leukoaraiosis (graded in anterior and posterior brain regions on a validated scale of 0 to 4). Leukoaraiosis was found to be an independent risk factor for warfarin-related ICH in survivors of ischemic stroke, including those in the commonly employed range of anticoagulation (Smith et al., 2010).

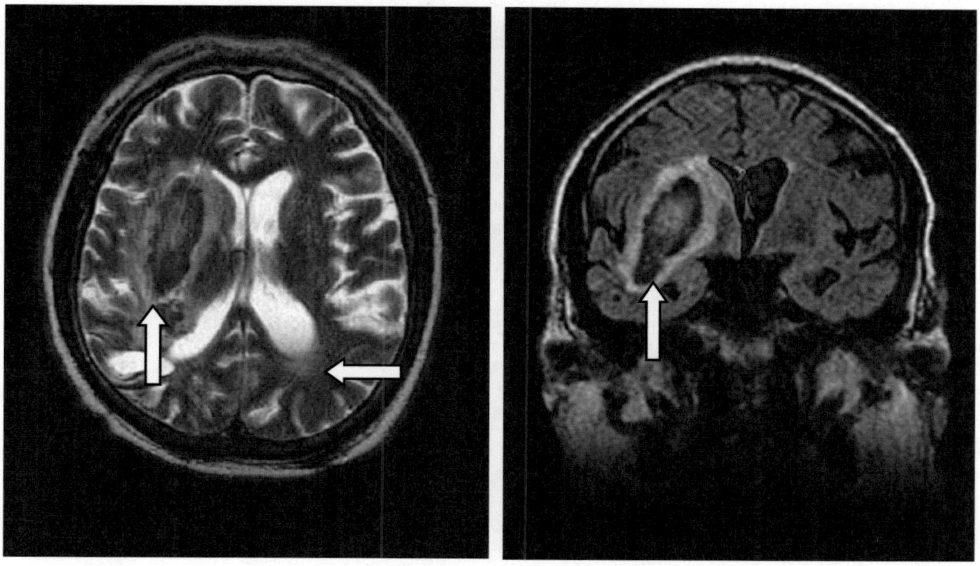

Fig. 7. Cerebral MRI scan (left: axial T2 weighted sequence; right: coronal FLAIR image) showing right temporo-parietal primary intracerebral hematoma (vertical arrow), mixed cerebral atrophy, leukoaraiosis (horizontal arrow), in a 65 years old male, known with untreated arterial hypertension, smoker, admitted for left hemiplegia suddenly occurred.

4.5 CADASIL

The distribution of white matter lesions in cerebral autosomal dominant arteriopathy with subcortical infarcts and leukoaraiosis (CADASIL) has been reported to be distinct from those in patients with ischemic leukoaraiosis and Binswanger's disease. In earlier European studies, diagnostic significance of white matter lesions in the temporopolar region (Tp), medial frontopolar region (Fp) and external capsule (EC) was stressed in diagnosing CADASIL (Tomimoto et al., 2005).

More recently, however, high sensitivity and specificity of Tp lesions have been demonstrated. Tomimoto et al examined the frequencies of CADASIL-associated lesions in 17 non-demented patients with ischemic leukoaraiosis and 20 patients with Binswanger's disease. The results indicated that Tp lesions were useful diagnostic marker in diagnosing CADASIL, whereas Fp and EC lesions were non-specifically observed (Tomimoto et al., 2005).

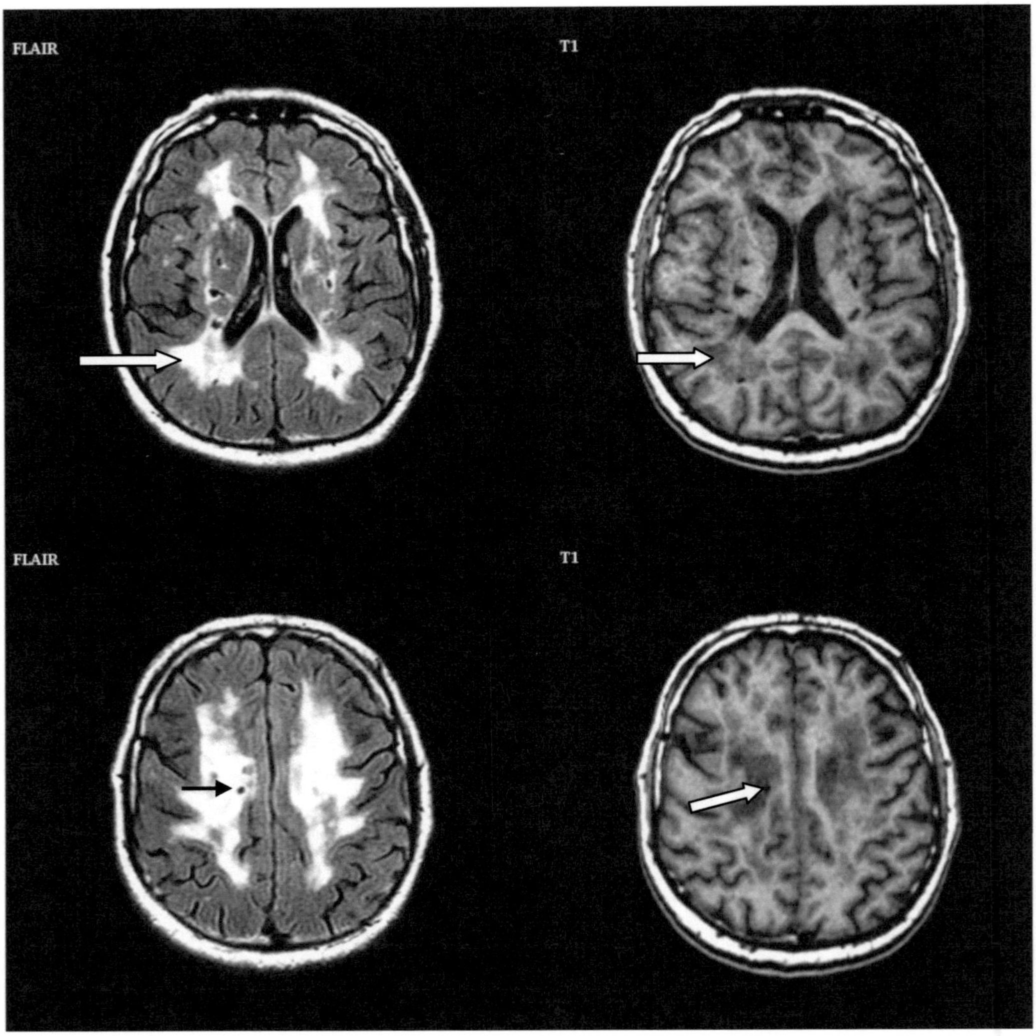

Fig. 8a. MR images from a 24-year old man with CADASIL; left: FLAIR diffuse hypersignal of the periventricular and deep white matter (leukoaraiosis) and small cerebrospinal fluid intensity area (lacunar subcortical infarction); right: T1 hyposignal (leukoaraiosis) and fluid intensity area (lacunar subcortical infarction) in the corresponding regions.

An intersting feature of leukoaraiosis, with possible relevance to the pathogenesis of the lesions, is the relatively conserved anatomic distribution across individuals and different vascular diseases. Exceptions are that in CADASIL, there is relative preferential involvement of the external capsule and anterior temporal white matter; and in cerebral amyloid angiopathy, there is relatively more posterior than anterior leukoaraiosis. Even so, in CADASIL and cerebral amyloid angiopathy patients, as well as others, the greatest burden of lesions is in the periventricular white matter around the frontal and occipital horns, with varying amounts of involvement of areas of subcortical white matter. The probability of subcortical white matter involvement varies inversely with the distance from the ventricular margin (Smith, 2010).

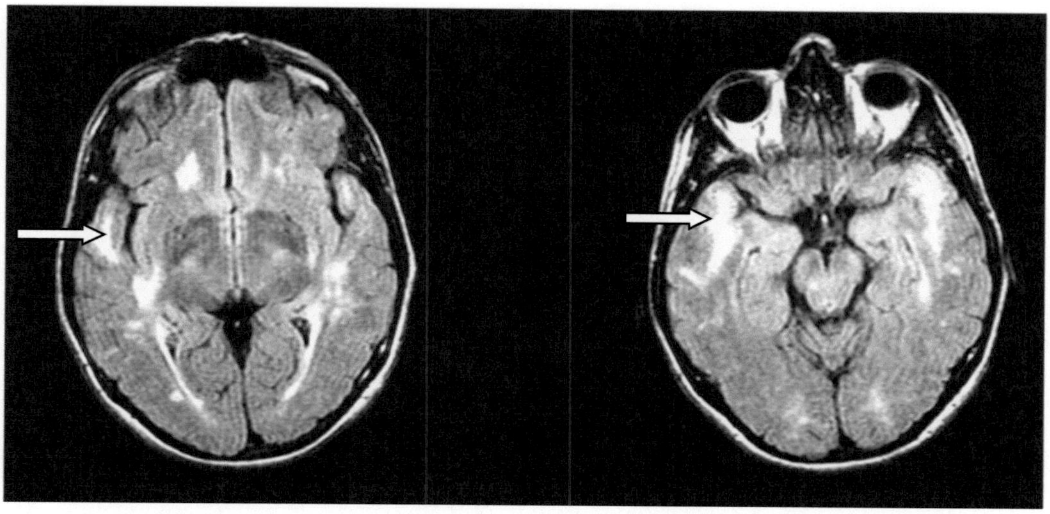

Fig. 8b. Same case: FLAIR hypersignal in the anterior pole of the temporal lobe, characteristic for CADASIL.

4.6 Amyloid angiopathy

Cerebral amyloid angiopathy affects the arteries of the leptomeninges and cortex, with little involvement of the penetrating arteries in the white matter and essentially no involvement of the perforating arteries at the base of the brain and brain stem (Smith 2010).

In Alzheimer's disease, and in patients with mild cognitive impairment, some of whom will have prodromal Alzheimer's, white matter changes correlate with serum levels of the $Ab_{1\text{-}40}$ peptide, which is the predominant peptide found in vessel deposits in cerebral amyloid angiopathy. But intriguingly, plasma Ab also correlates with the severity of white matter lesions in the population-based Rotterdam study. Given that cerebral amyloid angiopathy is a rare cause of leukoaraiosis at the population level, this suggests that Ab has an impact on white matter damage even in patients with arteriosclerotic small vessel disease and no pathological evidence of cerebral amyloid angiopathy. The underlying mechanisms of this association are not yet clear. Conversely, pathological studies in Alzheimer's disease suggest that arteriosclerotic small vessel disease can drive more extensive amyloid deposition and neurofibrillary tangle formation, which is consistent with epidemiological evidence that vascular risk factors are important, and suggests that the interaction may work in both directions (Gurol et al., 2006, van Dijk et al., 2004, Thal et al., 2003, as cited by O' Sullivan, 2008).

Leukoaraiosis is also increasingly recognised as a feature of sporadic cerebral amyloid angiopathy, without Alzheimer's disease.Amyloid deposits are found in more proximal portions of the small penetrating arteries than arteriosclerotic changes and it is not known whether these deposits alone, without downstream arteriosclerosis, are sufficient to cause leukoaraiosis. Notably, leukoaraiosis is found in some of the genetic amyloid angiopathies (for example, familial British dementia) suggesting that amyloid angiopathy alone is sufficient to cause this imaging appearance (Greenberg et al., 2004, as cited by O' Sullivan, 2008).

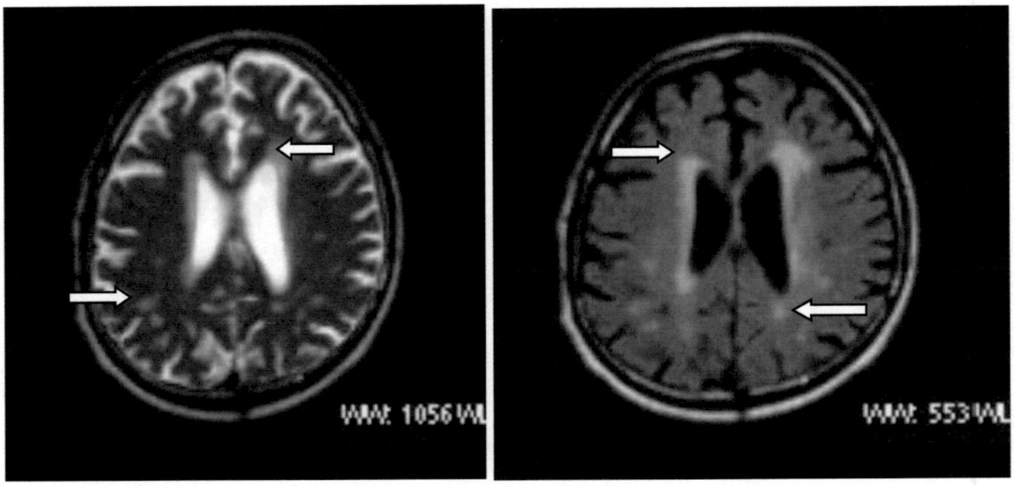

Fig. 9a. MR images from a 71-year-old man with probable cerebral amyloid angiopathy and leukoaraiosis; left: T2 hypersignal at the level of periventricular and deep white matter; right: FLAIR hypersignal at the level of the periventricular white matter.

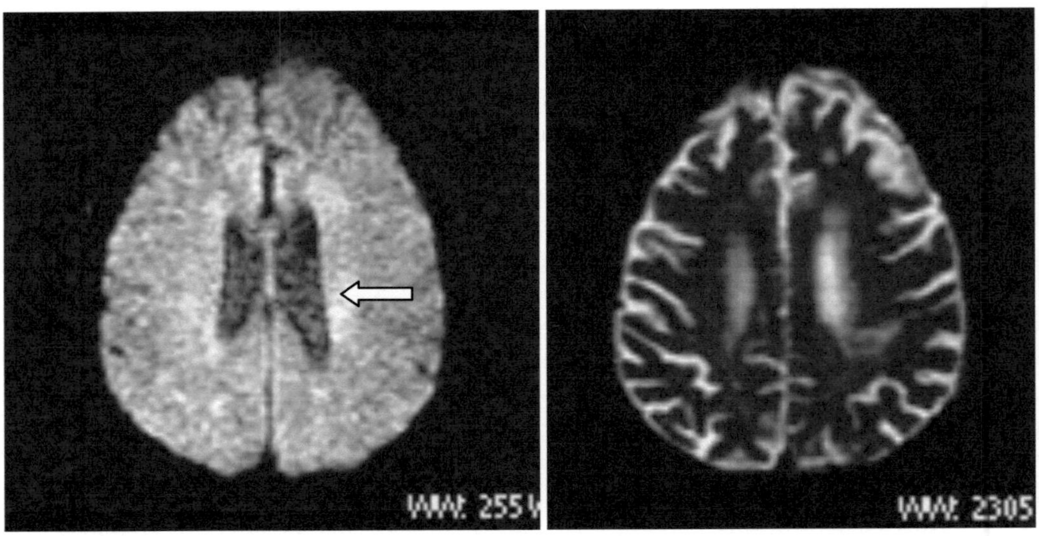

Fig. 9b. Same case: MR diffusion weighted image (DWI) and apparent diffusion coefficient (ADC) mapping; no apparent diffusion coefficient (ADC) restriction can be observed in the affected areas (leukoaraiosis).

4.7 Collagen arteritis

Neurologic manifestations are among the features of many multisystem autoimmune connective tissue disorders with various clinical presentations. Areas of patchy cortical or subcortical abnormality (hyperdensity on CT scan, T2 hyperintensity on MRI) may correspond to small vessel vasculitis or cerebritis (Ramachandran, 2011).

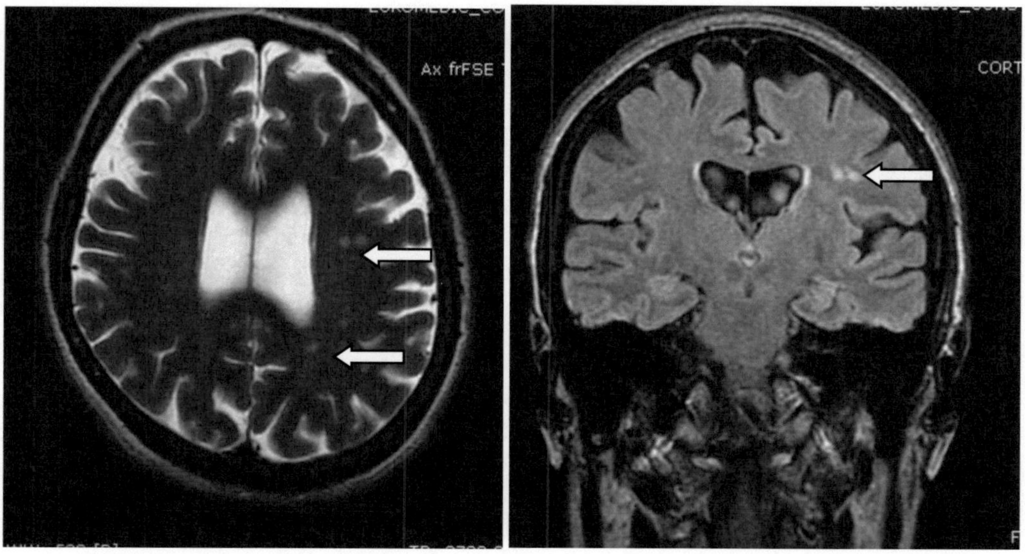

Fig. 10. MR images from a 51-year-old female with rheumathoid arthritis; T2 hypersignal (left) and FLAIR hypersignal (right) spots at the level of deep white matter can be seen.

5. Conclusions

Leukoaraiosis is a radiological finding whose pathogenesis or clinical significance is not completely acknowledged. LA predispose to stroke, independent of other stroke risk factors. Typically, leukoaraiosis predict a lacunar ischemic stroke but in patients with LA the risk of cortical infarct is also increased, as is that of vascular death. The presence of extensive LA predisposes to ICH, especially in patients treated with anticoagulants for secondary prevention after an ischemic stroke. Consequently, it is important for practicians to correctly assess LA in all patients presenting with cerebro-vascular pathology.

6. Acknowledgements

We are grateful to Dr. Virgil Ionescu and Dr. Mariana Bardaş for the images of this chapter.

7. References

Birns J. & Kalra L. (2008).Pathogenesis of Cerebral Small Vessel Disease, In: *Brain Hypoxia-Ischemia Research Progress*, O.M. Roux, (Ed.), 113-130, Nova Science Publisher Inc., ISBN: 978-1-60456-139-5, New York, USA

Bohnen, N.I.; Bogan C.W. & Muller M.L.T.M. (2009). Frontal and Periventricular Brain White Matter Lesions and Cortical Deafferentation of Cholinergic and Other Neuromodulatory Axonal Projections. *European Neurological Journal,* No. 1, pp. 1-7

Brown W.R., MoodyD.M., Challa V.R., Thore C.R. & Anstrom J.A. (2002). Apoptosis in leukoaraiosis lesions

Candelario-Jalil E., Thompson J., Taheri S., Grossetete M., Adair J.C., Edmonds E., Prestopnik J., Wills J., Rosenberg G.A. (2011). Matrix metalloproteinases are associated with increased blood-brain barrier opening in vascular cognitive impairment. Stroke, Vol. 42, No. 5, (May 2011), pp. 1345-50, ISSN 1524-4628

Chung C.P. & Hu H.H. (2010).Pathogenesis of leukoaraiosis: Role of jugular venous reflux. *Medical Hypotheses*, Vol. 75, No. 1, (July 2010), pp. 85-90

Debette, S., & Markus, H. (2010). The clinical importance of white matter hyperintensities on brain magnetic resonance imaging: systematic review and meta-analysis. BMJ, No. 341 (July 2010), c3666.

Smith E.E. (2010). Leukoaraiosis and Stroke. Stroke, Vol. 75, No. 1, (July 2010), pp. 85-90

Fazekas F., Kleinert R., Offenbacher H., Schmidt R., Kleinert G., Payer F., Radner H. & Lechner H. (1993). Pathologic correlates of incidental MRI white matter signal hyperintensities. *Neurology*, No.43, (September 1993), pp. 1683–9

Fernandez-Cadenas I, Mendioroz M, Domingues-Montanari S, Del Rio-Espinola A, Delgado P, Ruiz A, Hernandez-Guillamon M, Giralt D, Chacon P, Navarro-Sobrino M, Ribo M, Molina CA, Alvarez-Sabin J, Rosell A, Montaner J. (2010). Leukoaraiosis is associated with genes regulating blood-brain barrier homeostasis in ischaemic stroke patients. *European Journal of Neurology*, No. 18, (December 2010), pp. 826-35

Fujita S., Kawaguchi T., Uehara T. & Fukushima K. (2005). Progress of leukoaraiosis is inhibited by correction of platelet hyper-aggregability. *International psychogeriatrics,* Vol 17, No. 4, (December 2005), pp. 689-98, ISSN: 1041-6102

Gomes J.A. & Caplan L.R. White matter abnormalities in patients with cerebrovascular disease, In: MR imaging in white matter diseases of the brain and spinal cord, M. Filippi, (Ed.), 364-71, Springer, ISBN 3-540-40230-6, Heidelberg , Germany

Gorter J.W. (1999). For the Stroke Prevention in Reversible Ischemia Trial (SPIRIT) and European Atrial Fibrillation Trial (EAFT) Study Groups. Major bleeding during anticoagulation after cerebral ischemia: patterns and risk factors. *Neurology,* Vol. 53, (October 1999), pp. 1319–1327

Hachinski V.C., Potter, P. & Merskey, H. (1987). Leuko-araiosis. *Archives of Neurology,* No. 44, pp. 21-23

Hâncu A., Damian I., Popescu S., Davidescu B.H., Zguma D., Herțea C. & Kaivanifard M. (2009). Impact of imaging development upon leukoaraiosis detection in a group of vascular patients. *Romanian Journal of Neurology*, Vol. VIII, No. 3, (November 2009), pp. 109-114, ISSN 1843-8148

Inzitari D. Leukoaraiosis An Independent Risk Factor for Stroke? (2003). *Stroke,* Vol. 34, (June 2003), pp. 2067-2071 *Journal of the Neurological Sciences*, Vol. 203-204, (November 2002), pp. 169-171

Kurkinen M. (September 2009). Silent brain infarcts and leukoaraiosis in young patients with first-ever ischemic stroke. Available from https://helda.helsinki.fi

LeeS.J., Kim J.S., Lee K.S., An J.Y., Kim W., Kim Y.I., Kim B.S. & Jung S.L. (2008). The leukoaraiosis is more prevalent in the large artery atherosclerosis stroke subtype among Korean patients with ischemic stroke. *BMC Neurology,* Vol. 8, No. 1, (August 2008), pp. 31-33.

Lotz P.R., Ballinger W.E. Jr & Quisling R.G. (1986). Subcortical arteriosclerotic encephalopathy: CT spectrum and pathologic correlation. *American Journal of Roentgenology,* No. 147, (December 1986), pp. 1209–14

Martí-Fàbregas J., Valencia C., Pujol J., García-Sánchez C. & Martí-Vilalta J.L. (2002). Fibrinogen and the amount of leukoaraiosis in patients with symptomatic small-vessel disease. *European Neurology,* Vol. 48, No. 4, (January 2002), pp. 185-90.

Mijajlovic M.D., Pavlovic A.M., Mircovic M.M. & Sternic N. (2011). Connection Between Leukoaraiosis And Ischemic Stroke. *Current Topics in Neurology and Psychiatry Related Disciplines,* Vol. 19, No. 1, (March 2011), pp. 41-47

Murata T, Handa H, Mori K, Nakano Y. (1981). The significance of periventricular lucency on computed tomography: experimental study with canine hydrocephalus. *Neuroradiology,* No. 20, (January 1981), pp. 221-227

O' Sullivan M, Summers P.E., Jones D.K., Jarosz J.M., Williams S.C.R. & Markus H.S. (2001). Normal appearing white matter in ischemic leukoaraiosis: a diffusion tensor MRI study. *Neurology,* No. 57, (December 2001), pp. 2307–10

O' Sullivan, M. (2008). Leukoaraiosis. *Practical Neurology,* No. 8, pp. 26-38

O'Sullivan M., Lythgoe D. J., Pereira ., Summers P. E., Jarosz J. M., Williams S. C.R. & Markus H.S. (2002). Patterns of cerebral blood flow reduction in patients with ischemic leukoaraiosis. *Neurology,* No. 59, (August 2002), pp. 321–6

Ramachandran T.S. (29 june 2011). Neurologic Manifestations of Systemic Lupus. Available from http://emedicine.medscape.com/article/1146456-overview

Ropele S., Enzinger C., Söllinger M., Langkammer C., Wallner-Blazek M., Schmidt R. & Fazekas F. (2010). Impact of Sex and Vascular Risk Factors on Brain Tissue Changes with Aging: Magnetization Transfer Imaging Results of the Austrian Stroke Prevention Study. *American Journal of Neuroradiology, No.* 31, (August 2010), pp. 1297-1301

Rost N.S., Rahman R.M., Biffi A., Smith E.E., Kanakis A., Fitzpatrick K., Lima F., Worrall B.B., Meschia J.F., Brown R.D. Jr, Brott T.G., Sorensen A.G., Greenberg S.M., Furie K.L. & Rosand J. (2010). White matter hyperintensity volume is increased in small vessel stroke subtypes. *Neurology,* Vol. 75, No. 19, (November 2010), pp. 1670-1677

Saba L., Pascalis L., Sanfilippo R., Anzidei M., Bura R., Montisci R. & Mallarini G. (2011). Carotid Artery Wall Thickness and Leukoaraiosis: Preliminary Results Using Multidetector Row CT Angiography. *American Journal of Neuroradiology,* No. 32, (May 2011), pp. 955-61

Saba L., Sanfilippo R., Pascalis L., Montisci R. & Mallarini G. (2009). Carotid Artery Abnormalities and Leukoaraiosis in Elderly Patients: Evaluation with MDCT. *American Journal of Roentgenology, No.* 192, (February 2009), pp. W63-W70

Schneider R, Ringelstein EB, Zeumer H, Kiesewetter H, Jung F. (1987). The role of plasma hyperviscosity in subcortical arteriosclerotic encephalopathy (Binswanger's disease). *Journal of Neurology,* No. 234, (December 1987), pp. 67-73

Smith E.E., Rosand J., Knudsen K.A., Hylek E.M. & Greenberg S.M. (2002). Leukoaraiosis is associated with warfarin-related hemorrhage following ischemic stroke. *Neurology,* Vol.59, No. 2, (July 2002),pp. 193-197

Tomimoto H., Ohtani R., Wakita H., Lin J.X., Miki Y. & Mizuno T. (2005). Distribution of ischemic leukoaraiosis in MRI: a difference from white matter lesions in CADASIL. *Brain and nerve*, Vol. 57, No. 2, (February 2005), pp. 125-130

Wallin A. & Fladby T. (2010). Do white matter hyperintensities on MRI matter clinically?*BMJ*, Vol. 341, (July 2010), pp. C 3400

Xu H., Stamova B., Jickling G., Tian Y., Zhan X., Ander B.P., Liu D., Turner R., Rosand J., Goldstein L.B., Furie K.L., Verro P., Johnston S.C., Sharp F.R. & DeCarli C.S. (2010). Distinctive rna expression profiles in blood associated with white matter hyperintensities in brain. *Stroke*, No. 41, (October 2010), pp. 2744-49